Revision Notes

for the
MRCS Viva

Kanchana Sundaramurthy MBBS DNB (Surg) MRCSEd

Trust Senior House Officer, General Surgery
Prince Charles Hospital
Merthyr Tydfil, UK

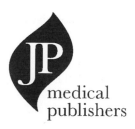

JP
medical
publishers

London • St Louis • Panama City • New Delhi

© 2010 JP Medical Ltd.
Published by JP Medical Ltd
83 Victoria Street, London, SW1H 0HW, UK
Tel: +44 (0)20 3170 8910
Fax: +44 (0)20 3008 6180
Email: info@jpmedpub.com
Web: www.jpmedpub.com

ISBN: 978-1-907816-01-7

British Library Cataloguing in Publication Data
A catalogue record for this book is available from the British Library

Library of Congress Cataloging in Publication Data
A catalog record for this book is available from the Library of Congress

JP Medical Ltd is a subsidiary of Jaypee Brothers Medical Publishers (P) Ltd, New Delhi, India with offices in Ahmedabad, Bengaluru, Chennai, Hyderabad, Kochi, Kolkata, Lucknow, Mumbai and Nagpur. Visit www.jaypeebrothers.com for more details.

Publisher:	Richard Furn
Development Editor:	Alison Whitehouse
Design:	Pete Wilder, Designers Collective Ltd
Copy Editor:	Robert Whittle

Typeset, printed and bound in India.

Preface

This is a unique book which aims to enable the MRCS viva candidate to score maximum marks. Though 18 out of 24 is the pass mark for the exam, being awarded the full 24 marks is what every candidate should aspire to, and what this book is all about.

Answering the MRCS viva is an art. Everything is timed, and the more you answer, the more marks you will score. Speed and accuracy are the two most important qualities examiners look for in your answer. This book will help you to practise for speed and accuracy with your friends before facing the actual examination.

The total number of achievable marks is 24, out of which the candidate must score a minimum of 18 to pass, 3 in each subject. If you score 2 in one, you can compensate by scoring 4 in another. But if you score 1 in any of the subjects, you cannot compensate by scoring 4 in two subjects, and you have failed even if your total score is 18 or more.

There are traditionally three sets of examiners, paired as Physiology and Critical Care, Pathology and Principles of Surgery, Anatomy and Operative Surgery. Each of them questions you for ten minutes, at the end of which the bell rings. You should aim to answer as many questions as possible in those ten minutes.

Three topics are taken in quick succession by each examiner, and three questions are asked in each topic. The first question is the basic one, where definitions are asked; the second one is more pointed and the third one is still more pointed. A fourth question is asked if you excel in answering the first three. As an example, in pathology, the first question might be: "What is an abscess?"; the second one might be: "Give me some examples of abscesses"; the third one: "What are the different types of peri-anal abscess?"; and if you are fast enough in answering those, there may be a fourth: "How will you treat them?". Then the examiner will switch abruptly to the next topic and start with another definition. If a sufficient number of fourth questions is asked, you are assured of four marks.

The topics given in this book are taken from the official MRCS syllabus of the Royal College of Surgeons, and the book is structured in such a way that each topic answers the four questions most likely to be asked by examiners. The purpose of this book is not to help you score three in each subject, but four. There are candidates who have prepared for the MRCS viva using material from this book and who have scored 23 out of 24, and this should be the aim of each candidate preparing for the exam.

Revising from this book will boost your confidence to such a degree that scoring 24/24 need no longer be a dream.

Any queries and comments may be addressed to kan_sundar@yahoo.co.in

Kanchana Sundaramurthy

Contents

Part 1

General principles

Chapter 1

General physiology

Body fluid compartments

Internal milieu (milieu interieur)

- Internal environment surrounding the cells, consisting of the functional extracellular fluid (ECF)
- Functions as medium for oxygen and nutrient intake and discharge of metabolic waste

Body weight

- Water:
  - Adult male – 60%
  - Adult female – 55%
  - Infant – 70%
  - Elderly – <60%
  - Intracellular fluid (ICF) – 55%
  - ECF – 45%
- Rest of the weight:
  - Proteins – 18%
  - Fat – 15%
  - Minerals – 7%

- ECF:
  - Plasma
  - Interstitial fluid
  - Transcellular fluid:
    - Gastrointestinal tract
    - Cerebrospinal fluid
    - Aqueous humour

Concentration of ions in ECF and ICF

- Na^+: 10 mM in the ECF; 140 mM in the ICF
- K^+: 150 mM in the ECF; 4.5 mM in the ICF
- Cl^-: trace in the ECF; 105 mM in the ICF

Actively transported across membranes by Na^+–K^+ pump, energy for which is derived from hydrolysis of ATP.

Fluid loss

- Urinary loss:
  - 1–2 L/day
  - Minimum volume necessary for adequate excretion of toxic waste material is 500 mL

Body fluid compartments, showing percentage of the total body fluid and the amount of fluid in each compartment. DCT, dense connective tissue; ISF, interstitial fluid; TCW, transcellular water; ECF, extracellular fluid; ICF, intracellular fluid

| 7.5% 3 L Bone | 7.5% 3 L DCT | | | |
| 7.5% 3 L Plasma | 20% 8.5 L ISF | 50% 23 L ICF | 2.5% 1 L TCW |

Functional ECF

- Insensible loss:
  - 500 mL/day
  - Evaporation of fluid from skin and airways
  - Increased in:
    - Ventilation
    - Laparotomy
- Loss by sweating:
  - Up to 5 L/day
  - Increased in:
    - Exercise
    - Environmental temperature
    - Fever

Intestinal loss:
  - 100 mL/day (faecal)
  - Increased in:
    - Vomiting
    - Diarrhoea
    - Intestinal obstruction

Colloid osmotic pressure

- Osmotic pressure generated by the presence of colloids on one side of a membrane that is impermeable to them
- Pressure necessary to prevent solvent migration
- Normal level – 25 mmHg

Osmolality

- The number of osmoles of solutes per kilogram of solvent
- Measure of the number of particles present in a unit weight of solvent (stated as milliosmoles/kg of solvent)
- Osmotic pressure across a selectively permeable membrane depends on the number of particles in the solution
- Directly measured by osmometer
- Normal osmolality of ECF is 280–295 milliosmoles/kg
- Tonicity is the osmolality of a solution relative to plasma

Osmolarity

- Number of osmoles of solute per litre of solution (milliosmoles/L)
- Calculated from a formula representing the solutes that, in ordinary circumstances, contribute to nearly all of the osmolarity of the solution, i.e. sodium, glucose and urea
- It is easy to calculate because it requires measurement of only three substances, which are all routinely measured in every hospital laboratory:
  $2 \times (Na^+ + K^+) + glucose + urea$ (mmol/L)
- Thirst centre in the hypothalamus is stimulated by increased osmolarity of ECF

Normal water balance

- Input:
  - Drink – 1500 mL
  - Food – 750 mL
  - Metabolic – 350 mL
  - Total input – 2600 mL
- Output:
  - Urine – 1500 mL
  - Faeces – 100 mL
  - Lungs – 400 mL
  - Skin – 600 mL
  - Total output – 2600 mL

Normal water requirement

- In adults:
  - 2 L/day
  - Sodium – 100 mmol/day
  - Potassium – 50 mmol/day
- In children:
  - First 10 kg – 4 mL/kg/hour
  - Next 10 kg – 2 mL/kg/hour
  - Next 10 kg – 1 mL/kg/hour
- Sodium and potassium requirement:
  - 1 mmol/kg/day

Safe rules for transfusing potassium

- Urine output at least 40 mL/hour
- Concentration of K^+ not more than 40 mmol/L
- Rate not more than 40 mmol/hour

Measurement of body fluids (by dilution method)

- Solute is introduced into the body and its relative proportion in the urine and plasma is measured

- For measurement of total body water (TBW):
  - Sucrose is used (called sucrose space) because it moves freely in all compartments and is not degradable
  - D_2O (heavy water) can also be used
- For measurement of plasma volume:
  - Evan's blue
  - Serum albumin tagged with radioactive iodine
- For measurement of ECF–ICF ratio:
  - Inulin
- For measurement of red blood cells:
  - Iron tagged with chromium or phosphate
- For measurement of ICF:
  - TBW minus ECF

Loss of ECF and TBW

- A man losing 1 L/day of water because he is marooned on a life raft will have lost, after 1 week, 7 L from his total body water of 42 L, i.e. 17%
  - Plasma volume will fall by 17%, which is survivable
- A man losing 1 L/day of water and electrolytes because of bowel obstruction, will have lost, after 1 week, 7 L from his functional ECF of 12 L, i.e. 58%
  - Plasma volume will fall by 58%, which is not compatible with life

Distribution of blood

Distribution of circulating blood volume at rest

- 50% – systemic veins (capacitance veins)
- 12% – heart cavities
- 18% – pulmonary circulation
- 2% – aorta
- 8% – arteries
- 1% – arterioles
- 5% – capillaries

When blood is transfused

- < 1% goes to the arterial system (high-pressure system)
- All the rest goes to systemic veins, pulmonary circulation and heart chambers other than left ventricle (low-pressure system)

Fluid shift – microcirculation

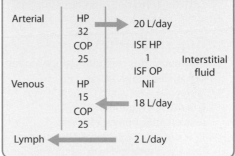

Fluid shifts in the microcirculation. HP, hydrostatic pressure, in mmHg; COP, colloid osmotic pressure; ISF HP, interstitial fluid hydrostatic pressure; ISF OP, interstitial fluid osmotic pressure

- Capillary pressure:
  - Arteriolar end: 32 mmHg
  - Venous end: 15 mmHg
- Pulse pressure:
  - Arteriolar end: 5 mmHg
  - Venous end: 0 mmHg
- Transit time of the blood from the arteriolar to the venular end is 1–2 seconds

Starling's forces causing fluid shift

- Arteriolar end:
  - The filtration pressure is more than the oncotic pressure
  - Therefore fluid moves into the interstitial space
- Venular end:
  - The oncotic pressure is more than the filtration pressure
  - Therefore fluid moves into the capillary

Starling's forces

Definition

- Starling's forces are forces that control fluid shift across the capillary membrane
- Explain the dynamics of fluid exchange between intravascular and interstitial spaces

- Starling's law of capillaries states that net filtration of water across a capillary wall is proportional to the difference between the hydraulic and osmotic forces across the vessel wall

Components

- Hydraulic forces: P_c and P_i
- Osmotic forces: p_p and p_i
- Net driving (filtration) pressure: $(P_c - P_i) - (p_p - p_i)$

Starling's equation

- Net filtration (flux) of fluid is proportional to net driving pressure
- $J_v = K_t (P_c - P_i) - s (p_p - p_i)$, where
  - J_v is the net filtration
  - K_t is the filtration co-efficient
  - P_c is the capillary hydrostatic pressure
  - P_i is the interstitial hydrostatic pressure
  - s is the reflection co-efficient
  - p_p is the capillary oncotic pressure
  - p_i is the interstitial oncotic pressure
- Increase in net driving pressure increases fluid flux out of the capillaries to interstitial space, and vice versa

Effects of vascular resistance

- R_a / R_v ratio is inversely proportional to P_c, where
  - R_a is arterial resistance
  - R_v is venous resistance
- An increase in the $P_c - P_i$ ratio or the $p_p - p_i$ ratio leads to oedema

Areas where Starling's forces are not in effect

- Glomerular capillaries:
  - Only filtration
  - No absorption
- Intestines:
  - Only absorption
  - No filtration

Crystalloids

- Normal saline – 6 L required to expand plasma by 1 L
- 5% dextrose solution – 13 L required to expand plasma by 1 L
- Lactated Ringer's solution – 3 L required to expand plasma by 1 L

Purpose of glucose in 5% dextrose water

- To maintain isotonicity of water

Normal fluid requirement per 24 hours

- 30–40 mL/kg of water
- 1 mmol/kg of sodium
- Requirement is met by transfusing 2000 mL of 5% dextrose solution plus 500 mL of normal saline or lactated Ringer's solution

Continuing abnormal losses above basal requirement

- Insensible loss
  - Increased in ventilated patients and during laparotomy
- Sweating and fever
  - Up to 5 L/day
- Intestinal excretion
  - 100 mL/day

Dehydration

- If both haematocrit and albumin are increased – loss of ECF
- If haematocrit is increased and albumin is normal – loss of plasma

Intra-operative fluid management

- Hartmann's solution – 5 mL/kg/hour
- Up to 2 L
- 5% dextrose is the ideal fluid for correction of cellular dehydration

Fluid and electrolyte derangements

Water lack

- Causes:
  - Poor water intake
  - Diabetes insipidus
- Results in:
  - Decreased total body fluid volume
  - No clinical dehydration because decreased ECF is balanced by decreased ICF
  - Increased levels of plasma sodium and urea

Water excess

- Increased total body fluid volume
- Causes:
  - Increased infusion of 5% dextrose
  - Syndrome of inappropriate ADH (SIADH)
- Biochemical results:
  - Increased ECF is balanced by increased ICF
  - Decreased levels of plasma potassium and plasma urea

ECF lack

- Caused by gastrointestinal losses, e.g. from vomiting or diarhoea, leading to diversion of transcellular water
- Increase in insensible loss
- Clinically:
  - Dehydration
  - Hypovolaemia
- Plasma urea is increased, with normal sodium levels maintained

ECF excess

- Caused by increased saline infusion with impaired excretion
- Clinically:
  - Increased central venous pressure
  - Cardiac failure
  - Oedema

Hypokalaemia

- Causes
  - Gastrointestinal losses
  - Diuretics
- ECG shows shallow T waves
- Precautions for K⁺ infusion:
  - 40 mmol/L
  - 40 mmol/hour
  - 40 ml/hour

Hyperkalaemia

- Causes
  - Acute renal failure
  - Increased potassium infusion
  - Diabetic ketoacidosis
- ECG shows peaked T waves
- Treatment:
  - 10 ml of 10% calcium chloride (cardiac protection)
  - 15 units of insulin with 50 mL of 50% glucose
  - 10 units of exchange resin (30 g/hour) enema (polystyrene sulphonate)

Plasma proteins

Functions

- Provide oncotic pressure that is crucial to the exchange of fluid across capillary membrane
  - Fluid exchange is disturbed in:
    - Decreased oncotic pressure – hypoalbuminemia
    - Increased hydrostatic pressure, e.g. in right heart failure or varicose veins
    - Increased capillary permeability, e.g. in sepsis
- Blood clotting
- Anticoagulation and inhibition of fibrinolysis by globulin fraction (antiproteinases):
  - Limit and localize thrombus
  - Fibrinolysis and inflammatory reaction
- Transport of:
  - Hormones
  - Bilirubin
  - Iron (transferrin)
  - Copper (ceruloplasmin)
  - Vitamins (retinol-binding protein)
  - Drugs
- Buffering of acid metabolites:
  - Carriage of CO_2 by venous blood decreases pH by increasing H⁺ ion concentration, but it is buffered by plasma proteins
- Acute phase response
- Defence against microbial invasion:
  - Complement system
  - Antibodies (by means of B lymphocytes)
  - Acute phase reactants, which are increased in acute infection and systemic inflammatory response syndrome (SIRS):
    - Ferritin
    - Fibrinogen
    - C-reactive protein (CRP), an important protein that is assayed for severity of illness

- Ceruloplasmin
- Alpha-2 antitrypsin
- Alpha-2 macroglobulin

Hereditary antiproteinase deficiencies

- Recurrent thrombus in deficiencies of:
  - Antithrombin III
  - Protein C
  - Protein S
- Bleeding tendency in deficiencies of:
  - Alpha-2 antiplasmin
  - Plasminogen inhibitor
- Pulmonary emphysema in deficiencies of alpha-1 antitrypsin
- Angioneurotic oedema in deficiencies of C1 inactivator

Thermoregulation

- The body temperature varies from central to peripheral areas
- The peripheral body temperature is subjected to substantial variations, while the central core temperature is relatively constant
  - For example, the peripheral temperature decreases in hypovolaemia and decreased colloid osmotic pressure
  - The peripheral temperature fluctuates with changes in either the environmental temperature or the type and quality of clothing being worn

Measurement of body temperature

- Central body temperature can be accurately measured in the:
  - Oesophagus
  - Rectum
  - Tympanic membrane
- Oral temperature may reflect core temperature but is affected by mouth breathing
- Axillary temperature is more unreliable
- Normal upper limit of core temperature is 37 °C (36.3–37.1 °C)
- Pyrexia is a core temperature of 38 °C or above

Regulation of body temperature

- Three components of regulation of body temperature:
  - Temperature receptors
  - Integration and control
  - Adjustment (behavioural and physiological)

Temperature receptors

- Peripheral receptors: A, delta and C fibres
- Central receptors: hypothalamic pre-optic nuclei
- Other receptors:
  - Great veins
  - Spinal cord
  - Abdominal viscera

Integration and control

- The hypothalamus sets the normal body temperature
  - Pre-optic nuclei detect the core temperature
  - Anterior hypothalamus controls the mechanisms for heat loss
  - Posterior hypothalamus controls the mechanisms of heat gain by comparing the core and peripheral temperatures and inducing appropriate actions to restore the body temperature to the set point

Adjustment

- Behavioural – individual activities mediated by higher cortical sensation:
  - Seeking shade
  - Drinking cool drinks
  - Wearing light clothes to reduce body temperature
  - Seeking warmth and shelter in cold season
  - Donning warm clothes to increase body temperature
- Physiological maintenance of balance between heat loss and heat gain
  - Regulation of heat loss, mediated by the anterior hypothalamus
    - Eccrine sweating, stimulated by cholinergic sympathetic fibres
    - Peripheral vasodilatation

- Regulation of heat gain, mediated by the posterior hypothalamus
  - Vasoconstriction
  - Pilo-erection, which causes air current by conduction and convection
  - Shivering, as a result of increased muscle tone)
  - Non-shivering thermogenesis, which occurs in brown fat in infants and newborns, and in the liver, intestines and muscles in adults), in response to increased catecholamines and thyroid hormones

Mechanisms of development of fever

Inflammatory mechanisms

- Inflammatory mediators
  - Endotoxins (lipopolysaccharides)
  - Circulating immune complexes
  - Tissue breakdown products
  - Inflammatory mediators
  - Other pyrogenic stimuli
- All react with monocytes, macrophages and Kupffer cells and cause release of cytokines – interleukin (IL)-1, IL-6 and tumour necrosis factor (TNF)
  - These act on preoptic hypothalamic nuclei
  - Synthesis and release of prostaglandin (PG)-E2 follows
  - Production of cAMP results
  - The hypothalamic temperature set-point is reset
  - The body senses that the core temperature is below the set-point (feels cold)
  - Activation of heat-production mechanisms until body temperature reaches the set-point
  - When the set point is reset to normal, the body feels hot
  - Heat-loss mechanisms are then activated until the temperature returns to normal

Metabolic mechanisms

- Increased metabolic rate leads to increased body temperature without any alteration in the set-point

- Exercise
- Ovulation
- Food (dynamic action)
- Increased endocrine activity (thyroid and adrenal medulla)
- Malignant hyperthermia (abnormal release of calcium from the sarcoplasmic reticulum to the cytosol in skeletal muscle)

Effects of fever

- Beneficial effects
  - Inhibits the growth of micro-organisms, e.g. pneumococci, anthrax
  - Increases antibody production
  - Slows the growth of some tumors
- Adverse effects
  - at 41 °C – permanent brain damage
  - > 41 °C – heat stroke, coma and death

Blood pressure

Definitions

- Systolic blood pressure: maximum value recorded during cardiac systole
- Diastolic blood pressure: minimum value recorded during cardiac diastole
- Pulse pressure: difference between systolic and diastolic pressures
- Mean pressure: the diastolic pressure plus one third of the pulse pressure

Control of blood pressure

Local (organ) control

- Myogenic autoregulation
- Metabolic autoregulation
  - Vasodilators
    - Prostacyclin
    - Nitric oxide
  - Vasoconstrictors
    - Thromboxane A2
    - Endothelin

Central or systemic control

- Long-term (hormonal) control
  - Vasodilators
    - Kinins
    - ANP
    - Epinephrine
  - Vasoconstrictors
    - Noradrenaline
    - Angiotensin II

- Short-term (neuronal) control
  - Vasomotor centre (the medulla)

Short-term control

- Control is through the nerve centres, i.e. the vasomotor centre and the baroreceptor reflex
- The receptors (nerve centres) act via afferent, stimulating the effectors (baroreceptors).
- Control can work either way, increasing or decreasing the blood pressure as situation demands
  - If the patient is hypotensive, the autoregulation begins to cause an increase in blood pressure up to twice the value within 5–10 seconds
  - If the patient is hypertensive, the autoregulation begins to cause a decrease in blood pressure up to 1 ½ times the value within 10–40 seconds
- Mechanism (baroreceptor reflex)
  - Negative feedback
  - Increase in blood pressure stimulates carotid sinus and aortic arch baroreceptors (pressoreceptors) and the walls of the right and left atria, which are stimulated by stretch
  - Impulses go through the glossopharyngeal nerve (Hering's nerve) and the vagus nerve to the nucleus of the tractus solitarius and to the vasomotor centre at the ventrolateral medulla
  - This results in inhibition of the vasoconstrictor centre and a decrease of tonic discharge of the vasoconstrictor nerves, stimulation of the vagal centre and excitation of the vagal innervation of the heart
  - Results in:
    - Vasodilatation of veins and arterioles
    - Decreased peripheral resistance
    - Decreased heart rate and contractility
    - Decreased cardiac output
  - Decreased firing from baroreceptors increases vasopressin and aldosterone and restores ECF volume
  - The reverse occurs when the blood pressure is decreased

Long-term control

- Hormonal control
- Control of ECF volume
- Mainly mediated by the kidneys
  - Renin–angiotensin system
  - Renal regulation of ECF volume

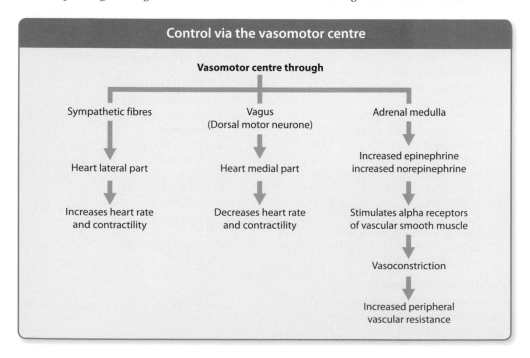

Vasomotor centre

- Found bilaterally in the reticular formation of the medulla and lower third of the pons
- Transmits parasympathetic and sympathetic impulses
  - Parasympathetic impulses through the vagus nerve to the heart
  - Sympathetic impulses through the spinal cord and peripheral sympathetic nerves to all blood vessels of the body
- Components
  - Vasoconstrictor area (C_1)
    - In anterolateral portion of upper medulla
    - Its neurones secrete noradrenaline
    - Its fibres travel to the spinal cord and stimulate sympathetic vasoconstrictor neurones, causing vasoconstriction
  - Vasodilator area (A_2)
    - In anterolateral portion of the lower medulla
    - Its fibres project upwards to inhibit the vasoconstrictor area, causing vasodilatation
  - Sensory area (A_2)
    - In the tractus solitarius in the posterolateral portion of the medulla and lower pons
    - Receives sensory nerve input signals from the vagus and glossopharyngeal nerves
    - Output signals control both vasoconstrictor and vasodilator areas
- Effects of the vasomotor centre
  - Effect on the heart
    - Lateral part through sympathetics – increases heart rate and contractility
    - Medial part through the vagus nerve – decreases heart rate and contractility
  - Effect on the adrenal medulla
    - Causes increased secretion of adrenaline and noradrenaline
    - Stimulates alpha receptors of vascular smooth muscle, causing vasoconstriction and increased peripheral vascular resistance

Receptors

- Baroreceptors in the carotid sinus and aortic arch
  - Carotid sinus
    - Hering's nerve to the glossopharyngeal nerve to the tractus solitarius (vasomotor centre)
  - Aortic arch
    - The vagus nerve to the vasomotor centre

Acid–base balance

Definitions

- An acid is a proton (H^+) donor
- A base is a proton (H^+) acceptor
- Buffer
  - Solution that contains a weak acid and its conjugate base or vice versa, i.e. conjugate pairs
  - Function is to minimise any change in pH by rapidly giving up or accepting hydrogen ions
- pH – negative logarithm to base 10 of the hydrogen ion concentration
- Anion gap
  - Sum of major cations (Na^+, K^+) minus the sum of major anions (HCO_3^-, Cl^-)
  - Normal: 12–20 mmol/L
- Base excess: measured in the laboratory by titrating the arterial blood sample using strong acid or base until a neutral pH is achieved
  - If a base is used to achieve neutrality, the sample is acidic, and base excess is reported as negative (-2 or -3)
  - If acid is used to achieve neutrality, the sample is alkaline, and the base excess is reported in positivity (+2 or +3, etc.)

Control of acid–base balance

- Acid–base buffers
  - Bicarbonate:
    - CO_2 excreted by the lungs
    - HCO_3 in the kidneys
  - Proteins
  - Phosphates
  - Haemoglobin
- Renal control (long-term)
- Respiratory control (short-term)

Excretion of acid

- By lungs: 16,000 mmol/day (as CO_2)
- By kidneys: 40–80 mmol/day (as H^+)
- $H^+ + HCO_3 \rightarrow H_2CO_3 \rightarrow H_2O + CO_2$
- Catalysed by carbonic anhydrase in red blood cells
- Equation can happen in either direction
- In acidosis
  - Increase in H^+ ion
  - Equation moves to right and CO_2 is excreted by lungs
  - Assisted by renal mechanisms (retention of HCO_3)
- Reverse occurs in alkalosis
- Proteins and phosphates contribute less towards control of acid base balance than HCO_3 and H^+ ions.

Renal control of pH

- Tubular secretion of H^+
- Absorption of HCO_3^-
- Step 1 (in renal tubular epithelial cells)
  - $H_2O + CO_2 \rightarrow H_2CO_3 \rightarrow H^+ + HCO_3^-$
- Step 2
  - H^+ goes to tubular fluid (active transport) and HCO_3^- goes to capillaries (diffusion)
- Step 3 (in tubular fluid)
  - $H^+ +$ (filtered) $HCO_3^- \rightarrow H_2O + CO_2$
- Step 4
  - CO_2 goes back to epithelium and H_2O is excreted in the urine
- End result
  - Filtered HCO_3^- is reabsorbed as CO_2
- In alkalosis
  - Increased plasma HCO_3^-
  - So increased urinary HCO_3^-
- In acidosis
  - Step 3 becomes $H^+ + HPO_4$ or NH_3^- in tubular fluid $\rightarrow H_2PO_4$ or $NH_4 \rightarrow$ excreted in urine
  - In step 4, filtered HCO_3^- goes back to capillaries and increases total HCO_3^-

Compensatory mechanisms in respiratory acidosis or alkalosis

- Mechanisms take several days
- Respiratory acidosis
  - Reaction as described above
  - Increase in step 3 and step 4

- Respiratory alkalosis
  - Decreased H^+ in plasma
  - So decrease in HCO_3^- absorption (step 3) and decreased plasma HCO_3^-

Respiratory control of pH

- $H_2O + CO_2 \rightarrow H_2CO_3 \rightarrow H^+ + HCO_3^-$
- So increased pCO_2 leads to increased H^+, which leads to decreased pH (equation moves to the right)
- Decreased pCO_2 leads to decreased H^+, which leads to increased pH (equation moves to the left)

Compensatory mechanism for metabolic changes

- Through chemoreceptors sensitive to H^+ ions, which alter the pCO_2
- Metabolic acidosis leads to increased ventilation, decrease in pCO_2 and increase in pH
- Metabolic alkalosis leads to decreased ventilation, increase in pCO_2 and decrease in pH
- Takes several hours to take full effect

Arterial blood gases (ABGs)

Normal values

- pH: 7.35–7.45 (H^+ ion concentration: 44–36 mmol/L)
- pCO_2: 4.5-5.5 kPa (35–45 mmHg)
  - p_aCO_2: 5.3 kPa (40 mmHg)
  - p_vCO_2: 6.1 kPa (46 mmHg)
- Base excess: –3 to +3
- pO_2: 10–13.3 kPa (75–100 mmHg)
  - p_aO_2: 13 kPa (95 mmHg)
  - p_aO_2: 5.3 kPa (40 mmHg)
- HCO_3^-: 22–26 mmol/L
- O_2 saturation: > 95%

Reading an ABG report

- Acidosis or alkalosis?
  - pH < 7.35 or > 7.45
- Respiratory component?
  - pCO_2 < 4.5 kPa suggests respiratory alkalosis if pH > 7.45 or attempted compensation of metabolic acidosis if pH < 7.35 and base excess < –3
  - pCO_2 > 5.5 kPa suggests respiratory acidosis if pH < 7.35 or attempted

compensation of metabolic alkalosis if pH > 7.45 and base excess > +3
- Metabolic component?
  - Base excess is always affected by metabolic acid–base changes
  - Metabolic acidosis causes base excess < –3
  - Metabolic alkalosis causes base excess > +3

Why bicarbonate should not be given in metabolic acidosis?

- Bicarbonate generates CO_2, which crosses easily into cells, making intracellular acidosis worse
- If ventilation is impaired, CO_2 is unable to escape via the lungs

Indications for bicarbonate therapy

- Acidosis due to diarrhoea
- Renal tubular acidosis
- Uraemic acidosis

Central venous pressure (CVP)

Measurement

- Electronic transducer
- Operates by connecting to an open-ended column of fluid; the height above zero is then measured

Zero point

- Fifth rib in the mid-axillary line, with patient supine
- Corresponds to position of the left atrium

Normal CVP

- 3–8 cmH_2O
- 1 mmHg = 1.36 cmH_2O

Fluid challenge

- 200 mL of colloid given over 5–10 minutes, or 1–2 L of crystalloid given over 20 minutes
- Response
  - Rises and falls to original value: dehydration
  - Sustained rise for 5 minutes of 2–4 cmH_2O: well-filled patient

- Rises by > 4 cmH_2O and does not fall again
  - Over-filling
  - Failing myocardium

Pulmonary capillary wedge pressure (PCWP)

- Measured by means of a balloon-tipped Swan–Ganz catheter in a branch of the pulmonary artery
- Assesses left ventricular function
- When the balloon is inflated to occlude the vessel, distal pressure is equal to left atrial pressure (the PCWP)
- Normal PCWP is 5–12 mmHg
- If CVP is high and PCWP is low, fluid challenge of PCWP is done and interpreted by similar changes in level (see above)
- Measures left ventricular end-diastolic pressure
- Also measures cardiac output and tissue oxygenation by means of mixed venous O_2 percentage

Technique

- Balloon is inflated as soon as the tip is in the superior vena cava
- Catheter guided with flow of blood through right side of heart to pulmonary artery
- Inflated balloon impacts in a pulmonary arteriole

Direct readings from pulmonary artery flotation catheter

- Right atrial pressure
- Pulmonary artery pressure
- PCWP
- Cardiac output
- Mixed venous O_2 saturation

Derived values from pulmonary artery flotation catheter

- Pulmonary vascular resistance
- Systemic vascular resistance
- O_2 extraction ratio: delivery and consumption
- Systemic O_2 consumption

Cardiopulmonary bypass

Definition

- Process by which the heart and lungs are stopped temporarily and their functions replaced by artificial means

Indications

- Cardiac surgery
- Non-cardiac surgery:
  - On great vessels
  - Lung transplant
  - Pulmonary embolectomy
- Cardio-pulmonary trauma
- Re-warming from profound hypothermia
- Resuscitation in severe respiratory failure

Initiation

- Arterial cannulation of the ascending aorta proximal to the brachiocephalic artery
- Venous cannulation into right atrium
- An alternative site is a femoro-femoral bypass for thoracic aortic procedures

The machine (pump)

- Blood is pumped from a venous reservoir and oxygenated with a membrane oxygenator that allows gas exchange across a silicone membrane
- Core systemic temperature is lowered in order to reduce metabolic demands
- Blood is filtered to remove particulate emboli and is then infused back into systemic arterial circulation via a roller pump (to produce a pulsatile flow)

Myocardial protection

- Cardioplegic arrest
  - Topical cooling
  - Intra-coronary infusion of cardioplegic solutions that contain K^+
- Intermittent cross-clamp ventricular fibrillation
- Total circulatory arrest

Discontinuing cardiopulmonary bypass

- Air is meticulously excluded from the cardiac chambers
- A direct current is used to initiate heartbeat
- The patient is re-warmed, acidosis is corrected, and ventilation is restarted
- The venous circulation is started first, then the arterial
- Protamine is given to reverse the effects of heparin

Complications of cardiopulmonary bypass

- Air embolism
- Bleeding disorders (disseminated intravascular coagulation)
- Infection
- Intestinal ischaemia or infarction
- Micro-embolisation
- Pancreatitis

Metabolic response to injury

Factors initiating the metabolic response to injury

- Volume depletion
  - Causes changes in plasma osmolality
  - Increases catecholamines, ADH and vasopressin
- Afferent nerve impulses (pain)
  - Increases sympathetic outflow
  - Increases pituitary hormones
- Bacteria and endotoxins – in gut reperfusion injury, damaged mucosal barrier and Gram-negative septicaemia

- Pro-inflammatory cytokine response – activates endogenic cascade system
- Inflammatory response:
  - Activated neutrophils and monocytes
  - Release of prostaglandins, kinins, complements and cytokines – interleukin (IL)-1, IL-6 and tumour necrosis factor (TNF)

Factors mediating the metabolic response to injury and features of the response

- See figure below

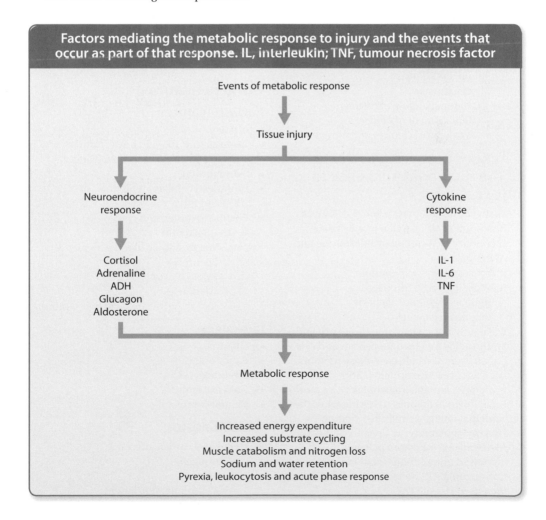

Factors mediating the metabolic response to injury and the events that occur as part of that response. IL, interleukin; TNF, tumour necrosis factor

Events of metabolic response

Tissue injury

Neuroendocrine response

Cytokine response

Cortisol
Adrenaline
ADH
Glucagon
Aldosterone

IL-1
IL-6
TNF

Metabolic response

Increased energy expenditure
Increased substrate cycling
Muscle catabolism and nitrogen loss
Sodium and water retention
Pyrexia, leukocytosis and acute phase response

Factors modifying the metabolic response to injury

- Factors that increase the metabolic response:
  - Severity of injury – the more severe the injury, the greater the metabolic response
  - Infection
  - Complications such myocardial infarction, deep vein thrombosis (DVT) and pulmonary embolism
  - Decreased ambient temperature
  - Some anaesthetics and drugs
    - Ether increases catecholamines and ADH
    - Morphine increases ADH
- Factors that decrease the metabolic response:
  - Co-existing diseases such as cancer and renal failure
  - Poor nutrition
  - Spinal anaesthesia
  - Miscellaneous:
    - Gentle handling of tissues
    - Replacement of fluid loss
    - Provision of calories and nitrogen

Changes occurring as a result of the metabolic response to injury

- Tachycardia and pyrexia for 24–48 hours
- Retention of Na and water for 2–3 days, secondary to secretion of aldosterone and ADH
- Increased energy expenditure
- Increased glucose turnover
  - Increased gluconeogenesis
  - Insulin resistance
- Breakdown of skeletal muscles to provide amino acids for gluconeogenesis and hepatic synthesis of acute phase proteins such as C-reactive protein (CRP), fibrinogen and macroglobulin
- Breakdown of adipose tissue becomes the principal energy source after trauma
- Hypercoagulability, as a result of increased ADH causing increased platelets, increased noradrenaline and increased fibrinogen for 12 hours, leading to an increased risk of DVT

- Hypocoagulability, caused by increased fibrinolysis, which can lead to the development of disseminated intravascular coagulation (DIC)

Urinary changes

- Oliguria in response to ADH secretion
- Decreased urinary Na^+ excretion, caused by renal retention of Na in response to aldosterone secretion
- Increased urinary K^+ excretion to avoid hyperkalaemia, because trauma releases intracellular K^+
- Increased urinary nitrogen excretion caused by breakdown of muscle protein

Shock

Definition

- Inadequate organ perfusion and tissue oxygenation
- State of inadequate cellular perfusion

Clinical features

Earliest features

- Anxiety
- Tachycardia: 100–120 beats/minute
- Tachypnea: 20–30 breaths/minute
- Skin mottling
- Prolonged capillary refill time (of > 2 seconds)
- Postural hypotension
  - 20–10–20 rule
    - Fall in systolic blood pressure of 20 mmHg
    - Fall in diastolic blood pressure of 10 mmHg
    - Rise in pulse rate of 20 beats/minute

Late signs

- Oliguria
- Pallor
- Sweating
- Cold extremities
- Mental confusion

Classification

- Decreased cardiac output:
  - Cardiogenic.
    - MI.
    - Ventricular fibrillation.
    - Cardiac arrest.

- Peripheral circulatory failure:
  - True hypovolaemia:
    - Blood loss.
    - Plasma loss.
    - Saline loss.
    - Dehydration.
  - Apparent hypovolaemia (vasodilatation):
    - Sepsis.
    - Adrenal insufficiency.
    - Neurogenic.
    - Anaphylaxis.

Pathophysiology of hypovolaemic shock

Cellular dysfunction

- Absence of O_2 → decreased ATP → decreased Na^+-K^+ pump
- Increased intracellular Na^+, Ca^{2+}, H_2O and decreased K^+ and Mg^{2+} ('sick cell syndrome')
- Mitochondrial swelling and disruption of the mitochondrial membrane
- Cellular swelling

Neurohumoral response

- Via sympathetic nervous system – vasoconstriction
- Via ADH – Na^+ and water conservation
- Via ACTH – cortisol, leading to Na^+ and water conservation
- Via the renin–angiotensin system – vasoconstriction
- Via histamine, kinin, complement components and arachidonic acid metabolites – alteration in vascular permeability and a pulmonary vascular response

Regional and microcirculatory flow disturbances

- Redistribution from skin, muscle and the gastrointestinal tract to the brain and the heart
- Failure of the gut barrier, with bacterial translocation
- Impairment of O_2 extraction
- Increased adhesiveness of red blood cells and platelets, causing increased blood viscosity

- Endothelial cell swelling, causing partial occlusion of capillary lumens
  - Decreased O_2 delivery
  - DIC
- Decreased intravascular hydrostatic pressure, causing influx of fluid from the interstitium

Approximate blood loss with fractures

- Pelvis: 1–5 L (about 2 L on an average)
- Femur: 1–2.5 L (about 1 L on an average)
- Tibia: 0.5–1.5 L (about 0.5 L on average)
- Humerus: 0.5–1.5 L
- Ribs: about 150 mL
- Volumes may be doubled in compound fractures

Assessment of circulation and control of haemorrhage

Parameters to assess

- Level of consciousness
- Heart rate
- Respiratory rate
- Blood pressure
- Capillary refill time

Beware

- Intra-abdominal or thoracic injury
- Femoral or pelvic fractures
- Arterial or venous penetrating injuries
- External haemorrhage
- Other causes of hypotension
  - Chest injuries
    - Cardiac contusion
    - Cardiac tamponade
    - Tension pneumothorax
    - Blunt thoracic trauma
  - Neurogenic shock (spinal cord transection)
  - Myocardial infarction
  - Septicaemia (especially if treatment has been delayed)

12-lead ECG features

- Tachycardia
- Premature ventricular beats
- ST changes
- Dysrhythmia

Sepsis

Definitions

- Bacteraemia: presence of micro-organisms in the bloodstream
- Septicaemia – acute toxic state produced by micro-organisms, their toxins or secondary mediators, in response to an invasive infection
- Systemic inflammatory response syndrome (SIRS): clinical features seen in a patient exhibiting systemic toxic response
  - Temperature > 38 °C or < 36 °C
  - Heart rate > 90 beats/minute
  - Respiratory rate > 20 breaths/minute or p_aCO_2 < 4.3 kPa (32 mmHg)
  - White cell count > 12×10^9/L (> 12,000/mm³) or < 4×10^9/L (< 4000/mm³) or > 10% immature forms
- Septic shock
  - Sepsis with systolic blood pressure < 90 mmHg or a drop of > 30 mmHg
  - Inadequate tissue oxygenation as a result of sepsis (usually Gram-negative sepsis)
- Sepsis – SIRS in a patient with confirmed infection

Haemodynamic response to sepsis

Peripheral circulation

- Decreased systemic vascular resistance as a result of:
  - Loss of vascular tone
  - Vasodilatation caused by nitric oxide
- Blood flow redistribution in favour of coronary and cerebral vasculature
- Other microcirculatory factors
  - Intravascular pooling (increased venous capacitance)
  - Microvascular sludging
  - Increased deformability of red blood cells
  - Increased platelet adhesiveness
  - Endothelial cell swelling, causing a decrease in vascular diameter
  - Interstitial oedema due to increased permeability:
    - Extrinsic capillary compression

- Acute respiratory distress syndrome (ARDS) – in pulmonary capillaries

Pulmonary circulation

- Increased pulmonary vascular resistance due to:
  - Endotoxins
  - Secondary mediators
- Neutrophil aggregation in lung capillaries
- Release of:
  - Oxygen free radicals
    - Superoxide
    - Peroxide
  - Proteases (elastase)
  - Leading to
    - Damage to basement membrane
    - Changes in permeability of the basement membrane
- Increased pulmonary vascular pressure, which may lead to right ventricular failure and right ventricular infarction

Direct myocardial effects

- Decreased myocardial contractility, caused by:
  - Increased myocardial oxygen demands
  - Left ventricular dilatation and decreased ejection fraction
  - Change in ventricular compliance, in ARDS and ventilation using positive end-expiratory pressure (PEEP)
  - Myocardial oedema, due to increased capillary permeability
  - Myocardial depressant substances released from the splanchnic bed
- Change in oxygen delivery
  - O_2 delivery = cardiac output × p_aO_2
  - In shock:
    - Cardiac output is decreased
    - Decreased oxygen content as a result of pulmonary oedema and intra-pulmonary shunts
    - So oxygen delivery is decreased
  - In sepsis, there is increased O_2 delivery, but it is inadequate because of:
    - Decreased arterial O_2 content due to ARDS
    - Splanchnic vasoconstriction
    - Microvascular sludging
    - Inability of cells to utilize O_2

Gut failure in sepsis

Definition

- Breakdown of the mucosal barrier to translocation of both endotoxins and intact organisms from the gastrointestinal into the portal circulation or the lymphatics

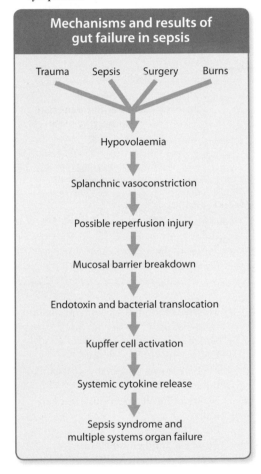

Mechanisms and results of gut failure in sepsis

Trauma   Sepsis   Surgery   Burns

↓

Hypovolaemia

↓

Splanchnic vasoconstriction

↓

Possible reperfusion injury

↓

Mucosal barrier breakdown

↓

Endotoxin and bacterial translocation

↓

Kupffer cell activation

↓

Systemic cytokine release

↓

Sepsis syndrome and multiple systems organ failure

Causes

- Acute
  - Hypovolemia
  - Ischemic hypoxic gut injury
- Chronic
  - Lack of enteral nutrition

Pathology

- Translocation of endotoxins and microorganisms
- Release of inflammatory mediators from reperfused ischaemic areas
- Failure of hepatic filtration of endotoxins
- Endotoxins and inflammatory mediators in the portal circulation, which activate Kupffer cells, leading to systemic release of cytokines

Clinical features

- Early features
  - Restlessness and slight confusion
  - Tachypnoea and tachycardia
  - Maintenance of CVP
  - Low systemic vascular resistance
  - High cardiac output
  - Normal or slightly decreased systolic blood pressure
  - Oliguria
  - Increased blood lactate
  - Warm, dry, effused extremities
- Late features
  - Decreased level of consciousness level
  - Tachypnea and tachycardia
  - Decreased CVP
  - High systemic vascular resistance
  - Low cardiac output
  - Systolic blood pressure < 90 mmHg
  - Oliguria
  - Increased blood lactate
  - Cold extremities

Acute respiratory distress syndrome (ARDS)

Definition

- Clinical syndrome characterized by type I respiratory failure, non-cardiogenic pulmonary oedema and hypoxia refractory to O_2 therapy

Events that lead to ARDS

These are shown in the figure overleaf

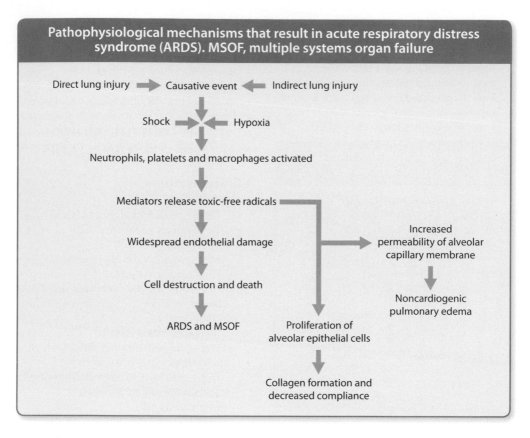

Pathophysiological mechanisms that result in acute respiratory distress syndrome (ARDS). MSOF, multiple systems organ failure

Aetiology

- Direct lung injury (local causes)
  - Blunt injury to the chest, leading to pulmonary contusion
  - Aspiration of gastric contents:
    - Coma
    - Post-operative status
  - Near-drowning
  - Embolism (fat, air or amniotic fluid emboli)
  - Inhalation of toxic fumes (e.g. from parquet)
  - Thermal injury to the respiratory tract
  - Pneumonia (bacterial, viral or drug-induced by bleomycin)
  - Radiation injury
  - O_2 toxicity
- Indirect (systemic) causes, as part of SIRS and multiple organ dysfunction syndrome
  - Severe generalised sepsis
  - Massive haemorrhage
  - Massive blood transfusion or repeated transfusions
  - Shock
  - DIC
  - Massive burns, especially with smoke inhalation
  - Major and multiple trauma or head injury
  - Pre-eclampsia
  - Amniotic fluid embolism
  - Acute severe pancreatitis
  - Cardiopulmonary bypass
  - Drug overdose or abuse
    - Tricyclic antidepressants
    - Narcotics, e.g. heroin
    - Salicylates

Phases

- Phase I
  - 16–24 hours after the initial event
  - Tachypnoea and tachycardia
  - Normal chest X-ray

- Phase II
  - 48 hours after the initial event
  - Dyspnoea and cyanosis
  - Hypoxaemia despite O_2 therapy
  - Inspiratory rhonchi
  - Normal chest X-ray
- Phase III
  - Marked tachypnoea and dyspnoea
  - High-pitched rhonchi
  - Chest X-ray shows bilateral fluffy infiltrates
- Phase IV
  - Lethargy and restlessness, leading to coma
  - Respiratory and metabolic acidosis
  - Severe hypoxaemia and hypotension
  - Urine output < 0.5 mL/kg/hour
  - Multiple organ failure
  - Chest X-ray shows white-out

Pathophysiology

- Pulmonary vasoconstriction (especially distal to the alveolar venules), leading to pulmonary hypertension, which causes neutrophil proliferation and fibrosis
- Increased pulmonary capillary permeability, leading to leakage of protein-rich fluid into the alveolar space, which also causes proliferation and fibrosis
- Less severe damage is called acute lung injury (ALI), whereas more severe damage is called ARDS
- p_aO_2–F_iO_2 ratio in ALI is 40 kPa (300 mmHg)
- p_aO_2–F_iO_2 ratio in ARDS is < 26.6 kPa (< 200 mmHg)

Treatment

- Respiratory support
  - High concentration of F_iO_2
    - If spontaneous breathing is present: continuous positive airway pressure (CPAP)
    - If on ventilator: intermittent positive pressure ventilation (IPPV)
  - Sedation
  - Large tidal volume
  - Positive end-expiratory pressure (PEEP) to reduce O_2 concentration
- Circulatory support

- Infusion of colloids, blood and cardiac tonics, e.g. dobutamine
- Monitored by Swan–Ganz catheter
- Other supportive measures
  - Elimination of infection
  - Nutritional support

Systemic inflammatory response syndrome (SIRS)

Definition

- A clinical syndrome that describes the systemic inflammatory response to a variety of severe clinical insults, manifested by two or more of the following:
  - Temperature > 38 °C or < 36 °C
  - Heart rate > 90 beats/minute
  - Respiratory rate > 20 breaths/minute or p_aCO_2 < 4.3 kPa (32 mmHg)
  - White cell count > 12×10^9/L (> 12,000/mm^3) or < 4×10^9/L (< 4000/mm^3) or > 10% immature forms

Multiple systems organ failure (MSOF)

Definition

- A clinical syndrome that describes the progressive dysfunction and ultimate failure of organs in response to a noxious stimulus, which may be trauma, infection, inflammation or their combination, leading to altered organ function in the acutely ill patient such that homoeostasis cannot be maintained without intervention
- Also known as multiple organ dysfunction syndrome (MODS)

Types

- Primary MSOF is directly attributed to the initiating insult, e.g. trauma
- Secondary MSOF is not directly attributable to the initiating insult but is a consequence of host response in organs remote from the initial insult, e.g. acute severe pancreatitis, severe burns

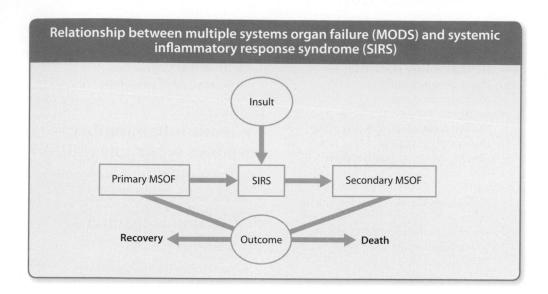

Relationship between multiple systems organ failure (MODS) and systemic inflammatory response syndrome (SIRS)

Conditions that lead to MSOF

- Prolonged inadequate perfusion
- Persistent infection
- Persistent inflammatory source
  - Pancreatitis
  - Dead tissue
- In trauma
  - Gut hypothesis: endotoxaemia
  - Two-hit model: initial injury followed by exaggerated response to a second insult

Mediators

- TNF
- IL-6 and IL-8
- Platelet activating factor

Pathology

- Adhesion of leukocytes to vascular endothelium
- Migration of white cells into the interstitial space
- Release of proteases and O_2 radicals
- Activation of arachidonic acid, leading to release of prostacyclin, thromboxane A and leukotrienes
- Vasoconstriction and microvascular thrombosis
- Mortality rate is 60%

Management

- Recognition and assessment of:
  - Underlying cause
  - Sepsis
  - Deteriorating organ functions
  - Progressive development
- Treatment involves:
  - Intravenous access
  - Infection screening
  - Haematological and biochemical screenings
  - Broad-spectrum antibiotics
  - Nutritional and organ support

Trimodal distribution of death

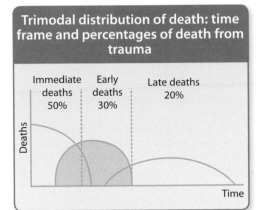

Trimodal distribution of death: time frame and percentages of death from trauma

- I – immediate deaths
- II – early deaths
- III – late deaths

Immediate deaths

- At the accident scene (40–50% of deaths from trauma)
- Seconds to minutes
- Causes
  - Primary CNS trauma
  - Brainstem laceration
  - Vascular trauma
  - Laceration to the aortic or other large blood vessels

Early deaths

- Early deaths now account for only 7% in countries where well equipped pre hospital care, field management and rapid action protocol is in place
- In areas where these are deficient, the early deaths still account for 30% of trauma mortality
- Minutes to hours
- Causes
  - Uncontrolled blood loss
  - Secondary CNS damage
- Timely intervention can prevent mortality (the 'golden hour')

Late deaths

- Account for 20% of deaths from trauma
- Days to weeks
- Causes
  - Mismanagement of stage II post-trauma
  - Sepsis
  - Systemic inflammatory response syndrome (SIRS) or multiple organ dysfunction syndrome (MODS)

Prevention of trauma

Primary prevention

- Elimination of trauma incidence, e.g. with better roads

Secondary prevention

- Reducing the severity of the incidence of trauma incidence: the 'triple Es'
  - Engineering
    - Safer vehicles
    - Head rest
    - Air cushions
  - Enforcement
    - Legislation
  - Education
    - Seat belts
    - Helmets

Tertiary prevention

- Optimisation of outcome by preventing:
  - Complications
  - Long-term disability
  - Death
- Treatment within the 'golden hour'
- Strategy for tertiary prevention
  - Protocol-based approach
  - Provision of emergency medical services (EMS)
  - Pre-hospital care, followed by hospital care, followed by trauma centre care, as required
  - Network of level 1, level 2 and level 3 hospitals
  - Research

Approach to a severely injured patient

- Establish patent airway, maintain adequate ventilatory exchange with supplementary O_2 via bag valve mask reservoir, giving 100% O_2 at 12–15 L/minute to maintain p_aO_2 of 80–100 mmHg or 95% O_2 saturation
- Establish adequate intravenous access with two wide-bore 16-gauge needle lines and assess tissue perfusion
- Take blood, and send blood for typing and cross-matching, and order baseline full blood count, electrolytes, blood glucose, alcohol level, toxicology tests and arterial blood gases if necessary; in females of child-bearing age, send urine for pregnancy testing
- Fluid challenge with crystalloids
- Brief neurological assessment: APVU (alert, response to voice, response to pain, unresponsive), examination of the pupils and Glasgow Coma Scale (GCS)
- Head-to-toe examination after initial resuscitation
- Gastric decompression and insertion of urinary catheter
- Initial fluid replacement: for each litre of blood loss, give 3 L of crystalloid replacement
- Evaluate fluid resuscitation and oxygen perfusion: if adequate, tachycardia settles down to near normal, the respiratory rate is down, the capillary refill time is down, and the hourly urine output is up

How does this approach differ from the usual approach to treat illness?

- Treat the greatest threat to life first (ABCD in that order – airways, breathing, circulation, disability assessment)
- The lack of a definitive diagnosis should not impede the application of indicated treatment, i.e. treat life-threatening situations before a definitive diagnosis is arrived at
- A detailed history is not a prerequisite to begin evaluation of a trauma patient, i.e., evaluate and treat simultaneously

Pre-hospital care

Definition

- The provision of access to the trauma system for the injured patient, and the provision of aid in the overall management by initiating evaluation and treatment by trained personnel at the scene of the accident

Goals

- Rapid access by well-equipped vehicles
- Appropriate field management by trained personnel
- Rapid transport to an appropriate hospital while providing good care en-route

Action

- Rapid assessment of the patient and the situation
- Appropriate airway management
- Field control of haemorrhage
- Stabilisation of fractures
- Initiation of volume replacement en-route
- Convey information to the hospital prior to arrival (MIVT)
  - M: mechanism
  - I: identified injuries
  - V: vital signs
  - T: treatment rendered

Emergency medical technicians (EMTs)

- Three levels of EMT: basic EMT, intermediate EMT and paramedic EMT
- Basic EMT
  - Basic life support skills, including cardiopulmonary resuscitation (CPR)
  - Splinting and bandaging
  - Extrication
  - Emergency childbirth techniques
  - Application of military anti-shock trousers (MAST)
  - Simple airway management
- Intermediate EMT
  - Basic EMT skills
  - Knowledge of the physiology of resuscitation
  - Evaluation and management of a critically injured patient, including administration of intravenous fluid therapy and endotracheal intubation

- Paramedic EMT
  - Intermediate EMT skills
  - Use of specific drugs, including adrenaline, glucose, insulin, naloxone, sodium bicarbonate, morphine, valium, calcium and frusemide

Treatment protocols

- Overall steps in patient care management taken by EMTs with every patient contact
- Established for almost every medical condition likely to be encountered
- Consists of specific standing orders
- Evaluation and emergency management is the primary emphasis when designing these protocols

Major incident triage

Definitions and patient groups

- Sorting and classification of casualties and determination of the priority of need and proper place of treatment
- Trauma patients are divided into three groups based on the extent of injury
  - Group I: rapidly fatal, within 10–15 minutes
  - Group II: potentially fatal
  - Group III: not fatal (minor injuries)
- Group II benefits most from triage
- Under-triage
  - Occurs when a patient not classified as being in group II actually belongs to it
  - Results in potentially preventable morbidity and mortality
- Over-triage
  - Occurs when a group III patient is wrongly classified as being in group II
  - Results in over-utilisation of resources

Field triage systems

- Use of physiological, anatomical and mechanism of injury data to make decisions that determine how a patient will be subsequently treated

Physiologic criteria-revised trauma score

- See table below

Anatomical criteria – abbreviated injury score (AIS)

- Penetrating injury to head, neck, torso or proximal extremity
- Two or more proximal long bone fractures
- Pelvic fracture
- Flail chest
- Amputation proximal to the wrist or ankle
- Limb paralysis
- > 10% burn or inhalation injury

Mechanism of injury

- Falls > 5 m
- Motor vehicle accident with a fatality at the scene
- Passenger ejection or a prolonged extrication (> 20 minutes)
- Major intrusion into the passenger compartment
- Pedestrians struck by a motor vehicle
- Motorcycle accident at a speed > 20 mph
- Penetrating injury to the head, neck, torso or proximal extremity

Other criteria

- Elderly patients
- Haemodynamic or respiratory dysfunction

Physiological criteria – revised trauma score. GCS, Glasgow Coma Scale			
GCS	Systolic BP (mmHg)	Respiratory rate	Coded value
13-15	>89	10-29	4
9-12	76-89	>29	3
6-8	50-75	6-9	2
4-5	1-49	1-5	1
3	0	0	0

Primary survey

Aims

- To prevent hypoxia
- To prevent hypercarbia
- To provide adequate tissue and organ perfusion
- To prevent further disability
- Plus initial neurological assessment and resuscitation

A – airway assessment

- Ask the patient's name (greet the patient)
- If the patient gives a logical response in a normal voice:
  - Airway is patent
  - Ventilation is intact
  - Cerebral perfusion is adequate
- Non-verbal response means partial or complete airway obstruction:
  - Foreign body
  - Tongue fallen back (hypopharyngeal obstruction)
  - Mandibular or maxillary fracture (genioglossus paralysis)
  - Tracheal or laryngeal disruption
- Manoeuvres
  - Triple airway manoeuvre
    - Chin lift
    - Jaw thrust
    - Mouth open
  - Cleaning of oropharynx by rigid metallic suction tube to prevent it travelling through a possible fracture of the cribriform plate into the cranial vault
- Role of the genioglossus muscle
  - Keeps the tongue up
  - In a fracture of the mandible, the genioglossus muscle is injured and the tongue falls back

Cervical spine

- 30% of polytrauma patients have cervical spine fractures
- Precautions to secure in-line immobilisation
  - Sand bag
  - Rigid collar
- Signs and symptoms of suspected cervical spine fracture
  - Quadriparesis
  - Paraparesis

- X-rays in suspected cervical spine fracture
  - Lateral cervical spine
  - Swimmer's view (for C7 and T1)
  - Open-mouth view (for C1 and C2)

B – breathing

- In an unconscious patient with no gag reflex: oropharyngeal airway (size 3)
- In a semiconscious patient: nasopharyngeal airway
- If airway is secure: give 100% O_2 in a tight fitting Hudson mask ($F_iO_2 > 0.8$) with a flow of 10–12 L/minute
- If airway is unstable: bag valve mask with reservoir bag attached and give 100% F_iO_2 with a flow of 10–12 L/minute flow ($F_iO_2 > 0.9$)
- Strip thorax
  - Look for marks, holes and movement
  - Respiratory rate
    - Normal rate is 12–18 breaths/minute
    - If < 9 breaths/minute or > 24 breaths/minute (likely if thoracic problems are haemorrhagic shock is present): assisted ventilation
- Assess pulse, blood pressure and ECG
- Look for:
  - Skin colour
  - Tracheal deviation
  - Chest movement
- Listen and percuss for:
  - Tension pneumothorax
  - Cardiac tamponade
  - Open chest wound of more than two thirds the tracheal diameter
  - Flail chest
  - Haemothorax
- Distinguishing between cardiac tamponade and tension pneumothorax (see table)
- Ensuring that oxygenation and ventilation is adequate
  - No cyanosis
  - Check neck for distended veins
  - Tracheal position – central
  - Symmetrical movement of chest
  - Percussion for bilateral air entry
  - Continuous oxygen saturation (pulse oximetry > 95%)
- When intubation ought to be performed depends on:
  - The stability of the airway
  - The patient's respiratory effort

Distinguishing between cardiac tamponade and tension pneumothorax

Features	Cardiac tamponade	Tension pneumothorax
Effects	Primary pathological effect: decreased cardiac output Respiratory impairment is a secondary effect Threat to life is due to cardiac impairment Acutely life-threatening Rapid therapy required	Primary pathological effect: decreased cardiac output Respiratory impairment is a secondary effect Threat to life is due to cardiac impairment Acutely life-threatening Rapid therapy required
Etiology and pathogenesis	Decrease in cardiac output due to accumulation of blood within pericardial sac sufficient to restrict the filling of ventricles	Air escapes from lung parenchyma raising pressure Ipsilateral lung compressed, collapses against mediastinum Mediastinum shift away from affected side Vena cava 'kinked', venous return to heart impaired Cardiac output compromised leading to circulatory collapse
Clinical features	Evidence of penetrating injury Dyspnoea Low-blood pressure, shock Distended neck veins Quiet heart sound Low-voltage electrocardiogram	Dyspnoea Distended neck veins Shock Cyanosis Mediastinal shift away from affected side Subcutaneous emphysema (air bubbles in tissues) Absent or quiet breath sounds Hyper-resonant percussion note (drum-like)

Classes of haemorrhagic shock

Parameter	Class I	Class II	Class III	Class IV
Blood loss (ml)	< 750	750-1500	1500-2000	> 2000
Blood loss (%)	< 15	15-30	30-40	> 40
Pulse rate/min	< 100	> 100	> 120	> 140
BP	Normal	Normal	↓↓	↓↓↓
Pulse pressure	Normal or ↑	Narrowed	Narrowed	Narrowed
Capillary refill	N (2 sec)	Delayed	Delayed	Delayed
Respiratory rate/min	14-20	20-30	30-35	> 35
Urine ml/hr	> 30	20-30	5-15	Negligible
CNS	Slightly anxious	Mildly anxious	Anxious, confused	Confused, lethargic
Fluid replacement	Crystalloid	Crystalloid	Crystalloid + blood	Crystalloid + blood

- How to monitor:
  - Pulse oximetry
  - Arterial blood gases: < 93% oxygen saturation (p_aCO_2 < 8.5 kPa) acts as a warning; < 90% means that the patient is in severe trouble
- Aims of assisted ventilation
  - To maintain:
    - p_aO_2 > 10 kPa (80 mmHg)
    - p_aCO_2 < 5.5 kPa (40 mmHg)
  - Ideally if p_aCO_2 is maintained at 4 kPa (30 mmHg), it will reduce cerebral oedema and intracranial pressure

C – circulation

- Look for bleeding
  - Capillary refill time > 2 seconds
  - Decreased pulse pressure
- Blood loss from fractures
  - Ribs: about 150 mL
  - Tibia or humerus: 0.5–1.5 L
  - Femur: 1–2.5 L (1 L average)
  - Pelvis: 1–5 L (2 L average)
  - Volumes may be doubled in compound fractures
- Assessment
  - Level of consciousness
  - Heart rate, respiratory rate and blood pressure
  - Capillary refill time
- Haemorrhagic shock class: see table, p. 27

Differential diagnosis of shock apart from haemorrhage

- Injuries above diaphragm
  - Myocardial contusion
  - Cardiac tamponade
  - Tension pneumothorax
- Blunt thoracic trauma
- Neurogenic shock (from spinal cord transection)
- Myocardial infarction
- Septicaemia (if treatment is delayed)

Action in haemorrhagic shock

- Two peripheral lines – 14–16 gauge (remembering Poiseuille's law: the rate of fluid flow through a pipe is directly proportional to the fourth power of radius and inversely proportional to the length)
- Blood drawn for baseline haematology, electrolytes, sugar, typing and cross-match

- Females of childbearing age: pregnancy test
- 12-lead ECG
  - Cardiac tamponade or tension pneumothorax may be shown by:
    - Tachycardia
    - Premature ventricular beats
    - ST changes
    - Dysrhythmia
    - Electromechanical dissociation
  - Hypoxia or hypoperfusion may be shown by:
    - Bradycardia
    - Aberrant conduction
    - Premature ventricular beats

Fluid challenge

- Warmed lactated Ringer's solution is used
  - Rapid intravenous infusion of either:
    - 200 mL colloid in 5–10 minutes (2 mL/kg in children), or
    - 1–2 L of crystalloid in 20 minutes (20 mL/kg in children)
- Assessment by urine output
  - Adult: 50 mL/hour
  - Child: 1 mL/kg/hour
  - Infant: 2 mL/kg/hour
- Response (see table)
  - Decrease in pulse rate, increase in blood pressure
  - Decrease in capillary refill time (to 2 seconds)
  - Patient well-orientated
  - Increase in urine output
  - Central venous pressure (CVP) rises to normal

CVP response (see figure)

- Normal CVP is 5–10 cmH$_2$O
- Normal pulmonary capillary wedge pressure (PCWP) is 10–15 mmHg
- A rapid CVP response indicates normovolaemia
- A transient CVP response indicates:
  - Ongoing haemorrhage
  - Inadequate resuscitation
- No CVP response indicates:
  - Massive haemorrhage (> 40% blood loss)
  - Pump failure
    - Myocardial contusion
    - Cardiac tamponade

Response to initial fluid resuscitation (200 mL of lactated Ringer's solution, or 20 mL/kg in a child)			
	Rapid response	**Transient response**	**No response**
Vital signs	Return to normal	Transient improvement Recurrence of ↓ BP and ↓ HR	Remain abnormal
Estimated blood loss	Minimal (10-20%)	Moderate and ongoing (30-40%)	Severe (>40%)
Need for more crystalloid	Low	High	High
Need for blood	Low	Moderate to high	High
Blood preparation	Type and crossmatch (1–2 hours)	Type specific (saline crossmatch – 10 min)	Emergency blood release (O negative)
Need for operative intervention	Possible	Likely	Highly likely
Early presence of surgeon	Yes	Yes	Yes

Central venous pressure (CVP) response to fluid challenge in hypervolaemia, normovolaemia and hypovolaemia

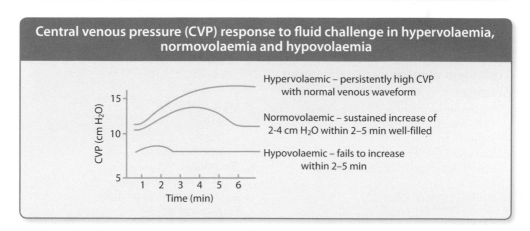

Blood transfusion

- Properly cross-matched blood available in 1–2 hours
- Saline cross-matched, type-specific blood available in 10 minutes
- Uncross-matched, O-negative blood available immediately
- Blood is ordered depending on the class of hypovolaemic shock

- Prevention of coagulopathy
  - 1 unit of fresh frozen plasma (FFP) for each unit of packed red blood cells (PRBCs) transfused
  - 10 units of platelets for each 6 units of PRBCs transfused
  - Calcium gluconate is given with the rapid infusion of 4 units of PRBC to provide cardiac protection in massive transfusion

Causes of unconsciousness

- Head injury
- Decreased oxygenation (hypoxia)
- Shock
- Alcohol and drugs
- Endocrine causes
  - Hypoglycaemia
  - Hyperglycaemia
  - Diabetic ketoacidosis
  - Myxoedema

D – disability

- Rapid neurological assessment
  - Aim is to prevent secondary brain damage
  - A: alert
  - V: response to verbal commands
  - P: response to pain
  - U: unresponsive
  - Plus pupillary size
- Glasgow Coma Scale (GCS)
  - Provides a quantitative measurement of the patient's level of consciousness
  - Mild impairment: GCS of 13–15
  - Moderate impairment: GCS of 9–12
  - Severe impairment: GCS < 8
  - It also assesses:
    - Pupillary function
    - Lateralised extremity weakness

Treatment of increased intracranial pressure

- Hyperventilation to decrease p_aCO_2 to 4 kPa (26–28 mmHg)
- Sedation and paralysis
- No hypo-osmolar intravenous fluids
- Mannitol 1 g/kg rapidly or frusemide 40–80 mg
- Monitor urinary volume

E – exposure

- Keep exposure to a minimum
- Prevent hypothermia

Secondary survey

History

- A: allergies
- M: medications
- P: past history
- L: last meal
- E: event mechanism

Head-to-toe examination

- Head
  - Eyes
  - Scalp
  - Head injury
- Maxillary–facial area
  - Airway
  - Cervical spine
  - Lacrimal ducts
- Neck
  - Oesophagus
  - Airway
  - Carotid arteries
- Chest
  - Pneumothorax
    - Tension pneumothorax
    - Open pneumothorax
  - Flail chest
  - Cardiac tamponade
  - Aorta
- Abdomen
  - Intraperitoneum
  - Retroperitoneum
  - Pelvis
- Perineum
  - Rectum
  - Urethra
  - Bladder
- Musculoskeletal
  - Spine
  - Digits
  - Vascular system
- Neurological
  - Intracranial pressure
  - Depressed skull fracture
- Fingers and tubes
  - Rectal examination to assess the rectal wall and prostate
  - Vaginal examination to assess the vaginal vault
  - Urinary catheter – beware of:
    - Blood in the meatus
    - Prostate
  - Nasogastric tube – beware of:
    - A mid-face fracture

Summary of the approach to an injured patient

- Primary survey – ABCDE
- Resuscitation and re-assessment
- Secondary survey – tubes and fingers
- Definitive care
- Approach to polytrauma
  - Establish a patent airway and maintain adequate ventilatory exchange with supplementary O_2 via bag valve mask reservoir, giving 100% O_2 at 10–15 L/minute to maintain p_aO_2 of 80–100 mmHg or 95% O_2 saturation
  - Establish adequate intravenous access with two intravenous lines with wide bore 16 gauge needles, and assess tissue perfusion
  - Fluid challenge with crystalloids
  - Brief neurological assessment
  - Head-to-toe examination after initial assessment

Head injury

Missile injury

- Causes a depressed fracture but does not enter the brain
- In a penetrating injury, the missile enters the skull but does not exit it
- In a perforating injury, the missile enters and leaves the skull

Non-missile injury

- Result mainly from road traffic accidents
- Primary brain damage is due to direct injury
  - Contusion
    - Coup
    - Contre-coup
  - Diffuse axonal injury
- Secondary brain damage is due to complications
  - Intracranial haemorrhage
  - Cerebral hypoxia
  - Cerebral oedema
  - Intracranial herniation
  - Infection

Sequelae of head injuries

- Death
- Persistent vegetative state
- Post-traumatic epilepsy
- Traumatic hemiplegia
- Post-traumatic dementia
- Cranial nerve palsies

Spinal cord injuries

Causes

- Road traffic accidents
- Falls
- Penetrating wounds
  - Incomplete (Brown–Séquard syndrome)
  - Complete
- Closed injuries
  - – Associated with fracture or fracture-dislocation of the vertebral column

Types of injury

- Primary damage
  - Contusion
  - Transection
  - Haemorrhage
  - Necrosis
- Secondary damage
  - Extradural haematoma
  - Infection
  - Infarction
  - Oedema

Pathogenesis

- Contusion and laceration causes oedema and increased tissue pressure
- If cord haemorrhage is added, it decreases blood supply
- The distribution of oedema, infarction and haemorrhage determines the neurological signs and symptoms

Complete transection

- Irreversible loss of voluntary movement distal to the level of transection
- Loss of all sensation distal to the level of transection

- Spinal shock
  - Loss of all reflexes, including bulbocavernosus and deep tendon reflexes
  - Lasts from a few hours to several weeks
  - Return of reflexes thereafter

Incomplete injury

- Some functions are preserved below the level of injury
- Anterior cord syndrome
  - Associated with flexion and rotation injuries to the spine with anterior dislocation, e.g. compression fracture of a vertebral body
  - Causes loss of power and of pain and temperature sensation below the lesion
  - Touch perception is unaffected
- Central cord syndrome
  - Associated with cervical spondylosis plus a hyperflexion injury
  - Causes flaccid (lower motor neurone) weakness of the arms
  - Perianal sensation and lower limb movement and sensation are preserved
- Posterior cord syndrome
  - Fracture of the posterior elements of a vertebra
  - Causes ataxia as a result of loss of proprioception
  - Power and pain and temperature sensation are preserved
- Brown–Séquard syndrome
  - Results from hemisection of the cord caused by a stab or a fracture of the lateral mass of a vertebra
  - Causes ipsilateral paralysis, with pain and temperature sensation lost on the contralateral side
- Cauda equina syndrome
  - Causes bowel and bladder dysfunction and leg weakness

Autonomic dysfunction

Vasomotor dysfunction

- Occurs in lesions above C5
- Interruption of sympathetic splanchnic control, leading to decreased venous return, which causes postural hypotension and syncope

- Initial period may be life-threatening due to autonomic dysfunction. Improves after the first few days

Dysfunction of temperature regulation

- Loss of thermoregulatory mechanisms below the level of the lesion
- Loss of shivering and sweating

Loss of bladder control

- In spinal shock, acute retention can occur
- In an upper motor neurone lesion above the sacral segments, 'automatic bladder' occurs after the initial spinal shock
- In a lower motor neurone lesion, an autonomous bladder occurs, causing overflow incontinence

Loss of bowel function

- Injuries above the sacral segments result in automatic bowel emptying
- In an upper motor neurone lesion, the external sphincter is hypertonic
- In a lower motor neurone lesion, there is an autonomous bowel with intrinsic contractility and a lax external sphincter

Autonomic dysreflexia

- Occurs in lesions above T5
- Occurs after the period of spinal shock
- Distension of the bladder
- Sympathetic over-activity below the level of injury, causing vasoconstriction and hypertension, and leading to stimulation of the carotid and aortic baroreceptors, increased vagal tone and bradycardia

Peripheral nerve injuries

- Neuropraxia
  - Temporary block in the conduction of nerve impulses caused by blunt trauma to a nerve that leaves the axonal transport system intact
- Axonotmesis
  - Axonal transport is interrupted but endoneural tubes are intact and the axon grows distally
- Neurotmesis
  - Complete disruption of the nerve
  - No regeneration is possible

- See tables overleaf for summaries of peripheral nerve injuries in the limbs

Penetrating trauma

- Results from gunshot and stab wounds
- Clinical consequences are dependent on:
  - Energy transfer
  - Anatomical factors

Energy transfer

- Energy transfer varies according to:
  - Kinetic energy of the weapon or missile
  - Mean presenting area of the weapon or missile
  - The tendency of the weapon or missile to deform and fragment
  - The density of the tissue penetrated
  - The mechanical characteristics of the missile
    - High-velocity missiles have a high kinetic energy
    - A knife used in a stabbing has a low kinetic energy
  - The neighbouring tissues that are injured as a result of the transfer of kinetic energy; the maximum injury occurs when the missile fragments and fails to exit

Cavitation

- Neighbouring tissues are pushed away from the missile track, forming a temporary cavity that is 30–40 times the diameter of the missile (depending on the energy transfer)
- Lasts a few milliseconds
- Tissues retract back to a permanent cavity, owing to the immediate destruction of tissue in the direct path of the missile
- Consequences
  - Functional and mechanical disruption of neighbouring tissues (disruption is more with solid organs)
  - Core of clothing can be carried with the missile into the cavity, leading to contamination and infection
  - If the missile traverses a narrow part of the body, such as the arm, the exit wound is larger than the entry wound because of cavitation
  - If the missile traverses a larger part of the body, such as the abdomen, the exit wound is smaller than the entry wound because cavitation occurs within the part of the body that has been traversed

Anatomical factors

- A stab wound heals like a clean incised wound, with minimal scarring
- Consequences depend on the type and extent of organs involved, e.g. if the heart is penetrated it is fatal

Blast injuries

- Sudden release of considerable energy
- Initial instantaneous increase in pressure in the surrounding air, called a shock front or blast wave
- Moves through the air in all directions and becomes weaker at the periphery
- Blast wind
  - Movement of air at the periphery of a blast wave
  - Carries fragments from bomb or debris, which may cause high-energy transfer wounds

Types of injuries

- Primary effects
  - Caused by the shock front
  - Affects air containing organs, e.g. the lung ('blast lung'), the bowel ('blast gut'), the ears ('blast tympanic membrane')
  - Blast lung
    - Haemorrhage into the alveolar spaces
    - Damage to the alveolar septums
    - Stripping of the bronchial epithelium
    - Emphysematous blebs on the pleural surface
  - Blast gut
    - Contusion of the gut wall and leakage of blood into lumen, leading to perforation
  - Blast tympanic membrane
    - Rupture or congestion of the tympanic membrane
  - Ventilation–perfusion mismatch may occur, leading to hypoxia

Summary of peripheral nerve injuries – upper limb

Nerve	Branches to	Level of injury	Deformity	Sensory loss	Test
Upper brachial plexus (Erb-Duchenne) C5–7	Biceps, brachialis, brachioradialis, supinator, deltoid		Internal rotation, elbow extended, forearm pronated, wrist flexed (waiter's tip)	Lateral aspect of arm	
Lower brachial plexus (Klumpke) C8, T1	Small muscles of hand		Claw hand (median & ulnar) & Horner's syndrome	Medial aspect of forearm & medial 1½ fingers	
Axillary (C5, C6)	Deltoid	Surgical neck of humerus	Flattening of shoulder	Badge area of the upper arm	Abduction of shoulder 30–90°
Long thoracic nerve of Bell (C5–7)	Serratus anterior	Mastectomy	Winging of scapula	-	Abduction of shoulder > 90° Pushing against wall
Radial (C5–8, T1)	Triceps, brachioradialis, extensor carpi radialis longus	Axilla	Paralysis of triceps Wrist drop	Dorsum of forearm Anatomical snuff box	Extension of wrist
		Radial groove	Wrist drop	Anatomical snuff box	
		Below elbow	Wrist drop	-	
Ulnar (C8, T1)	Flexor carpi ulnaris, inner half of flexor digitorum profundus, small muscles of hand except thenar	Elbow	Wasting of ulnar side of forearm & hypothenar muscles Ulnar claw hand	Medial 1½ fingers Hypothenar eminence	Paper test for adduction of fingers
		Wrist	Ulnar claw hand	Medial 1½ fingers	

Median (C5–8, T1)	All flexors of forearm except flexor carpi ulnaris & medial half of flexor digitorum profundus	Elbow	Pointing index Wasting of thenar eminence Simian (ape) hand	Radial 3½ fingers	Hand deviates to ulnar side when flexed Oschner's clasping test Pen test for abduction of thumb
		Wrist	Wasting of thenar eminence. Simian (ape) hand.		

Summary of peripheral nerve injuries – lower limb

Nerve	Branches to	Level of injury	Deformity	Sensory loss	Test
Common peroneal (lateral popliteal)	Extensors & peroneal muscles	Neck of fibula	Talipes equinovarus Foot drop	Lateral aspect of leg & dorsum of foot except skin of 1st web space	High-stepping gait
Tibial nerve (medial popliteal)	All plantar flexors	Open leg wounds	Talipes calcaneovarus Claw toes	Sole of foot	Plantar flexion of foot
Femoral nerve	Quadriceps	Groin	Paralysis & wasting of quadriceps	Medial aspect of lower $1/3$ of leg	Inability to extend knee
Sciatic nerve	All flexors of knee Hamstrings	Above branch to hamstrings	Paralysis of hamstrings Foot drop	Below knee except medial aspect of leg	Absent ankle jerk
		Below branch to hamstrings	Foot drop only	Same	Same

- Multiple air emboli can cause sudden death
- Secondary effects
  - Caused by the direct impact of fragments carried in the blast wind
  - The patient presents with multiple extensive wounds of varying depth, which are grossly contaminated
- Tertiary effects
  - Result of the dynamic force of the wind itself, which may be great enough to carry all or part of the patient with itself
    - Impact (deceleration) injuries
    - Traumatic amputations
  - Injuries from falling masonry, fires, toxic chemicals and flash burns
  - Acute and chronic psychological disturbances

Hypothermia

Definition

- Condition in which the temperature of the body drops below the level required for normal metabolism and for bodily functions to take place

Stages

- Stage I: drop of 1–2 °C
  - Shivering
  - Tachypnoea
- Stage II: drop of 2–4 °C
  - Shivering is more severe
  - Peripheral vasoconstriction
- Stage III: body temperature < 32.2 °C
  - Failure of major organs, owing to shutdown of cellular metabolism

Treatment

- Emergency treatment: bathe in medium-temperature water with clothes on
- Warming blankets, warming devices, warm intravenous fluids, and warm lavage of bladder, stomach, chest and abdominal cavities
- High risk of arrhythmia, so jostling and other disturbances should be minimised

Induced hypothermia

- Used as preparation for surgery on the heart
- Can be used during artificial coma to increase survival chances after cardiac arrest or severe trauma
- Occurs during anaesthetic induction due to vasodilatation

Heat exhaustion

Definition

- Mild-to-moderate dysfunction of temperature control associated with elevated ambient temperature; it may rapidly progress to heat stroke
- Definition of heat stroke
  - Extreme hyperthermia (> 40 °C) associated with a systemic inflammatory response, which leads to end-organ damage and universal involvement of the CNS

Types

- Exertional: in young people after severe exercise
- Classic: in elderly people, caused by high environmental temperatures

Pathophysiology

- Rate of heat gain exceeds the ability of the body to dissipate heat
- Normal heat acclimatisation results in:
  - Earlier onset of sweating, increased sweat volume and dilute sweat
  - Increased cardiovascular performance
  - Activation of renin–angiotensin–aldosterone axis, leading to salt conservation and increased plasma volume
  - Increased glomerular filtration rate
  - Ability to resist rhabdomyolysis
- However, failure of the normal mechanism of heat acclimatisation results in:
  - Acute-phase response
  - Production of cytokines and mediators
  - Fever and shunting of splanchnic blood to periphery
  - Endotoxaemia
  - Heat stroke
- Patients at the extremes of age are more susceptible

Clinical features

- Heat exhaustion, with non-specific symptoms and signs
- Heat stroke
  - Hyperdynamic cardiovascular system
  - Delerium, seizures and coma
  - Disseminated intravascular coagulation and other coagulation disorders

Treatment

- ABC of resuscitation
- Immediate cooling
  - Tepid water bath and fan
  - Ice packs

- Correction of dehydration
- Laboratory work-up should be done to detect end-organ damage
- Support of organs

Radiation injury

- Natural radiation injury
  - Cosmic radiation
  - Radar gas from rocks and minerals
- Man-made radiation injury
  - Nuclear weapons and tests
  - Medical tests and treatments
- Radiation damage depends on:
  - Amount of radiation
  - Duration of exposure
  - Exposed area
  - Type of tissue (the gastrointestinal tract, bone marrow and gonads are particularly radiosensitive)

Clinical features

- Acute radiation damage
  - Haemopoietic abnormalities with aplastic anaemia as a result of damage to the bone marrow, spleen and lymph nodes
  - Gastrointestinal tract damage
    - Nausea, vomiting and diarrhoea, causing dehydration
    - Gut barrier failure, causing severe septicaemia
  - CNS
    - Confusion
    - Seizures
    - Coma leading to death
- Chronic radiation damage
  - Abnormalities of cell growth, leading to cancer
  - Birth defects

Effects of radiation therapy given for cancer

- Nausea, vomiting and loss of appetite

- Skin: hair loss, redness, thinning and spider naevi
- Mouth and jaw: dental abscesses and osteoradionecrosis of the mandible
- Lungs: radiation pneumonitis and fibrosis
- Heart: pericarditis and fibrosis
- Spinal cord: paralysis
- Abdomen: radiation enteritis
  - Chronic ulcers
  - Scarring
  - Stricture
  - Perforation
- Gonads
  - Amenorrhoea
  - Infertility
- Kidneys: renal failure, with anaemia and hypertension
- Muscles: atrophy, calcification and malignancy
- Thyroid: cancer

Diagnosis

- Blood counts
- Geiger counter: swabs from the nose, the throat and wounds

Outcome

- Cerebrovascular: usually fatal
- Gastrointestinal and haematopoietic: survival depends on dosage of radiation

Treatment

- Depends on severity
- Isolation
- Removal of radioactive material from the body using:
  - Potassium iodide
  - Diethylene triamine penta-acetic acid (DTPA) or ethylene diamine tetra-acetic acid (EDTA)
  - Penicillamine
- Growth factors, erythropoietin colony stimulating factors, bone marrow transplantation

Chapter 4

General pathology

Cell growth and development

Definitions

- Hyperplasia: increased number of cells as a result of inflammation, work load, endocrine drive or metabolic demand
- Hypertrophy: increase in cell size but not number, caused by a demand for increased function
- Metaplasia: reversible replacement of one differentiated cell type with another
- Dysplasia:
  - Disordered cellular development, caused by increased mitosis or pleomorphism (pre-neoplastic)
  - Degree of failure of maturation of tissue
- Hamartoma: overgrowth of mature cells with disordered architecture
- Teratoma: growth of cells originating from more than one cell line
- Neoplasia: abnormal mass of tissue when growth is unco-ordinated, exceeds that of normal tissue and persists in the same manner after cessation of the evoking stimulus
- Latent period: time required for a single cell to proliferate into a clinically detectable mass
- Growth fraction: proportion of cells within a tumour mass that are in replicative pools (20% in rapidly growing tumours)
- Hypoplasia: reduction in frequency of cell division relative to the normal rate for that tissue or organ
- Aplasia: complete cessation of cell growth and multiplication

Cell cycle

Definition

- Interval between each cell division

Phases

- G0: resting phase
- G1: first gap phase (synthesis of proteins)
- S: synthesis of DNA (requires epidermal growth factor)
- G2: second gap phase (preparation for mitosis)
- M: mitosis

Restriction point

- Point at G1 when the cell becomes committed to enter S phase
- Growth factors are required before the restriction point but not after it
- Growth factors at G1 check point:
  - Platelet-derived growth factor (PDGF)
  - Epidermal growth factor (EGF)
  - Insulin-like growth factor (IGF) 1 and 2

Cell types in relation to cell cycle

- Labile cells: cells that are constantly renewed, e.g. skin cells
- Stable cells: quiescent cells but can be stimulated to divide, e.g. liver cells
- Permanent cells: cells that do not undergo mitosis, e.g. cells in the brain

Duration of cell cycle

- Only the duration of G1 varies, e.g. 12 hours for intestinal epithelial cells; > 1 year for hepatocytes
- Other phases are constant:
  - M: 1 hour
  - S: 6–8 hours
  - G2: 3–4 hours
- Mitotic index: percentage of cells in mitosis at a given time

Response of cell to damage

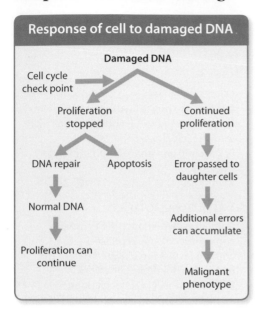

Response of cell to damaged DNA

Damaged DNA

Cell cycle check point → Proliferation stopped → Continued proliferation

Proliferation stopped → DNA repair / Apoptosis

DNA repair → Normal DNA → Proliferation can continue

Continued proliferation → Error passed to daughter cells → Additional errors can accumulate → Malignant phenotype

Apoptosis

Definition

- Degradation of a cell to balance mitosis in regulating the size and function of the tissue, or to eliminate unwanted or damaged cells that have abnormal DNA
- Also known as programmed cell death

Events

- A series of genetically controlled steps causing chromatin condensation, fragmentation and cell shrinkage
- Resultant material is engulfed by neighbouring cells without inflammatory reaction (unlike death by lysis, which causes an inflammatory reaction)
- Inability to undergo apoptosis promotes cancer growth
  - Genetic instability
  - Resistance to chemotherapy and radiotherapy
  - Increased rate of cell growth

Regulation (control) of apoptosis

- *bcl*-2 decreases apoptosis by mediating apoptosis inhibitors, e.g. growth factors, oestrogens and androgens
- bax protein increases apoptosis by mediating apoptosis stimulators, e.g. glucocorticoids and cytotoxic drugs
- *bcl*-2–bax protein ratio determines the cell's decreased susceptibility to apoptosis
- This ratio is otherwise called molecular switch
- Its clinical importance lies in the possibility of finding therapeutic agents to enhance cell death in the treatment of malignant neoplasms

Inflammation

- Definition: physiological response to tissue injury
- Classification is according to its time course:
  - Acute
    - Initial and transient series of tissue reactions to injury
    - Lasts from a few hours to a few days
  - Chronic
    - Subsequent and prolonged tissue reactions that occur after the initial response

Acute inflammation

- Features
  - Initial vasodilatation and increased permeability
  - Exudative phase: fluid and cells escape from permeable vessels
    - Neutrophils
    - Mast cells
    - Macrophages
  - Outcomes
    - Regression (resolution)
    - Suppuration leading to abscess
    - Organisation and repair
    - Progression to chronic inflammation
- Causes
  - Microbial infections
    - Pyogenic bacteria
    - Viruses
  - Hypersensitivity reactions
    - Parasites
    - Tuberculosis
  - Physical agents
    - Trauma
    - Ionising radiation

- Heat
- Cold
- Chemicals
  - Corrosives
  - Acids and alkalis
  - Reducing agents
  - Bacterial toxins
- Tissue necrosis: ischaemic infarction
- Macroscopic appearance
  - Redness (*rubor*)
  - Heat (*calor*)
  - Swelling (*tumor*)
  - Pain (*dolor*)
  - Loss of function
- Microscopic appearance
  - Changes in vessel calibre and flow (triple response)
    - Momentary arteriolar vasoconstriction
    - Flush, caused by capillary dilatation
    - Flare, caused by arteriolar dilatation
    - Wheal, caused by exudation
  - Increased vascular permeability, causing exudates (protein leak)
    - Increased colloid osmotic pressure of interstitial fluid
    - Increased fluid leak, causing oedema
  - Cellular exudates, caused by neutrophil emigration
    - Rich in immunoglobulin, fibrinogen (fibrin exudates)
    - Neutrophil margination, adhesion and emigration produced by inflammatory mediators, e.g. interleukin (IL)-1, tumour necrosis factor (TNF), complement and bradykinin
- Role of neutrophil polymorphs
  - Chemotaxis towards inflammation
  - Opsonisation of micro-organisms (rendering them more amenable for phagocytosis)
  - Phagocytosis of micro-organisms and intracellular killing
- Suppurative inflammation
  - Production of pus, which consists of degenerate neutrophils, organisms and liquefied tissues
  - Walled off by granulation and/or fibrosis, leading to abscess formation
  - Inaccessible to antibiotics

- If deep, may cause sinus or fistula formation
- If longstanding, may lead to dystrophic calcification
- Constitutional symptoms, e.g. fever, malaise and anaemia

Chronic inflammation

- Features
  - Predominance of lymphocytes, plasma cells and macrophages
  - May be primary or may follow recurrent acute inflammation
  - Granulomatous inflammation is a specific type: a granuloma is an aggregate of epithelioid histiocytes
  - May be complicated by secondary amyloidosis
- Causes
  - Primary chronic inflammation, e.g. tuberculosis, brucellosis
  - Transplant rejection
  - Progression from acute in bacterial infections as a result of defence mechanisms to phagocytosis
    - Outer capsule
    - Exotoxin
    - Binding to non-phagocytic cells
- Macroscopic appearance
  - Chronic ulcer
  - Chronic abscess cavity
  - Thickening of wall of a hollow viscus
  - Granulomatous inflammation
  - Fibrosis
- Microscopic appearance
  - Cellular infiltrate
    - Lymphocytes
    - Plasma cells
    - Macrophages, which fuse to form multinucleated giant cells
  - Production of new fibrous tissue from granulation tissue
  - Evidence of continuing tissue destruction with regeneration and repair
- Role of lymphocytes
  - B lymphocytes: production of antibody
  - T lymphocytes: cell-mediated immunity
    - Recruitment of macrophages
    - Production of inflammatory mediators

- Recruitment of other lymphocytes
- Destruction of target cells
- Interferon production
- Role of macrophages
  - Derived from blood monocytes
  - Can ingest and kill bacteria (mononuclear phagocyte system)
  - Produce important cytokines – IL-1, IL-6, IL-8, interferon (IFN)-alpha, IFN-beta and TNF
  - Specialised macrophages
    - Epithelioid histiocytes in granulomatous inflammation
    - Histiocytic giant cells, caused by indigestible bacterial accumulation inside macrophages
    - Langhan's giant cells (seen in tuberculosis)
    - Foreign body giant cells
    - Touton's giant cells

Systemic effects of inflammation

- Pyrexia
  - Caused by endogenous pyrogens acting on the hypothalamus to set thermoregulatory mechanism at a higher temperature
  - Stimulated by:
    - Phagocytosis
    - Endotoxins
    - Immune complexes
- Constitutional symptoms
  - Malaise
  - Anorexia
  - Nausea
- Weight loss, caused by negative nitrogen balance
- Reactive hyperplasia of the reticuloendothelial system
  - Lymph nodal enlargement
  - Splenomegaly
    - Malaria
    - Infectious mononucleosis
- Haematological changes
  - Increased erythrocyte sedimentation rate (ESR)
  - Leukocytosis
    - Neutrophilia (in pyogenic inflammation)
    - Eosinophilia (in allergic inflammation)
    - Lymphocytosis (in chronic inflammation)
    - Monocytosis (in infectious mononucleosis)
  - Anaemia
    - Blood loss, e.g. in ulcerative colitis
    - Haemolysis, caused by toxins
    - Toxic depression of bone marrow
- Amyloidosis
  - Chronic inflammations elevate serum amyloid A protein, causing secondary (reactive) amyloidosis

Chemotaxis
Definition

- Process of movement of cells towards the site of insult
- An example is the movement of neutrophils towards an inflammatory site

Mechanism

- Contraction of cytoplasmic microtubules
- Changes in cytoplasmic fluidity
- Both result in directional movement

Control of chemotaxis

- Calcium ions, which increase chemotaxis
- Increased intracellular concentration of cyclic nucleotides, which increases chemotaxis

Cytokines
Definition

- Low-molecular-weight peptides that act on or are produced by lymphocytes

Classification

- Interleukins – IL-1 to IL-13
- Interferons – IFN-alpha, IFN-beta, IFN-gamma
- Colony stimulating factors (CSFs)
  - Macrophage CSF (M-CSF)
  - Granulocyte CSF (G-CSF)
  - Granulocyte–macrophage CSF (GM-CSF)

Functions

- Initiation of inflammatory process
- Promotion of cell recruitment to damaged area during repair
- M-CSF enhances ability of macrophages to ingest micro-organisms
- Short-range messenger system of communication between the cells of the immune response

Cell injury

Definition

- An alteration in cell structure or function that results from stress and that exceeds the ability of the cell to compensate through normal physiological adaptive mechanisms

Causes

- Genetic derangements
  - Inherited or acquired mutations in genes lead to altered synthesis of crucial cellular proteins
    - Developmental defects
    - Abnormal metabolic functioning
    - Abnormal cell differentiation and replication, causing cancer
- Hypoxia
  - Depletes ATP
  - Generates O_2-derived free radicals
- Nutritional imbalance
  - A deficiency or excess of cellular substrates, carbohydrates, proteins, minerals or vitamins, e.g. in obesity, malnutrition or scurvy
  - Causes cellular injury and disease
- Chemical agents (poisons)
  - Drugs or their metabolites
  - Toxins from micro-organisms
  - By-products of normal metabolism, e.g. lactic acid or O_2-derived free radicals
  - Environmental chemical agents (organic agents, inorganic agents or ions)
- Physical agents
  - Mechanical injury
    - Crush
    - Fractures
    - Laceration
    - Haemorrhage
  - Thermal (extremes of temperature)
    - Freezing, e.g. frostbite or hypothermia
    - Heating, e.g. burns, heat stroke or heat exhaustion
  - Ionising or non-ionising radiation
    - X-ray
    - Ultraviolet radiation
    - Radioactive elements
  - Electric injury
  - Sudden change in atmospheric pressure
    - Blasts
    - Diving
  - Noise trauma
- Infective agents
  - Pathogenic viruses
  - Bacteria
  - Fungi
  - Protozoa
  - Helminths
  - Mechanisms include:
    - Replication inside cells, causing disruption, e.g. herpes virus
    - Toxin production, e.g. *Clostridia* species, diphtheria
    - An inflammatory or immune response that leads to cells being caught in a cross-fire between the immune system and invading micro-organisms, e.g. rheumatic fever
- Immunological causes
  - Exaggerated immune reactions, e.g. anaphylaxis
  - Inappropriate activation of the immune system, e.g. autoimmunity causing inflammation and cell injury
  - Abnormal suppression of the immune system, e.g. immunodeficiency causing increased vulnerability to microbial invasion

Non-infective cellular injury

Definition

- Occurs when a cell has been exposed to an influence that has left it alive but functioning at less than optimum level
- Can result in recovery, permanent impairment or death

Morphology

- Hydropic change: swelling caused by damage to membrane-bound ion pumps
- Fatty change, caused by damage to energy-generating mechanisms and protein synthesis
- Eosinophilic change, caused by loss of ribosomes and diminution in cytoplasmic RNA
- Nuclear changes
  - Pyknosis: condensation of the nucleus
  - Karyorrhexis: dilatation of the endoplasmic reticulum
  - Karyolysis: fragmentation of the nucleus
- All of these changes lead to apoptosis

Causes

Trauma

- Freezing
  - Ice crystals
  - Cutting macromolecules
- Heating
  - Vibration
  - Breaking of macromolecules

Ionising radiation

- Radiation induced DNA damage
  - Strand breakage
  - Base alteration
  - Formation of new cross-links
- Consequences
  - Cell death
  - Repair
  - Permanent change in genotype
- The most rapidly dividing tissues are the most sensitive
- Acute effect: cell death resulting from decreased mitosis
- Chronic effect: atrophy and fibrosis causing:
  - Vascular endothelial cell loss
  - Platelet adhesion and thrombosis
  - Intimal proliferation, causing endarteritis obliterans
  - In bone marrow: suspension of renewal of all cell lines
  - In skin:
    - Desquamation and hair loss
    - Hyperpigmentation
    - Thinning of dermis
    - Telangectasia

- In the intestines, causes loss of surface epithelium, leading to:
  - Diarrhea
  - Malabsorption
  - Strictures
- In the gonads:
  - Sterility
  - Teratogenecity
- In the lung – progressive pulmonary fibrosis
- In the kidney:
  - Loss of parenchyma, leading to renal failure
  - Intra-renal stenosis, leading to hypertension
- In the haemopoietic system: carcinogenesis

Cellular injury by poisons

- Definition of poisons: chemical agents that have a deleterious effect on living tissue
- Mechanism of action
  - Modification of activities of enzymes by:
    - Binding inappropriately to active sites
    - Altering conformation of enzyme molecule
    - Direct reaction with critical molecular cellular components
- Examples
  - Heavy metals and cyanide, which bind to sulfhydryl group of respiratory enzymes, blocking respiration and so increasing acidity, which leads to decreased ATP level and accumulation of free radicals, finally resulting in membrane damage and loss of ionic control
  - Carbon monoxide, which binds strongly to haemoglobin to form carboxy-haemoglobin
  - Paracetamol, which acts indirectly through a metabolite

Molecular basis of cell injury

- Injury producing stress particularly affects four biochemical cellular systems
  - Cell membranes
  - Energy metabolism
  - Protein synthesis
  - Genetic apparatus
- Cell membrane damage

- Plasma membrane
  - Damage to Na^+– K^+ pump causes Na^+ and water to enter the cell, which swells and may rupture (lysis)
  - K^+ leaks out of the cell, causing loss of resting membrane potential
  - Ca^{2+} moves from the extracellular fluid and intracellular storage site to the cytoplasm
  - The protein kinase system and other enzymes are activated
  - Attack and breakdown critical cell components ensues, e.g. lipid membranes, ATP, cytoskeletal proteins and DNA
- Mitochondrial membrane
  - Impairment of energy metabolism
- Lysosomal membrane
  - Release of hydrolytic enzymes into the cytoplasm
  - Autodigestion of cellular proteins
- Endoplasmic reticulum
  - Interferes with intracellular protein synthesis and transport
- Energy metabolism
  - Hypoxia and mitochondrial damage cause decreased generation of adequate ATP
    - Interferes with nutrient and protein synthesis
    - Shift of energy metabolism to anaerobic glycolysis, leading to accumulation of lactic acid and inorganic phosphate, which causes acidosis and so disturbs the enzyme function and damages nuclear DNA
  - Accumulation of O_2-derived free radicals
    - Lipid peroxidation leads to damage to cell membrane
    - Polypeptide fragmentation impairs enzyme function
    - Breakage or abnormal cross-linking of DNA strands
- Protein synthesis
  - Denaturation of enzymes
    - Impairment of intracellular metabolic reactions
  - Destruction of structural proteins
    - Impairment of the intracellular transport mechanism

- Disruption of the supportive protein cytoskeleton
- Genetic apparatus
  - DNA damage leads to:
    - Interference with cell replication
    - Decreased synthesis of structural and functional proteins

Giant cells

Definition

- Very large cells that may have a single nucleus, although they are most often multinucleated or multilobed

Classification

Normal giant cells

- Skeletal muscle cells – largest
- Neurones – largest
- Cardiac muscle cells
- Osteoclasts
- Cytotrophoblasts (syncytiotrophoblasts)
- Oocytes
- Megakaryocytes (single, multilobed nucleus)

Abnormal giant cells

- Many nuclei in a large cell is an indication of abnormal nuclear division during mitosis or a sign of cell fusion
- Macrophage-related giant cells
  - Foreign body giant cells, caused by fusion of phagocytes in an attempt to phagocytose the foreign body)
  - Langhans' giant cells
- Giant cells related to specific diseases
  - Tuberculosis
  - Sarcoidosis
  - Crohn's disease
- Virus-induced giant cells (the 'mulberry cells' of viral infection)
  - Warthin–Finkeldey giant cells in measles, derived from lymphocytes
  - Cytomegalovirus and herpes simplex multinucleate giant cells, derived from epithelial cells
- Tumour-induced giant cells
  - Reed–Sternberg cells (modified B lymphocytes), the mirror-image twin nucleated giant cell in Hodgkin's lymphoma

- – Bizarre epithelial giant cells in anaplastic carcinoma
- – Bizarre glial giant cells in grade 4 astrocytoma
- Other giant cells
  - – Megaloblasts in folates and vitamin B12 deficiency
  - – Giant cells in adrenal cytomegaly
  - – Giant cells in thyroid cytomegaly

Accumulations and depositions

Definition

- Accumulation of intermediates of metabolic pathway caused by a defective step, which is due either to a genetic factor or to trauma
- Examples include lactate causing acidosis and carbon tetrachloride causing liver damage

Amyloid

- Extracellular material
- Extra active circulating proteins from chronic inflammation are removed and stored as inactive and inert beta-pleated sheets, which cannot be metabolised by the body's enzymes
- Accumulates around vessels of various organs and causes progressive vascular occlusion and organ failure

Calcification

- Seen physiologically in developing or healing bone
- Occurs pathologically when calcification is present outside the sites where the mineral is normally deposited

Hemochromatosis

- Abnormal deposition of iron in the body

Amyloidosis

Definition

- A set of disorders characterised by extracellular deposition of one of a group of fibrillar proteins – amyloid, a starch-like material in inert, twisted beta-pleated sheet form, which is not normally found in human tissue and which cannot be metabolised

Types

Primary amyloidosis

- Absence of any recognisable preceding or concurrent disease
- Predilection for mesenchymal tissue, heart, lung, skin, nerves and joints
- Manifestations
  - – Peripheral neuropathy
    - Glove and stocking parasthesia
    - Pain
  - – Restrictive cardiomyopathy with amyloid pulmonary infiltration
  - – Skin manifestations
    - Pinch purpura
    - Wax nodules
    - Areas of thickness
    - Loss of hair and baldness
  - – Polyarthropathy of large joints
  - – Macroglossia
  - – Idiopathic carpal tunnel syndrome
  - – Bleeding tendency, caused by isolated factor X deficiency (Stuart–Prower syndrome)
  - – Autonomic neuropathy
    - Disturbed gastrointestinal motility
    - Impotence
    - Orthostatic hypotension
    - Dyshidrosis

Secondary amyloidosis

- Follows or co-exists with a wide variety of disease processes
- Predilection for parenchymal tissue, liver, kidney, spleen and adrenals
- Conditions that can be associated with secondary amyloidosis
  - – Chronic inflammation resulting from infection
    - Tuberculosis
    - Leprosy
    - Bronchiectasis
    - Syphilis
    - Chronic osteomyelitis
  - – Chronic inflammation associated with possible infection

- Reiter's syndrome
- Whipple's disease
- Chronic inflammation of unknown aetiology
  - Rheumatoid arthritis and its variants
  - Inflammatory bowel disease
  - Other connective tissue disorders
- Neoplasms
  - Hypernephroma
  - Medullary thyroid carcinoma
  - Plasma cell myeloma
  - Endocrine tumours
- Neurodegenerative disorders
  - Alzheimer's disease
  - Longstanding paraplegia, probably as a result the risk of recurrent renal infections

Systemic (generalised) amyloidosis

- Inherited or familial amyloidosis
- Acquired amyloidosis
  - Immune amyloidosis
  - Reactive amyloidosis

Localised amyloidosis

- Acquired amyloidosis
- Organ-limited amyloidosis
- May be of immune origin

Chemical amyloidosis

- Different manifestations of amyloidosis are caused by different types of amyloid protein, which have diagnostic and therapeutic implications

Pathogenesis of secondary amyloidosis

- At the end of inflammatory process, the excess acute-phase reactant proteins are converted into an inert material that the body has no enzymes to metabolise
- Purpose of this conversion is to remove the active protein from the circulation
- In acute inflammation, this conversion is short-lived and advantageous but in chronic inflammation, it is prolonged and dangerous
- Excess acute-phase proteins lead to excess amyloid, resulting in:
  - Excess deposition around the vessels
  - Progressive vascular occlusion
  - Failure of tissues and organs

Diagnosis

- Biopsy
  - Gingival
  - Rectal submucosal
  - Internal organ biopsy
    - Liver
    - Spleen
    - Kidney
  - Fine-needle aspiration of periumbilical subcutaneous fat
  - Bleeding is a serious complication
- Staining
  - Lugol's iodine plus dilute sulphuric acid
    - Amyloid stains blue–black or blue–violet
  - Methyl violet
    - Normal tissue is stained violet
    - Tissue with amyloid stains rose pink
    - Best seen using frozen sections
  - Congo red and Sirius red stain
    - Measurement of disappearance of a known dose of Congo red, given intravenous
    - Fatal anaphylactic reaction can occur
    - Amyloid stains orange–red in light microscopy
    - Amyloid seen as apple-green birefringence in polarised light microscopy
  - Thioflavin T stain
- Immunohistochemistry
  - Immunofluorescent and immunoperoxidase methods
  - Using anti-AA amyloid antibody or anti-AL amyloid antibody
- Serum amyloid-A (SAA) protein level
- Serum amyloid-P (SAP) scanning (done in the UK)
  - Radionuclide imaging using 123-I labeled human SAP
  - Most reliable method

Treatment

- No known treatment
- In secondary amyloidosis, the cause should be treated
- In immune disorders, stem cell transplantation (a recent treatment) or chemotherapy can be used
- If an isolated organ is affected, transplantation may be offered

Calcification

- Seen physiologically in developing or healing bone
- Occurs pathologically when calcification is present outside the sites where the mineral is normally deposited
- Metastatic calcification
  - Occurs in structurally and functionally normal tissues
  - Associated with excessively high levels of plasma calcium
  - Causes
    - Hyperparathyroidism
    - Hypervitaminosis D
    - Excessive dietary intake of calcium
    - Multiple myeloma
    - Sarcoidosis
    - Breast cancer (paramalignant calcification)
- Pathological calcification with normal circulating calcium (dystrophic calcification)
- Calcinosis – a form of dystrophic calcification
  - Calcifying tendinitis
  - Systemic calcinosis and CREST syndrome (systemic sclerosis with calcinosis: calcinosis, Raynaud's syndrome, oesophageal dysmotility, sclerodactyly and telangiectasia)
  - Idiopathic calcinosis of the scrotum (calcification of multiple epidermoid cysts)
  - Tumour calcinosis, affecting the soft tissues in front of shoulder (a familial trait seen in young Afro-Caribbeans)

Haemochromatosis

Definition

- Abnormal deposition of iron in the body

Causes

- Primary (hereditary) haemochromatosis
  - Caused by abnormal metabolism of iron in the presence of normal serum iron levels
  - Four types (I, II, III and IV)
  - Caused by chromosomal abnormalities
- Secondary (acquired) haemochromatosis

- Associated with iron overload leading to increased serum levels of iron
- Causes
  - Iron-loading anaemia, e.g. thalassaemia major and chronic haemolytic anaemia
  - Dietary iron overload
  - Parenteral overload from multiple blood transfusions
  - Long-term haemodialysis
  - Chronic liver disease
  - Portocaval shunt

Clinical features

- Solid organ failure
- Haemoptysis
- Arthritis

Thrombosis and clot formation

Definition

- Solid mass formed in the living circulation from the components of the streaming blood
- Can occur in the heart, arteries, veins and capillaries

Stages of clot formation

- Platelets adhere to damaged endothelium
- Fibrin and leukocytes adhere to platelets
- Clot (composed of red blood cells and fibrin) develops on this layer of platelets, fibrin and leukocytes
- A secondary layer of platelets collects
- Organisation occurs with adherence to wall of vessel as mural thrombosis
- Further batch of platelets laid down on this layer
- Repeat of cycle

Virchow's triad

- Damage to vessel wall
  - Atherosclerotic plaques, caused by:
    - Smoking
    - Hypercholesterolaemia
    - Diabetes mellitus
  - Synthetic wall (prosthesis)
- Alterations in blood flow, caused by:
  - Prolonged inactivity
    - Surgery

- Trauma
- Myocardial infarction
  - Heart failure
  - Proximal occlusion of venous drainage
- Alterations in constituents of blood
  - Increased number of platelets following:
    - Surgery
    - Injury
  - Increased adhesiveness of platelets
  - Fluid loss, causing increased viscosity of blood
  - Thrombophilia, an abnormal balance of clotting factors and natural anticoagulants, seen in:
    - Protein C and protein S deficiencies
    - Antithrombin III deficiency
    - Heparin use

Fate of thrombi

- Resolution
- Organisation leading to scar formation
- Recanalisation
- Embolisation in whole or in part

Coagulation factors

- Factor I: fibrinogen
- Factor II: prothrombin
- Factor III: tissue thromboplastin
- Factor IV: calcium
- Factor V: pro-accelerin (labile factor)
- No factor VI
- Factor VII: prothrombin conversion factor (stable factor)
- Factor VIII – Anti-haemopoietic factor
- Factor VIII A: von Willebrand's factor
- Factor IX: Christmas factor
- Factor X: Stuart–Prower factor
- Factor XI: plasma thromboplastin antecedent
- Factor XII: Hageman's factor
- Factor XIII: fibrin stabilizing factor
- Pro-kallikrein – Fletcher's factor
- High-molecular-weight kininogen – constant activation factor

Coagulation cascade

- See figure below

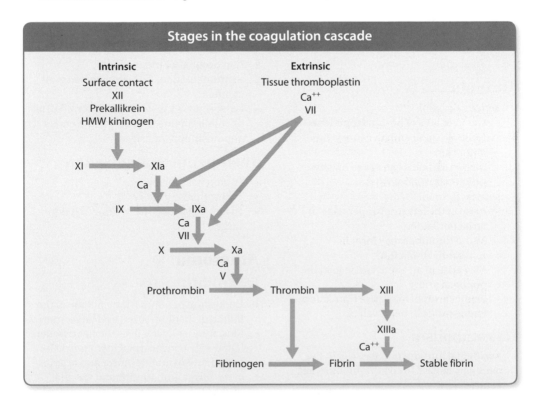

Stages in the coagulation cascade

Tests for coagulation

- Prothrombin time (PT), for the extrinsic and common pathways
- Activated partial thromboplastin time (aPTT), for the intrinsic pathway
- Kaolin–cephalin clotting time (KCCT) – for intrinsic and common pathways

Embolism

Definition

- Occurs when an embolus, an abnormal mass of undissolved material, passes in the bloodstream from one part of the circulation to another, lodging in a vessel too small to allow it to pass

Types

- Thrombus
- Gas (air, nitrogen)
- Fat
- Tumour
- Amniotic fluid
- Foreign body
- Therapeutic emboli
  - Gel foam
  - Muscle
  - Steel coil

Thrombi

- Venous thrombi
  - Occur in 30% of hospital inpatients
  - Multiple small emboli cause pulmonary embolism
  - A large embolus can cause massive pulmonary embolism
- Arterial thrombi
  - Arise in the left atrial appendage in atrial fibrillation
  - Mural thrombus may form in myocardial infarction
  - May arise in an aneurysm, e.g. in the popliteal artery
  - Septic thrombi may arise from infective endocarditis in heart valves

Gas embolism

- Accidental introduction gas, e.g. in the neck can cause a frothy thrombus in left ventricle

- Decompression sickness (Caisson's disease): nitrogen embolism with gas bubbles in the circulation, causing severe pain

Fat embolism

- Pulmonary fat embolism
  - Rarely causes death
  - Causes respiratory distress and haemorrhagic skin eruptions
- Systemic fat embolism can affect the brain, skin, kidneys and other organs
- Causes respiratory distress and haemorrhagic skin eruptions

Tumour embolism

- Tumour cells can become coated with thrombus and embolise

Amniotic fluid embolism

- Causes respiratory distress that disproportionate to the volume of fluid embolised
- Mechanism of respiratory distress is due to chemical composition of the amniotic fluid

Foreign body embolism

- Can occur after intravenous instrumentation, from broken pieces of cannula
- Can occur as a result of undissolved drugs or contaminants following intravenous administration of drugs

Therapeutic embolisation

- To stop haemorrhage
- To thrombose aneurysms
- To reduce vascularity of tumour before surgery

Atheroma

Definition

- Deposition of fibrous–fatty plaque in the intima of medium-sized and large arteries
- Most frequently involves the heart (where it may cause myocardial infarction), the brain (stroke) and the aorta and arteries of the lower limb (peripheral vascular disease)

Lesions

- Fatty streaks: intracellular lipid deposits in smooth muscle and macrophages
- Gelatinous plaques: elevations in the aorta and large arteries
- Fibrous–lipid plaques, which can lead to:
  - Rupture
  - Thrombosis
  - Haemorrhage
  - Calcification
  - Necrosis
  - Thinning of the media

Risk factors

- Ethnic and demographic factors
  - Age (more common in advanced age)
  - Sex (more common in males)
  - Familial – a true genetic predisposition
  - Race: more common in Caucasians
- Environmental factors
  - Smoking
  - Hypertension
  - Diabetes mellitus
  - Hyperlipidaemia

Pathogenesis

- Fatty streaks raise the intima, causing turbulence of the bloodstream and slowing of the blood flow as well as increased viscosity, which promotes thrombogenesis
- Loss of endothelial cells as a result of the fatty streaks causes loss of intrinsic fibrinolytic activity of the endothelial cells and so deposition of fibrin, platelets and atheromatous plaque

Ischaemia

Definition

- Condition of an organ or tissue in which the supply of oxygenated blood is inadequate for the metabolic needs

Causes

- General causes
  - Sudden decrease in cardiac output
  - Myocardial infarction
- Local cause
  - Arterial obstruction
    - Atherosclerosis
    - Intra-arterial thrombosis
    - Embolism
  - External pressure
    - Adhesive band
    - Compartment syndrome
    - A light cast
  - Venous obstruction (engorgement can cause secondary arterial block)
    - Strangulated hernia
    - Mesenteric venous thrombosis
    - Phlegmasia cerulea dolens
  - Small vessel obstruction
    - Vasculitis
    - Frostbite
    - Microembolism
    - Precipitated cryoglobulins
    - Thrombocythaemia

Factors that determine the severity of ischaemia

- Speed of onset
- Extent of obstruction
- Extent and patency of collateral vessels
- Metabolic requirements of the ischaemic tissue

Infarction

Definition

- Death of tissue following acute ischaemia when irreparable damage has occurred

Sequence of events

- Blood seeps out through damaged capillaries
- Dead tissue undergoes autolysis of cells and haemolysis of red blood cells
- Surrounding living tissue undergoes acute inflammatory response (demolition phase)
- Ingrowth of granulation tissue and organisation into a fibrous scar (repair phase)
- Some dystrophic calcification may take place

Systemic effects

- Fever
- Increased white blood cell count
- Increased ESR

Infarction of specific organs

- CNS
  - Cell death within few minutes
  - Liquefaction necrosis
- Lungs
  - Caused by emboli
  - Wedge-shaped infarct with base on the pleural surface, which causes pleuritic pain and a pleuritic rub
  - Oedema and bleeding into alveoli
- Intestines
  - Mechanical
    - Strangulated hernia
    - Adhesive band
  - Superior mesenteric artery thrombosis and embolism
  - If less severe – only mucosal infarction, which may repair itself but cause a stricture
- Skeletal muscle
  - Fibrous replacement
  - If veins and arteries are affected, e.g. following a supracondylar fracture of the humerus, Volkmann's ischaemic contracture may ensue

Anaemia

Definition

- Clinically, a reduction in the red blood cell mass leading to a lowered haemoglobin and haematocrit levels in the blood that are below the normal range for the person's age and sex, meaning that the O_2 demands of the tissues cannot be met without the use of compensatory mechanisms
- Strictly speaking, a patient is said to be anaemic when the haemoglobin level falls below the lower end of normal range, i.e. 13.3 g/dL in men and 11.8 g/dL in women
- Clinically relevant anaemia (symptomatic anaemia) occurs at much lower haemoglobin values – 8.0 g/dL because with haemogloblins lower than this, the O_2 carrying capacity of the blood is reduced

Classification

- Decreased production of red blood cells
  - Haematinic deficiency
    - Iron

- vitamin B12
- Folic acid
  - Marrow failure
    - Aplastic anaemia
    - Leukaemia
    - Red blood cell aplasia
- Decreased red blood cell maturation
  - Myelodysplasia
  - Sideroblastic anaemia
- Increased red blood cell destruction
  - Inherited haemolytic anaemia
    - Sickle cell anaemia
    - Thalassaemia
  - Acquired haemolytic anaemia
    - Autoimmune disease
    - Disseminated intravascular coagulation (DIC)
- Effect of disease
  - Chronic illness
  - Renal, endocrine or liver disease

Aetiological classification

Blood loss

Acute blood loss
- Revealed bleeding from a body orifice, e.g. haematemesis, bleeding per rectum or epistaxis
- Concealed bleeding into a body cavity, e.g. the retro-peritoneum, the gluteal region or the thigh

Chronic blood loss
- Genital tract, e.g. menorrhagia or haematuria
- Gastrointestinal tract, e.g. varices, peptic ulcer, hookworm infestation or malignancy

Decreased red blood cell production or function

Haematinic deficiency
- Iron (decreased input, decreased absorption or increased requirement)
- Folic acid (decreased intake, malabsorption, alcoholism or liver failure)
- Vitamin B12 (lack of intrinsic factor or Crohn's disease)

Bone marrow failure/depression
- Marrow failure
  - Aplasia
    - Aplastic anaemia
    - Red cell aplasia

- Leukaemia
  - Abnormal red cell maturation
    - Myelodysplasia
    - Sideroblastic anaemia
  - Toxic injury
    - Radiotherapy
    - Chemotherapy
    - Sepsis
- Marrow infiltration
  - Myeloproliferative disorders
    - Myelofibrosis
    - Multiple myeloma
  - Lymphoma
  - Metastases
- Drugs
  - Immunosuppressive drugs, cytotoxic agents and chemotherapy agents
  - Corticosteroids
  - Antithyroid drugs
- Anaemia of chronic disorders
  - Chronic systemic disease
    - Renal
    - Hepatic
    - Infection and sepsis
  - Multisystem disease, e.g. collagen disease
  - Endocrine disease – hypothyroidism or hyperthyroidism
  - Malignancy

Increased or premature red cell destruction
- Congenital haemolytic anaemias
  - Red blood cell membrane defects
    - Hereditary spherocytosis
    - Hereditary elliptocytosis
  - Red blood cell enzyme defects
    - Glucose-6-phosphate dehydrogenase deficiency
    - Pyruvate kinase deficiency
  - Haemoglobinopathy
    - Sickle cell disease
    - Thalassaemia
- Acquired haemolytic anaemias
  - Immune haemolytic anaemia
    - Autoimmune
    - Haemolytic disease of newborn
    - Blood transfusion reaction
    - Drug induced
  - Non-immune haemolytic anaemia
    - Microangiopathic haemolytic anaemia

- Infections
- Prosthetic valves
- Extracorporeal circuits
- Haemolytic uraemic syndrome
- Hypersplenism
- Spurious anaemias
  - Dilutional anaemia, caused by excessive crystalloids
  - Physiological anaemia, in pregnancy
  - Caused by a sampling error

Polycythaemia

Primary polycythaemia (normal erythropoietin)
- Polycythaemia vera (myeloproliferation)
- Myelofibrosis
- Chronic myeloid leukaemia
- Essential thrombocythaemia

Secondary polycythaemia
- Appropriate erythropoietin excess
  - Emphysema and other lung diseases causing hypoxia
  - Congestive heart failure
  - Hemoglobinopathies causing high-affinity haemoglobin
- Inappropriate erythropoietin excess
  - Renal neoplasms
  - Cerebellar haemangioblastoma
  - Phaeochromocytoma
  - Hepatocellular carcinoma
  - Prostatic adenocarcinoma
  - Uterine leiomyoma
  - In athletes

Relative polycythaemia
- Apparent, caused by plasma volume loss, e.g. in burns
- Stress polycythaemia, caused by contraction of the volume of the extracellular fluid

Jaundice

Definition
- Yellowing of the skin, sclera and mucus membranes because of the presence of bilirubin (bilirubin levels > 40 mmol/L are associated with clinical jaundice)

Features of pre-hepatic, hepatic and post-hepatic jaundice. ALP, alkaline phosphatase			
	Pre-hepatic (hemolytic)	Hepatic	Post-hepatic (obstructive)
Jaundice	Mild	Variable	Variable
Colour of urine	Normal	Normal	Dark
Colour of faeces	Normal	Normal	Pale
Serum bilirubin	Unconjugated	Both	Conjugated
Transaminases	Normal	↑↑	Normal or mild ↑
Serum ALP	Normal	Mild ↑	Gross ↑

Classification

- Jaundice can be:
  - Pre-hepatic (haemolytic)
  - Hepatic
  - Post-hepatic (obstructive)
- See table

Hyperuricaemia

Definition

- Increase in serum uric acid

Pathogenesis

- Purine is metabolised to xanthine and hypoxanthine and then to uric acid by xanthine oxidase
- Disturbance in this mechanism causes hyperuricaemia

Causes

- Primary hyperuricaemia
  - Absolute or relative abnormality in xanthine–hypoxanthine handling
- Secondary hyperuricaemia
  - Increased purine breakdown as a result of increased cell turnover or decreased apoptosis
    - Psoriasis
    - Sickle cell disease
    - Malignant tumours, especially after chemotherapy
  - Decreased uric acid excretion
    - Chronic renal failure
    - Thiazide diuretics

Complications

- Joint disease, leading to osteoarthritis
- Urinary tract calculi, leading to renal failure
- Deposition in skin (gouty tophi)
- Radiological appearance may be mistaken for malignancy

Oedema

Definition

- Abnormal excessive accumulation of tissue fluid, mainly in the interstitial space but also in the intracellular space
- Represents a breakdown of balanced fluid transport with net accumulation of tissue fluid

Classification

- Localised, resulting from increased vascular permeability and Starling's forces
  - Inflammatory oedema
  - Neurogenic oedema
  - Local hypersensitivity reaction
- Generalised, due to failure to excrete salt and water
  - Cardiac oedema
  - Renal oedema
  - Hepatic oedema

Causes

- Increased hydrostatic gradient, in cardiac failure

- Increased osmotic gradient, in hypoproteinaemia
- Increased endothelial permeability, in inflammatory exudate
- Lymphatic obstruction, e.g. in malignancy
- Oedema of critical illness
  - Increased crystalloid infusion
  - Increased capillary permeability
  - Decreased oncotic pressure
  - Interstitial space sequestration, resulting from inflammatory mediators causing increased permeability of membranes

Mechanisms

- Generalised oedema in chronic disease
  - Excessive water and salt retention
  - Disease specific factors:
    - Hypoalbuminaemia in chronic liver disease
    - Secondary hyperaldosteronism in cirrhosis
  - Increased venous pressure leading to decreased absorption on venous side
  - Decreased oncotic pressure due to hypoproteinaemia:
    - Nephrotic syndrome, causing increased filtration of protein
    - Chronic liver disease, causing decreased protein synthesis
    - Protein malnutrition
- Generalised oedema in critically ill patients
  - Increased crystalloid infusion
  - Third space losses
  - Decreased cardiac output
  - Increased capillary permeability
  - Decreased oncotic pressure, due to dilution
- Localised oedema
  - Pathology
    - Vasodilatation
    - Increased permeability of capillary endothelium
  - Inflammatory oedema
    - Escape of fluid and albumin, causing increased interstitial oncotic pressure and more escape of fluid
    - Commonly occurs in anastomotic leaks

- Limb oedema
  - Previous deep venous thrombosis and post-phlebitis syndrome
  - Lymphoedema, which is prone to infection and may be primary or result from trauma, surgical excision, radiotherapy
- Disuse or local gigantism
- Angioneurotic oedema
  - Congenital absence of C1 esterase inhibitor

Rhabdomyolysis

Definition

- Clinical syndrome caused by the release of potentially toxic muscle cell components into the circulation following skeletal muscle injury

Causes

- Ischaemia and/or injury
  - Blunt trauma to muscle
    - Crush injury
    - Compression injury
  - Massive burns
  - Compartment syndrome
  - Vascular injury
  - Arterial embolism causing acute ischaemia
  - Acute reperfusion injury
  - Prolonged limb tourniquet
  - Prolonged immobilisation
- Increased muscle activity
  - Strenuous and prolonged muscle exercise
  - Prolonged seizures
  - Electric shocks and lightening injuries
- Infection
  - *Escherichia coli*
  - *Salmonella* species
- Metabolic disease
  - Diabetes mellitus, causing ketoacidosis or a hyperosmolar non-ketotic state
  - Hypothermia
  - Hyperthermia and hyperpyrexia
- Drugs
  - Alcohol
  - Cocaine
  - Amphetamines
  - Lipid-lowering drugs

Molecular pathophysiology

- Impairment of sarcolemmic Na^+– K^+ pump, resulting in:
  - Decreased Na^+ extrusion
  - Decreased Ca^{2+} and water efflux
  - Myofibril disruption and muscle damage, mainly to type 2 (red) muscle fibres, which causes:
    - Myoglobin release
    - Purine release
    - K^+ release
    - Phosphate release

Complications

- Hypovolaemia, as a result of:
  - Injured muscle sequestrating massive amounts of fluid
  - Haemorrhage into the necrotic muscle
- Acute renal failure in up to 30% of patients, due to:
  - Myoglobinuria, which arises because the iron content is toxic to renal tubules and from mechanical blockage
  - Hypovolaemia
- Electrolyte disturbances
  - Metabolic acidosis
  - Hyperkalaemia, from release of intracellular K^+, renal failure and acidosis
  - Hyperphosphataemia, from release of phosphate from damaged muscle
  - Hyperuricaemia, from increased hepatic conversion of released purines
  - Early hypocalcaemia and late hypercalcaemia, leading to Ca^{2+} deposition in necrotic muscle
- Compartment syndrome
  - Swelling of injured muscle
  - Increase in intra-compartmental pressure
  - Worsening of ischaemia
- DIC, caused by pathological activation of the coagulation cascade by the released muscle components

Clinical picture

- Non-specific features
  - Malaise
  - Fever and tachycardia
  - Nausea and vomiting

- Muscular symptoms
  - Pain and tenderness
  - Weakness and stiffness
- Urinary symptoms
  - Dark urine (not always present)

Investigations

- Serum enzymes
  - Creatine kinase (CK), creatine phosphokinase (CPK), muscle CK (CK-MM)
    - Increased to up to five times the upper limit of normal
    - Increase begins 2–12 hours after the muscle injury, peaks in 1–3 days and declines in 3–5 days
  - Lactate dehydrogenase (LDH): increased, non-specific
  - Carbonic anhydrase III: increased; more specific marker than serum CK or myoglobinuria
- Urine analysis
  - Myoglobinuria: positive dipstick for blood in the absence of haematuria
  - Proteinuria
  - Haematuria
- Arterial blood gases: metabolic acidosis
- Serum electrolytes
  - Hyperkalaemia
  - Hyperphosphataemia
  - Hypocalcaemia

Treatment

- Hydration
  - Large quantities of intravenous fluids to ensure:
    - Adequate hydration
    - Urine output > 300 mL/hour
    - Myoglobin-free urine
  - Monitor fluid balance
    - Central venous pressure
    - Pulmonary artery occlusion pressure
- Correction of electrolyte disturbances
  - For hyperkalaemia: insulin and glucose
  - For hyperphosphataemia: oral phosphate-binding agents, e.g. calcium carbonate
- Diuretics
  - Osmotic diuresis, e.g. with mannitol 30 mL/hour, to dilute and clear myoglobin from the kidneys

- Alkalinisation of urine
  - Maintenance of a urine pH > 6.5
  - Sodium bicarbonate infusion helps to prevent dissociation of myoglobin into nephrotoxic metabolites
- Renal replacement therapy may be needed in:
  - Established oliguric renal failure
  - Uncontrolled hyperkalaemia
  - Fluid overload

Reperfusion injury (reperfusion syndrome)

- Revascularisation of a non-viable, acutely ischaemic lower limb showing paraesthesia, complete paresis, muscle turgor, fixed mottled pigmentation
- Associated with a sudden release of toxic anaerobic metabolites from infracted muscle to the systemic circulation, causing:
  - Acidosis
  - Hyperkalaemia
  - Rhabdomyolysis, leading to myoglobinuria
- Myoglobinuria is a potent cause of acute renal failure, and its iron content (rather than mechanical blockage) is the likely cause of tubular damage

---

Ascites

Definition

- Abnormal collection of free fluid in the peritoneal cavity

Causes

- Transudative ascites
  - Hydrostatic changes (increased fluid)
    - Cirrhosis
    - Right heart failure
    - Budd–Chiari syndrome
    - Obstruction to the thoracic duct
  - Plasma oncotic changes (decreased protein)
    - Hypoproteinaemia of liver failure
    - Protein-losing enteropathy
    - Starvation
    - Nephrotic syndrome
  - Metabolic changes (increased retention)
    - Secondary hyperaldosteronism
    - Hypothyroidism
- Exudative ascites
  - Inflammatory causes
    - Peritonitis
    - Peritoneal secondaries
    - Uraemia
    - Pancreatitis
  - Iatrogenic causes
    - Abdominal surgery
    - Continuous ambulatory peritoneal dialysis

Investigations on ascitic fluid

- Microscopy
  - Bacteria
  - White blood cells
  - Red blood cells
- Culture and sensitivity
- Cytology
  - Carcinoma (primary or secondary)
  - Lymphoma (non-Hodgkin's lymphoma)
- Cytogenetics
- Biochemistry
  - Amylase (increased in pancreatitis)
  - Protein

Transudative ascites

- Caused by imbalance between hydrostatic and oncotic pressures (Starling's forces), resulting in fluid of low protein content traversing the intact epithelial surface
- Examples
  - Increased hydrostatic pressure, e.g. congestive heart failure or renal failure
  - Decreased oncotic pressure in hypoproteinaemia
  - Lymphoedema

Exudative ascites

- Caused by inflammation resulting in a fluid of relatively high protein content traversing a damaged endothelial surface
- Examples
  - Serous, e.g. in malignant ascites
  - Fibrinous, e.g. in pericarditis
  - Purulent, e.g. in *Escherichia coli* peritonitis
  - Haemorrhagic, e.g. in tuberculosis
  - Pseudomembranous, e.g. in clostridial infection

Blood transfusion

Constituents of products for transfusion

Whole blood

- Components
  - Red blood cells
    - Plasma-reduced
    - Leukocyte-poor
    - Frozen
    - Phenotyped
  - Platelets
  - White cells (buffy coat)
  - Fresh frozen plasma
  - Cryoprecipitate, which contains:
    - Factor VIII
    - von Willebrand's factor
    - Fibrinogen
- Plasma products
  - Human albumin
  - Coagulation product concentration
  - Immunoglobulin
    - Specific immunoglobulins
    - Human immunoglobulin

Indications for transfusion

Red blood cells

- Haemorrhage
- Anaemia
- Bone marrow failure

Platelets

- Surgical reasons
  - Bleeding and thrombocytopenia
  - Cover for operations
    - Count $< 50 \times 10^9/L$
    - Platelet dysfunction
  - Acute DIC
  - Massive blood transfusion
  - Following surgery requiring cardiopulmonary bypass
- Medical reasons
  - Bone marrow suppression
  - Aplastic anaemia

Fresh frozen plasma

- Isolated deficiency of factor II, V, VII, X, XIII, XI, pseudocholinesterase or antithrombin III
- Reversal of oral anticoagulation with warfarin
- Liver disease, major hepatic resections and liver injuries (given with vitamin K)
- Haemolytic–uraemic syndrome
- DIC
- Bleeding diathesis after massive transfusion or cardiopulmonary bypass
- Thrombotic thrombocytopenic purpura

Cryoprecipitate

- Fibrinogen deficiency
- Bleeding associated with uraemia
- von Willebrand's disease

Complications

- Acute complications
  - Allergic
  - Anaphylaxis
  - Haemolysis
  - Metabolic disturbances
  - Transfusion-related acute lung injury
  - Circulatory overload
  - Non-haemolytic febrile transfusion reaction
  - Haemostatic dilution of clotting factors and thrombocytopenia
  - Septic shock (from bacterially infected units)
- Late complications
  - Delayed haemolytic transfusion reaction
  - Sensitisation and allo-immunisation
  - Haemolytic disease of the newborn
  - Immunosuppression
  - Graft-versus-host disease
  - Transfusion-related iron overload (haemosiderosis)
- Infective complications
  - Bacterial
    - Brucellosis
    - Syphilis
    - Chagas disease
  - Helminthic
    - Filariasis
  - Protozoal
    - Babesiosis
    - Kala-azar
    - Malaria
    - Trypanosomiasis

- Toxoplasmosis
  - Rickettsial
    - Relapsing fever
    - Rocky Mountain spotted fever
  - Viral
    - Human parvovirus B19
    - Cytomegalovirus
    - Epstein–Barr virus
    - Yellow fever
    - HIV-1, HIV-2
    - Human T-lymphotropic virus (HTLV)-1 and HTLV-2
    - Hepatitis A, hepatitis B, hepatitis G

Massive blood transfusion

- Definition: transfusion of a volume of blood greater than the recipient's blood volume in < 24 hours
- Indications
  - Major trauma
  - Gastrointestinal bleed
  - Obstetric complications
- Complications
  - Underlying coagulopathy
  - Thrombocytopenia
  - Lack of factors V and VIII
  - Hyperkalaemia
  - Hypothermia (prevented by blood warmers)
  - Acute respiratory distress syndrome (ARDS) (prevented by microaggregate filters with pore size of 40 micrometres)
  - Hypocalcaemia caused by citrate in the transfused blood
  - Decreased 2,3-diphosphoglycerate, resulting in increased haemoglobin affinity to O_2 (which is temporary, lasting only 48 hours)

Alternatives to blood transfusion

- Substances with O_2-carrying capacity to replace blood and its products in the therapy of shock

Advantages

- Free of contamination, eliminating infective risks
- Longer shelf life
- Universal ABO compatibility

- Similar O_2-carrying capacity to that of blood

Agents

- Human free haemoglobin
  - Obtained from outdated blood
  - Possible side effects resulting from retained erythrocyte stromal elements
    - Allergic reactions
    - Renal failure
    - Coagulopathies
    - Immune dysfunction
- Human stroma free haemoglobin (SFH)
  - Purification of human free haemoglobin from erythrocyte stromal elements, thus eliminating side effects
  - Disadvantages
    - High affinity for O_2
    - Short plasma half-life
    - Available only from human sources
- Bovine SFH (polymerised bovine haemoglobin)
  - Advantage of being from an animal source
  - Binding with other molecules or incorporation into liposomes can reduce the O_2 affinity and improve plasma retention time
- Perfluoro chemical compounds, e.g. perfluorocarbons and perfluorodecalin
  - Unique enhanced ability to dissolve gases, but require emulsification to be water-soluble
  - Contain electrolytes, bicarbonates and starch to obtain a pH balance with plasma
  - Have a lower O_2-carrying capacity than haemoglobin, but this can be corrected by higher F_iO_2
  - Potential side effects
    - Acute pulmonary oedema
    - Activation of complement and coagulation cascade
    - Acute respiratory failure
    - Depression of the reticuloendothelial system
  - Other potential disadvantages
    - Expensive
    - Special storage is needed to prevent gelatinisation

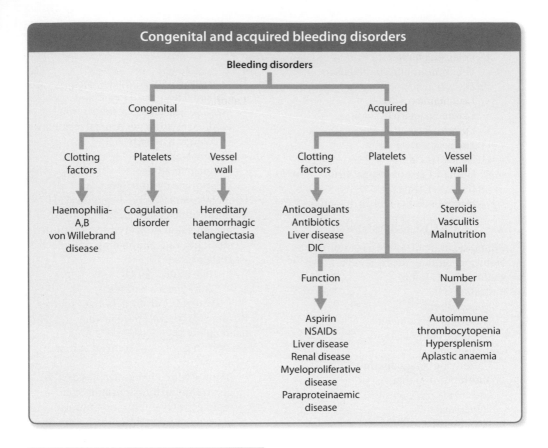

Congenital and acquired bleeding disorders

Bleeding disorders

- See figure above

Inherited bleeding disorders

- Vascular disorders
  - Hereditary haemolytic telangiectasia
  - Ehlers–Danlos syndrome
  - Marfan's syndrome
  - Osteogenesis imperfecta
- Coagulation disorders
  - Hemophilia A
    - Inherited deficiency of factor VIII
    - X-linked-recessive inheritance, so affects males and is carried by females
    - PT is normal, aPTT is prolonged
  - Hemophilia B (Christmas disease)
  - von Willebrand's disease
    - Deficiency of von Willebrand's factor, causing vascular endothelium to release decreased levels of factor VIII

- Autosomal-dominant inheritance
- Platelet count is normal but platelet interaction with endothelium is decreased due to the deficiency of von Willebrand's factor
  - Afibrinogenaemia
  - Dysfibrinogenaemia
  - Specific factor deficiencies
- Disorders of platelet function
  - Glanzmann's thrombasthenia (defective platelet aggregation)
  - Grey platelet syndrome
- Disorders of fibrinolysis

Acquired bleeding disorders

- Disorders of the platelets
  - Decreased number (thrombocytopenia)
    - Idiopathic thrombocytopenic purpura
    - Hepatic disease
    - Tumours
    - DIC

- Blood transfusion
- Drugs
  - Decreased function (thrombasthenia)
    - Uraemia
    - Hepatic disease
    - Leukaemia
    - Extracorporeal circulation
    - Drugs
- Defective coagulation
  - Hepatic disease
  - Tumours
  - DIC
  - Anticoagulants
  - Massive transfusion
- Coagulation inhibition
  - Heparin
  - Lymphoma
- Excessive fibrinolysis
  - DIC
  - Drugs

Vitamin K deficiency

- Vitamin K is present in green vegetables and is synthesised by intestinal bacteria
- Requires bile for its absorption
- Required for formation of factors II, VII, IX and X
- Deficiency is found in:
  - Obstructive jaundice
  - Antibiotics that alter the intestinal flora
  - Prolonged total parenteral nutrition without supplement

Hepatic disease

- Failure of clotting factor synthesis
- Production of abnormal fibrinogen
- In addition, thrombocytopenia may be present as a result of hypersplenism

DIC

- Simultaneous activation of coagulation and fibrinolytic systems
- Formation of microthrombi in many organs with consumption of clotting factors and platelets, leading to haemorrhage
- Causes
  - Septicaemia
  - Malignancy
  - Trauma
  - Shock
  - Liver disease

- Acute pancreatitis
- Obstetrical problems
  - Toxaemia
  - Amniotic fluid embolism
- Clinically causes widespread haemorrhage
- Laboratory findings
  - Thrombocytopenia
  - Decreased fibrinogen
  - Increased fibrin degradation products
- Treated with heparin

Tests for bleeding disorders

- Platelet count
  - Normal: $160–450 \times 10^9/L$
  - Thrombocytopenia: $\leq 100 \times 10^9/L$
- Bleeding time
  - Normal: 1–8 minutes
  - Prolonged in:
    - Thrombocytopenia
    - Platelet defect
    - Failure of vascular contraction
- Clotting time
  - Normal: 5–15 minutes
- Prothrombin time (PT):
  - Tests extrinsic and final common pathway
  - Prolonged in defects of factor I, II, V, VII or X
- Activated partial thromboplastin time (aPTT)
  - Reflects all intrinsic clotting mechanisms
  - Tests all factors except factor VII
- Thrombin time (TT)
  - Prolonged if there is inadequate fibrinogen (seen in heparin use)
- Fibrin degradation products
  - Products released from fibrinogen and fibrin by plasmin
  - Increased in DIC

Platelet disorders

Decreased number (thrombocytopenia)

- Decreased production of platelets
  - Aplastic anaemia
  - Drugs:
    - Tolbutamide
    - Alcohol
    - Cytotoxic agents

- Viral infections
  - Epstein–Barr virus
  - Cytomegalovirus
- Myelodysplasia
- Bone marrow infiltration
  - Carcinoma
  - Leukaemia
  - Myeloma
- Megaloblastic anaemia
- Hereditary thrombocytopenia
- Decreased platelet survival
  - Idiopathic thrombocytopenic purpura
  - Drugs
    - Heparin
    - Quinine
    - Sulphonamides
  - Infection
  - Post-transfusion
  - DIC
  - Thrombotic thrombocytopenic purpura
- Hypersplenism (sequestration)

Decreased function (thrombasthenia)

- Glanzmann's disease
- Uraemia
- Hepatic disease
- Leukaemia
- Extracorporeal circulation
- Drugs

Hypercoagulable states (thrombotic disorders)

- Otherwise called thrombophilia
- Predispose to venous thromboembolism

- Caused by deficiency or inactivity of key proteins that regulate the activation of blood coagulation
  - Antithrombin III
  - Protein C
  - Protein S

Antithrombin III

- Provides protective mechanism against activation of intravascular coagulation
- Deficiency may be familial
- Clinically, deficiency is seen as recurrent deep venous thrombosis starting in the teenage years
- Diagnosis is by low antithrombin III levels
- Treatment is with lifelong oral anticoagulation

Proteins C and protein S

- Vitamin K dependant factors synthesised in the liver
- Protein C (activated)
  - Inhibits factors V and VIII
  - Low levels cause recurrent deep venous thrombosis
  - If warfarin is given in protein C deficiency, causes further decrease in action and results in extensive acute skin necrosis, owing to thrombosis of the cutaneous vessels
- Protein S
  - Co-factor for activated protein C
  - Also regulates coagulation

Hypersensitivity reactions

Gell and Coomb's classification – types

- Gell and Coomb's classification covers types I, II, III and IV
- Type I: anaphylactic or immediate reaction
  - First exposure leads to IgE formation
  - IgE binds to mast cells and basophils
  - Second exposure releases mediators from mast cells and basophils
    - Histamine
    - Leukotrienes
    - Chemotactic factors
    - Platelet-activating factors
  - Examples of type I reactions
    - Hay fever
    - Asthma
    - Anaphylaxis
- Type II: cytotoxic reaction
  - Complement-dependent or antibody-dependent
  - Mediated by antibodies against intrinsic or extrinsic antigens on the cell surface
  - Examples of type II reactions
    - Transfusion reaction
    - Graft rejection
- Type III: immune complex-mediated reaction
  - Complement activation leads to neutrophil activation and lysosomal enzyme release
  - Examples of type II reaction
    - Systemic lupus erythematosus (SLE)
    - Acute glomerulonephritis
- Type IV: cell-mediated or delayed hypersensitivity reaction
  - Release of lymphokines by sensitized T-lymphocytes
  - Examples of type IV reaction
    - Tuberculosis
    - Transplant rejection
- Type V: stimulatory reaction
  - Stimulation of cell function by antireceptor antibodies
  - Examples of type V reaction
    - Graves' disease
    - Myasthenia gravis

Complement

Definition

- The complement system is a soluble enzymic cascade that focuses and amplifies the activity of the specific and innate immune systems as well as having lytic activity against bacteria

Pathways

- Classical pathway, triggered by antigen–antibody complexes
- Alternative pathway, triggered by contact with exposed bacterial capsules

Activation of the complement cascade

- Tissue necrosis
- Infection
- Kinins

Important complement products

- C5a
  - Chemotactic for neutrophils
  - Increases vascular permeability
  - Promotes release of histamine from mast cells
- C3a
  - Similar to C5a but less active
- C567
  - Chemotactic to neutrophils
- C56789
  - Cytolytic
- C4b, C2a and C3b
  - Opsonisation of bacteria, i.e. facilitates phagocytosis by macrophages

Immunoglobulins

Types of immunoglobulin

- IgG, IgA, Ig M, Ig D and Ig E
- IgG
  - Most abundant type
  - Major antibody during secondary response
  - Neutralises toxins and binds micro-organisms

- IgA
  - Found in secretions: saliva, nasal secretions, tears, gastrointestinal secretions, bronchial secretions and genitourinary secretions
  - Prevents bacterial adhesion to these epithelial surfaces
- IgM
  - Also known as macroglobulin
  - Induces agglutination and cytolysis
  - Found in the intravascular compartment when it contains bacteraemia
- IgD
  - Bound to the surface of lymphocytes
  - Controls lymphocyte proliferation and suppression
- IgE
  - Confined to mucosal surfaces
  - Acts in association with mast cells to defend mucosal surfaces
  - Involved in allergic reactions, e.g. extrinsic asthma and hay fever

Structure and general function of immunoglobulins

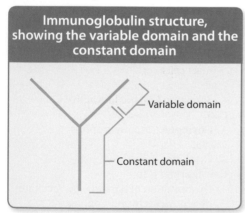

Immunoglobulin structure, showing the variable domain and the constant domain

— Variable domain

— Constant domain

- The constant domain connects with the host's defence effector system
- The variable domain binds with antigens

Autoimmune disease

Definition of autoimmunity

- Reaction and damage of host's tissues by immune mechanisms

Mechanisms to prevent autoimmunity

- Clonal deletion in early life: destruction by the thymus of T cells that express self-recognizing receptors
- Clonal anergy: functional suppression (inactivation) of self-reactive T-cell receptors (B-cell clones) on surface of thymocytes, in the absence of T cells which are already destroyed by thymocytes
- Other suppressor mechanisms involving cytotoxic T cells

Mechanisms of autoimmunity

- Alteration of ratio of T-helper cells to cytotoxic T cells in the peripheral blood
- Alteration in target organs, e.g. the thyroid and the pancreas, that express non-self-antigens
  - These alterations are induced by:
    - Infection
    - Physiological triggering, e.g. lactation
    - Action of interferons and tumour necrosis factor (TNF)-alpha

Classification of autoimmune disorders

- Organ-specific disorders
  - Graves' disease
  - Hashimoto's disease
  - Addison's disease
  - Type I diabetes mellitus
  - Pernicious anaemia
    - Megaloblastic anaemia
    - Atrophic gastritis
    - Achlorhydria
- Non-organ-specific disorders
  - Rheumatoid arthritis
  - SLE
  - Chronic active hepatitis
  - Primary biliary cirrhosis

Mechanisms of organ damage

- Cytotoxicity of macrophages, natural killer (NK) cells and B cells primed with auto-antibodies
- Cytotoxic T cells

Examples of auto-antibodies

- Graves' disease: long-acting thyroid stimulator, an IgG auto-antibody to thyroid stimulating hormone
- Rheumatoid arthritis: rheumatoid factor, an IgM auto-antibody to the patient's own IgG
- SLE: antinuclear factor, an auto-antibody to double-stranded DNA

Immunodeficiency

Definition

- Condition in which the patient is unable to mount an appropriate defence against invading organisms and is thus liable to serious infections

Types

- Global: affecting T cells, B cells and phagocytes
- Specific: affecting one or more components of specific or non-specific defence

Causes

- Primary immunodeficiency
  - Phagocyte deficiency
  - Leukocyte adhesion deficiency
  - Myeloperoxidase deficiency
  - Primary antibody deficiency
- Secondary immunodeficiency (the more common sort)
  - Malnutrition
  - Infection
  - Blood or plasma loss
  - Lymphoproliferative disease
  - Surgery
  - Renal or hepatic failure
  - Splenectomy
  - Hypercatabolic state, e.g. trauma or burns
  - Foreign bodies
  - Cytokines, prostaglandins or complement
  - Drugs
  - Malignancy

Stratification of risk

- Low risk
  - Patients are more susceptible than normal to infection by pathogenic organisms
- Moderate risk
  - Patients are additionally susceptible to infection by commensal organisms
- High risk
  - Patients are high risk of fatal infection by both pathogenic organisms and commensal organisms
  - Therefore the patient requires isolation and prophylactic antibiotics

Risk factors

- Age: increased risk at the extremes of age
- Metabolic factors: chronic renal disease and chronic hepatic disease
- Drugs, e.g. antibiotics, non-steroidal anti-inflammatory drugs and steroids
- Specific disorders, e.g. diabetes mellitus, advanced malignancy, collagen disease and rheumatoid arthritis
- Malnutrition
- Invasive procedures, e.g. bladder catheterisation, intravenous cannulation, endotracheal intubation and surgical procedures
- Congenital neutropenia, congenital deficiencies in cell-mediated immunity

Immunosuppression

Definition

- Disruption of the immune response to a specific antigen
- Controlled reduction of an immune response to foreign antigen on a transplanted tissue (the graft)

Modalities

- Partial lymphocyte irradiation
- Chemical immunosuppression
  - Corticosteroids and azathioprine
    - Depress circulating T cells

- Cyclosporin
  - Suppression of both antibody production and cell-mediated immunity
  - Selective inhibitory effect on T-cell-dependent responses
  - Not profoundly lymphotoxic or myelotoxic

Side effects of immunosuppressive drugs

- Corticosteroids
  - Avascular necrosis
  - Diabetes mellitus
  - Obesity
  - Cushing's syndrome
  - Pancreatitis
  - Cataract
  - Skin problems
  - Psychosis
  - Increased risk of infection
- Azathioprine
  - Bone marrow suppression
  - Polycythaemia
  - Hepatotoxicity
  - Increased risk of infection
- Cyclosporine
  - Nephrotoxicity and hepatotoxicity
  - Increased risk of infection

Transplantation

Definition

- Transfer of an organ or tissue from one part of the body to another, either in the same individual, or to another tissue type matched individual or from a tissue type matched animal to a human

Forms of transfer

- Transfer of tissue
  - Blood
  - Bone marrow
- Transfer of solid organ
  - Skin
  - Cornea
  - Kidney
  - Heart
  - Liver
  - Pancreas

Types of transplantation

- Autograft: transfer of one part of the body to another in the same person, e.g. skin graft
- Allograft: transfer of one part of the body to another person, e.g. blood transfusion, bone marrow graft or kidney transplant
- Xenograft: transfer of one part of the body from an animal source

Requirements

- Compatibility
  - ABO compatibility
    - Chromosome 9
    - Donor–recipient compatibility is an absolute requirement
    - Incompatibility leads to early irreversible rejection
  - Human leukocyte antigen (HLA) compatibility
    - Chromosome 6
    - Involved in both humoral and cellular mechanisms of rejection
    - HLA cross-match negativity is an absolute requirement: if it is positive, i.e. if it causes agglutination, it leads to hyperacute rejection if transplanted

Rejection

- Hyperacute rejection
  - Occurs within hours
  - Immediate antibody-mediated graft rejection in sensitised recipients as a result of preformed cytotoxic antibodies
- Acute rejection
  - Occurs in a few days or weeks
  - Mediated almost exclusively by T lymphocytes in response to major histocompatibility complex (MHC) or transplantation antigens
- Chronic rejection
  - Occurs over months or years
  - Caused by deposition of anti-histocompatibility antibodies resulting in a slow, gradual loss of function

Avoidance of rejection

- Tissue typing
- Immunosuppression

Individual organ transplantation

Kidney transplant

- Performed in those aged 5–70 years
- Indication: chronic renal failure, including renal failure due to glomerulonephritis, pyelonephritis and polycystic kidney disease
- Infections, peptic ulcer and metabolic bone disease must be treated prior to transplant
- Conditions such as previous abdominal operations, peripheral vascular ischaemia and ileal conduits need to be taken into account
- Donor kidney is implanted extraperitoneally, in the iliac fossa
- The renal artery and the renal vein are anastomosed to the iliac artery and the iliac vein
- The ureter is anastomosed to the bladder
- Signs of rejection
  - Decreased urinary output
  - Increased urea and creatinine
  - Biopsy findings

Heart transplant

- Indications
  - Cardiomyopathy
  - Terminal ischemic heart disease
  - Congenital cardiac disease
- The donor atria are anastomosed to the posterior wall of the corresponding chamber
- The pulmonary artery and the aorta are anastomosed

Combined heart and lung transplant

- Indications
  - Pulmonary hypertension
  - Cystic fibrosis
  - Emphysema

- Infection is common and so immunosuppression must be rigorously managed
- Domino procedure: if the recipient of a heart–lung transplant has a good functioning heart, it is transplanted to another recipient
- 2-year survival is 60%

Liver transplant

Indications

Common

- Acute liver failure
  - Seronegative hepatitis (sporadic nonA nonB hepatitis)
  - Drugs
    - Paracetamol
    - Isoniazid
  - Viral
    - Hepatitis B
  - Metabolic
    - Neonatal haemochromatosis
    - Wilson's disease
- Chronic liver disease
  - Viral hepatitis B and C
  - Autoimmune hepatitis
  - Cholestatic disorders
    - Primary sclerosing cholangitis
    - Primary biliary cirrhosis
    - Extra-hepatic biliary atresia
  - Alcoholic liver disease
  - Metabolic disorders
    - Wilson's
    - Haemochromatosis
    - Deficiency of α_1 antitrypsin
  - Non-alcoholic steatohepatitis
- Cryptogenic cirrhosis
- Hepatocellular carcinoma
- Polycystic liver disease
- Budd–Chiari syndrome, veno-occlusive disease

Uncommon

- Familial hypercholesterolaemia
- Primary hyperoxaluria
- Protoporphyria
- Crigler-Najjar syndrome
- Deficiencies in the urea cycle
- Glycogen storage disease

- Lysosomal storage disease
- Tyrosinaaemia
- Galactosaemia
- Haemophilia A & B
- Cystic fibrosis
- Deficiencies of protein C & S
- Amyloidosis
- Sarcoidosis
- Severe graft versus host disease
- Alagille syndrome
- Hepatic trauma

Contraindications

- Absolute
  - Severe cardiopulmonary disease
  - Uncontrolled sepsis
  - Current extrahepatic malignancy
  - Psychiatric or neurological disorders
  - Active alcoholism
- Relative
  - Age >70 years
  - Extensive thrombosis of the portal vein and/or superior mesenteric vein
  - Severe hyponatraemia (risk of pontine myelinosis)
  - Severe malnutrition
  - Lack of financial and social support
  - Active sepsis
  - Untreated HIV infection

The ideal donor must

- Be less than 60 years
- Have normal biochemistry
- Not have an episode of ongoing sepsis
- Not have received a high dose of inotropes
- Not have a prolonged episode of cardiorespiratory arrest recorded
- Not have evidence of severe macrovascular steatosis
- Have been in the ITU for <5 days
- Not have malignant disease

- Be HIV negative
- Not have ischaemic heart disease

Procedure

- Liver placed orthotopically after removal of diseased organ
- Veno-venous bypass to reduce physiological effects

1-year survival

- 1-year survival is 85%

Graft-versus-host reactions

In transplant patients

- Graft-versus-host disease (GvHD) may develop if the graft contains component T cells that react against host cells that are incapable of rejecting them
- GvHD is most likely following bone marrow transplant and small bowel transplant
- Skin and gut are predominantly affected

In blood transfusion

- GvHD is caused by transfusion of T lymphocytes into a severely immunosuppressed host
- Cellular components are irradiated prior to transfusion in these patients

Types of reaction

- Acute GvHD
  - Occurs < 100 days post-transplant
  - Resolves with conservative management
- Chronic GvHD
  - Occurs > 100 days post transplant
  - Causes acute immune-like features, multiple organ involvement and fibrosis

Cancer

Definition

- Process of uncontrolled cell proliferation with invasion and metastases

Features of cancer cells

- Absence of contact inhibition
- Alteration in cell surface glycoprotein
- Lack of differentiation
- Alteration in restriction point of cell cycle

Epidemiological definitions

- Prevalence: proportion of population with a condition at a given time
- Incidence: proportion of population developing a condition in a given time
- Risk factor: an agent or characteristic predisposing to the development of the condition
- Relative risk: association between risk factor and condition
- Disease-free survival: time from diagnosis to recurrence

Chromosomal abnormalities associated with neoplasia

- Translocation
- Deletion
- Extra chromosome (trisomy)
- Abnormal configuration (ring chromosome)

DNA abnormalities

- Polyploidy: multiples of normal number of chromosomes
- Aneuploidy: abnormal number of chromosomes (not multiples)

Histological manifestations of cancer

- Hyperchromatism
- Variable nuclear size
- Multiple or enlarged nucleoli
- Abnormalities of chromatin distribution

Classification of tumours

- The classification of tumours by cell tupe into benign and malignant is tabulated overleaf

Difference between benign and malignant neoplasms

- The difference between benign and malignant neoplasms is tabulated overleaf

Complications of benign neoplasms

Obstruction

- Direct obstruction
  - Biliary, caused by an adenoma of the biliary duct
  - Obstruction to the cerebrospinal fluid, caused by a meningioma or ependymoma
- Indirect obstruction
  - Intussusception, from a polyp

Pressure effects

- Venous obstruction
  - Uterine myoma
  - Retrosternal goitre

Haemorrhage

- From a large bowel tumour
- From an endometrial polyp
- From a capillary hemangioma (in an infant)

Infection

- Large bowel polyp
- Biliary system, as a result of obstruction

Infarction

- Torsion of submucosal fibroid or appendix epiploicae

Classification of tumours by cell type into benign and malignant

Tissue/cell type	Benign	Malignant
Epithelial		
Glandular	Adenoma	Adenocarcinoma
Squamous	Squamous papilloma	Squamous carcinoma
Mesenchymal		
Fibrous tissue	Fibroma	Fibrosarcoma
Smooth muscle	Leiomyoma	Leiomyosarcoma
Skeletal muscle	Rhabdomyoma	Rhabdomyosarcoma
Vascular	Angioma	Angiosarcoma
Nerve sheath	Neurofibroma	Neurogenic sarcoma
Fat	Lipoma	Liposarcoma
Bone	Osteoma	Osteosarcoma
Cartilage	Chondroma	Chondrosarcoma
Lymphoreticular		
Lymphocytes or lymphoid tissue	–	Lymphoma (HL, NHL)
Primitive/embryonal		
Kidney	–	Nephroblastoma
Autonomic nerve	–	Neuroblastoma
Cerebellum	–	Medulloblastoma
Liver	–	Hepatoblastoma
Others		
Neuroendocrine		
Pancreatic islet cells	–	Insulinoma, glucagonoma, gastrinoma
Gut and bronchial	–	Carcinoid
Thyroid C cells	–	Medullary thyroid carcinoma
Melanocytes	Naevi	Melanoma
Germ cell	Mature teratoma	Immature teratoma, seminoma

Differences between benign and malignant neoplasms

Benign	Malignant
Non-invasive	Invades surrounding tissue
Does not metastasise	Capable of metastases
Necrosis rare	Necrosis common
Ulceration rare	Ulceration common
Slow-growing	Rapid-growing
Histologically resembles tissue of origin	Variable resemblance to tissue of origin
Nuclear morphology normal	Nuclear morphology abnormal
Border circumscribed	Border irregular

Ectopic hormone secretion

- Pituitary tumours, which may secrete growth hormone, ACTH, thyroid stimulating hormone, follicle stimulating hormone or luteinising hormone
- Adrenal tumours, which may secrete cortisol or aldosterone
- Ovarian tumours, which may secrete oestrogen
- Parathyroid tumours, which may secrete parathyroid hormone
- Phaeochromocytomas, which secrete catecholamines

Electrolyte loss

- From large bowel polyps

Polycythaemia

- Associated with large uterine fibroids

Tumour-like lesions

- Benign, non-neoplastic masses arising as simple developmental abnormalities (errors), the growth of which is co-ordinated with that of the person, i.e. is under the normal growth controls of the body
- Two types
  - Hamartomas – arise at the site of origin of the tissue
  - Choristomas – arise at an ectopic site

Hamartomas

- Tumour-like malformations composed of a haphazard arrangement of one or more mature, well-differentiated tissue or cell types, normally found at the site from which they arise
- Examples
  - Benign melanocytic naevi (moles)
  - Pulmonary (bronchial) hamartomas
  - Haemangioma of the vessels
  - Peutz–Jeghers polyps of the bowel
  - Osteochondroma of the long bones
  - Neurofibromatosis of von Recklinghausen's disease
  - Bizarre neuroepithelial cells of tuberous sclerosis

- Overgrowth of any developmental remnants
- Complications
  - Obstruction
  - Pressure (direct or indirect)
  - Infection
  - Infarction
  - Haemorrhage
  - Fracture
  - Mistaken diagnosis as malignancy, with over-treatment and consequent morbidity and mortality
  - Malignant transformation
    - Chondrosarcoma arising in an osteochondroma
    - Neurofibrosarcoma arising in von Recklinghausen's disease
  - Association with neoplasm without arising from a hamartoma, e.g. the ovaries in a patient with Peutz-Jeghers syndrome may contain fibromas

Choristomas

- Tumour-like malformations composed of a perfectly formed mature tissue in an ectopic site (rests)
- Examples
  - Ectopic adrenal tissue in the ovary
  - Ectopic pancreatic tissue in the wall of the gut

Epidemiology of cancer

Uses of cancer epidemiology by the surgeon

- Definition of size of the problem
  - Incidence: rate of development of new cases in a defined period as a proportion of the whole population
  - Prevalence: the number of cases in the population at any one time
- Identification of high-risk groups
  - To develop strategies for early detection and prevention
  - As a guide to resource allocation
- Identification of poor prognostic groups
  - By using variable characteristics of the tumour and the patient
  - To enable logical planning of treatment for an individual case

- Indication of aetiological factors, especially leading to positive identification of carcinogens; for example:
  - Smoking as a cause of lung cancer
  - Diet and infective agents studied for carcinogenesis

Oncogenes

- Derived from proto-oncogenes
- Proto-oncogenes are normal cellular genes that function as positive regulators of growth
- Converted to oncogenes by mutation
- Oncogenes encode proteins that stimulate abnormal cellular growth
  - Growth factors
  - Growth factor receptors
  - Transcription factors
- Oncogenes are dominant genes
- Examples
  - k-*ras*
    - In chromosome 11
    - Colorectal cancer
    - Pancreatic cancer
    - Leukaemia
  - *erb*-b2
    - In chromosome 17
    - Breast cancer
    - Ovarian cancer

  - *myc*
    - In chromosome 8
    - Burkitt's lymphoma
    - Small-cell lung cancer
  - *ret*
    - thyroid
  - *src*
    - in chromosome 20

Tumour suppressor genes

- Also known as recessive oncogenes
- Normally suppress cell proliferation and promote cell loss (apoptosis)
- Mutation causes loss of function, leading to increased cell proliferation
- Since the gene is recessive, mutation of a single gene leads to a carrier state
- Mutation in both genes leads to cancer
- Examples
  - *p*53 (normal function: apoptosis)
    - On chromosome 17
    - Colorectal cancer
    - Breast cancer
    - Gastric malignancy
  - *RB*-1
    - On chromosome 13
    - Associated with retinoblastoma, but affects more than one tissue: people with the defective gene who survives

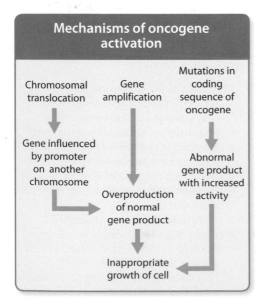

Mechanisms of oncogene activation

Chromosomal translocation → Gene influenced by promoter on another chromosome → Overproduction of normal gene product → Inappropriate growth of cell

Gene amplification → Overproduction of normal gene product → Inappropriate growth of cell

Mutations in coding sequence of oncogene → Abnormal gene product with increased activity → Inappropriate growth of cell

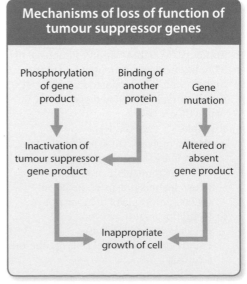

Mechanisms of loss of function of tumour suppressor genes

Phosphorylation of gene product → Inactivation of tumour suppressor gene product → Inappropriate growth of cell

Binding of another protein → Inactivation of tumour suppressor gene product → Inappropriate growth of cell

Gene mutation → Altered or absent gene product → Inappropriate growth of cell

childhood retinoblastoma have a high incidence of osteosarcoma in adolescence
- Retinoblastoma
- Osteosarcoma
- *APC* and *DCC*
  - On chromosome 5
  - Colorectal cancer
- *BRCA*-1
  - Breast cancer
  - Ovarian cancer
- *BRCA*-2
  - Breast cancer
- *bcl*-2
  - On chromosome 18
  - B-cell lymphoma

Carcinogenesis

Definition of a carcinogen

- Any external influence that can be shown to cause cancer

Classification of carcinogens

- Polycyclic aromatic hydrocarbons, e.g. benzopyrene in tobacco smoke
- Viruses
  - Human papilloma virus
    - Cancer of the cervix
  - Epstein–Barr virus
    - Burkitt's lymphoma
    - Hodgkin's lymphoma
  - Hepatitis B virus, hepatitis C virus
    - Hepatocellular carcinoma
  - Human T lymphocyte virus (HTLV)
    - T-cell leukaemia
  - HIV
    - Kaposi's sarcoma
- Genetic
  - Due to mutation of genes which regulate growth and proliferation, e.g. oncogenes
- Miscellaneous
  - Ultraviolet light
    - Skin cancer
  - X-rays
    - Bone marrow tumours
    - Thyroid cancer

- Alcohol
  - Oesophageal cancer
- Asbestos
  - Cancer of the pleura
- Oestrogen
  - Breast cancer
- Nickel, chromate, arsenic
  - Lung cancer

Definition of carcinogenesis

- Multistep process by which cancer forms due to any external influence, leading to successive genetic mutations
- See figure overleaf

Types of carcinogens

- Remote carcinogen: precursor of a carcinogenic agent that may be found in the environment
- Proximate carcinogen: metabolite of a remote carcinogen that may be modified further in the body
- Ultimate carcinogen: active carcinogen that interacts with DNA and causes cancer

Gompertzian pattern of tumour development

- Small tumours grow rapidly
- As a tumour increases in size, the rate of growth decreases, owing to:
  - Decreased blood supply
  - Decreased nutrition
  - Necrosis
  - Pressure effects
  - Decreased growth fraction

Tumour markers

Definition

- Substances produced by the tumour that can be detected in the blood, lymph or serous fluid and within solid tumours

Uses

- Focused investigation in a symptomatic patient
- Assessment of response to treatment
- Detection of relapse

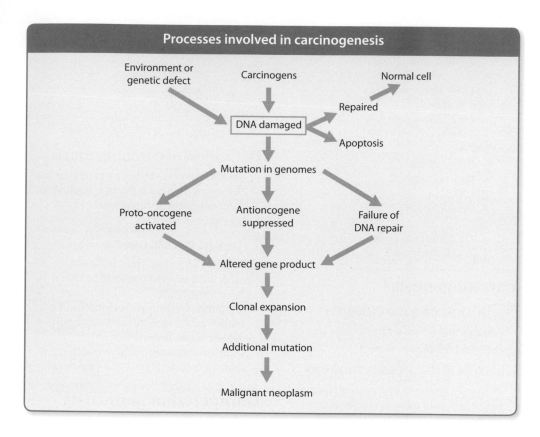

Processes involved in carcinogenesis

Types

- Oncofetal proteins
  - Carcinoembryonic antigen (CEA)
    - Colorectal cancer, pancreatitis
  - Alpha-fetoprotein
    - Hepatocellular carcinoma
    - Teratoma
  - Carbohydrate antigen (CA) 19-9
    - Gastrointestinal cancers
  - CA 125
    - Ovarian cancer
  - Prostate-specific antigen (PSA)
    - Prostate cancer
- Hormones:
  - Human chorionic gonadotropin (hCG)
    - Choriocarcinoma
  - Calcitonin
    - Medullary carcinoma of the thyroid
  - 5-Hydroxyindoleacetic acid (5-HIAA)
    - Carcinoid
- Enzymes
  - Alkaline phosphatase
    - Bone metastases

Definitions related to tumour markers

- Sensitivity: indicates how commonly a tumour marker level is elevated in the presence of tumour
  = {[True positive/(True positive + False positive)] × 100}
- Specificity: proportion of true negatives, i.e. patients without tumours with normal marker levels
  = {[True negative/(True positive + False positive)] × 100}
- Positive predictive value: percentage of true positives
  = [(True positive/All positive) × 100]
- Negative predictive value: percentage of true negatives
  = [(True negative/All negative) × 100]

Ideal tumour marker

- Should be present in the blood
- Should be undetectable in health
- Should be produced by malignant tissue

- Should be organ-specific
- Circulating concentration should be proportional to tumour mass

Screening

Definition

- Application of a test in order to detect a tumour while it is still asymptomatic

Criteria

- Well understood natural history
- Recognisable early stage of tumour
- Test must be sensitive, specific, safe and inexpensive, and acceptable to the population being screened

Bias

- Types
  - Lead-time bias: early diagnosis advances the time of diagnosis
  - Length bias: slow-growing tumours are more likely to be detected
  - Selection bias: type of person who will agree to be screened
- Elimination of bias
  - Randomised controlled trials
  - Target population

Available screening programmes

- Colon
- Stomach
- Breast
- Cervix
- Prostate
- Ovary

Definitions related to screening

- Sensitivity: proportion of people with the disease who have a positive test
- Specificity: proportion of people without the disease who have a negative test
- Targeted screening: investigation of the siblings of an index case of a heritable disease, e.g. familial adenomatous polyposis, hereditary non-polyposis colorectal cancer, breast cancer

Invasion and metastases

Invasion

- Increased cell proliferation caused by increased growth factors
- Decreased cell adhesion caused by:
  - Loss of cellular proteins that mediate adhesion
  - Failure of extracellular matrix glycoproteins
- Increased motility caused by abnormalities of actin cytoskeleton
- Proteolytic enzymes, e.g. metalloproteinases, causing degradation of extracellular matrix

Metastases

- Definition: breaking off of cells or clumps of cells from the primary tumour, movement of the cells to a distant site, and growth of secondary tumour at that site
- Routes of metastasisation
  - Blood
  - Lymphatics
  - Body cavities
  - Cerebrospinal fluid (in the case of CNS tumours)
- Mechanism: retraction of endothelial cells by metalloproteinases, which causes vascular invasion

Common pattern of metastases

- Liver: from gastrointestinal, pancreatic, lung, breast and genitourinary tumours and malignant melanoma
- Skeletal: from lung, breast, prostate, kidney and thyroid tumours
- Brain: from lung tumours and malignant melanoma
- Adrenal glands: from lung and breast tumours
- Trans-coelomic: from gastric, colonic and ovarian tumours
- Lung: from kidney, breast, colorectal and ovarian tumours

Staging of tumours

Definition

- Process by which the extent of tumour, in terms of both local and metastatic spread, is estimated, by means of a combination of clinical, radiological and histopathological examinations

Uses

- Estimation of prognosis
- Useful in treatment planning
- Allows for case mix when evaluating the outcome of treatment
- Allows for comparative trials in patients from different centres

Types

- International Union against Cancer (Union Internationale Contre le Cancer: UICC): TNM staging
- American Joint Committee on cancer (AJCC) : stages 0–4

TNM staging

- T: extent of the primary tumour
- N: degree of spread to regional nodes
- M: distant metastases
- T1 to T4 represents increasing extent of primary tumour in terms of size and degree of penetration
- N1 to N3 represents increasingly distant sites of lymph node metastases and/ or increased number of involved lymph nodes
- Prefix 'p', e.g. pT3, pN1 indicates TNM staging based on histopathology

AJCC system – stages 0–4

- Based on:
  - Size of primary tumour
  - Presence of affected lymph nodes
  - Presence of metastases

Stage shift

- Patients with identical clinical stage may have very different outcomes because staging is dependent on availability and accuracy of investigations, e.g. chest CT scan versus chest X-ray

Grading of tumours

Definition

- Histopathological examination to grade the tumour in terms of its degree of differentiation

Types

- Invasion of basement membrane
  - *In situ*
  - Invasive
- Pleomorphism in an invasive carcinoma
  - Well differentiated
  - Moderately differentiated
  - Poorly differentiated

Differentiation

- Definition: degree to which neoplastic cells resemble their tissue of origin
- Based on:
  - Nuclear pleomorphism
  - Cellularity
  - Necrosis
  - Cellular invasion
  - Number of mitoses
- Features of poor differentiation
  - Increased nuclear pleomorphism
  - Atypical mitoses
  - Hyperchromatic nuclei
  - Increased ratio of nuclear size to cytoplasmic size
  - Presence of giant cells

Nottingham prognostic index (NPI)

- Definition: pathological system that combines tumour grade, node status and tumour size to give a prognostic score
- Mainly used for breast cancer
- NPI is the grade plus the lymph node score plus (size of tumour in centimetres × 0.2)
- Vascular invasion adds 1 further point to the score
- Prognosis based on the score
  - 2.0–2.4: excellent prognosis
  - 2.4–3.4: good prognosis
  - 3.4–5.4: moderate prognosis
  - > 5.4: poor prognosis

Specific staging systems

Melanoma

- Breslow's thickness
  - Stage I: < 0.75 mm
  - Stage II: 0.76–1.5 mm
  - Stage III: 1.5–4.0 mm
  - Stage IV: > 4 mm

Nottingham prognostic index		
Points	Grade	Lymph nodes
1	Well-differentiated	No nodes
2	Moderately differentiated	1–3 nodes
3	Poorly differentiated	>3 nodes

- Clarke's levels
  - Level I: involving only the epidermis
  - Level II: involving the papillary dermis
  - Level III: invading the papillary dermis up to the interface
  - Level IV: involving the reticular dermis
  - Level V: invading the reticular dermis up to the subcutaneous fat
- TNM classification
  - TX: cannot be assessed
  - T0: no primary
  - T_{IS}: melanoma *in situ* (equivalent to Clarke's level I)
  - T1: up to papillary dermis (equivalent to Clarke's level II)
  - T2: up to reticular dermis (equivalent to Clarke's level III)
  - T3: invading reticular dermis (equivalent to level Clarke's IV)
  - T4: up to subcutaneous fat (equivalent to level Clarke's V)
  - NX: nodes cannot be assessed
  - N0: no nodes involved
  - N1: regional nodes involved
  - N2: second level drainage involved
  - N3: distant nodes ± in-transit metastases
  - MX: metastatic spread cannot be assessed
  - M0: no metastases
  - M1: distant metastases
- AJCC staging
  - Stage IA: localised, < 0.75 mm, no nodes, no metastases (T1 N0 M0)
  - Stage IB: localised, 0.76–1.5 mm, no nodes, no metastases (T2 N0 M0)
  - Stage IIA: localised, 1.5–4.0 mm, no nodes, no metastases (T3 N0 M0)
  - Stage IIB: localised, > 4.0 mm, no nodes, no metastases (T4 N0 M0)
  - Stage III: regional or in-transit metastases, no systemic metastases (T_{ANY} N2 M0)
  - Stage IV: systemic metastases (T_{ANY} N_{ANY} M1)

Colorectal carcinoma

- Dukes' staging
  - Stage A: confined to the bowel wall, no lymph nodes
  - Stage B: outside bowel wall; no lymph nodes
    - Stage B1: into the muscularis propria
    - Stage B2: through the muscularis propria
  - Stage C: lymph node involvement
    - Stage C1: regional nodes
    - Stage C2: highest nodes
  - Stage D: distant metastases
- TNM
  - TX: cannot be assessed
  - T0: no primary tumour
  - T_{IS}: carcinoma *in situ*
  - T1: invasion of the submucosa
  - T2: invasion of the muscularis propria
  - T3: through the muscularis propria into the subserosa or into the non-peritonealised pericolic or perirectal tissues
  - T4: perforation of visceral peritoneum or direct invasion of other organs or structures
  - NX: nodes cannot be assessed
  - N0: no nodes
  - N1: involvement of one, two or three pericolic or perirectal lymph nodes
  - N2: involvement of four or more pericolic or perirectal lymph nodes
  - N3: involvement of any lymph nodes along the course of named vascular trunks

- MX: metastatic spread cannot be assessed
- M0: no distant metastases
- M1: distant metastases
- AJCC staging and comparison with Duke's, with 5-year survival rates:
  - Stage 0 = TIS N0 M0.
  - Stage I:
    - T1 N0 M0 ⎤ Duke's A.
    - T2 N0 M0 ⎦ 80% 5-year survival.
  - Stage II:
    - T3 N0 M0 ⎤ Duke's B.
    - T4 N0 M0 ⎦ 60% 5-year survival.
  - Stage III:
    - T_{ANY} N1 M0 ⎤ Duke C.
    - T_{ANY} N2,3 M0 ⎦ 30% 5-year survival.
  - Stage IV:
    - T_{ANY} N_{ANY} M1 – Duke's D, 5% 5-year survival.

Biopsy

Definition

- Removal of representative sample of tissue for histological diagnosis

Types

- Excisional biopsy: whole tumour removed
- Incisional biopsy: a small portion removed from the edge of an inoperable tumour
- Core needle biopsy ('tru-cut'), which may be direct or guided by ultrasound or CT
- Fine-needle aspiration biopsy, via a 21–23 gauge needle; may be direct or guided by ultrasound or CT
- Endoscopic biopsy, using special biopsy forceps, or may be a brushing or a washing
- Frozen section
- Sentinel lymph node biopsy

Staining techniques

- Eosin and haematoxylin, for tissue structure
- Special stains
  - Alcian blue, for mucus
  - Gieson's stain, for connective tissue
  - Congo red, for amyloid
  - Ziehl–Neelsen stain, for melanin and neuroendocrine tissue

- Immunohistochemistry
  - For antigen–antibody system
  - For undifferentiated tumours
- Polymerase chain reaction (PCR)

Frozen section biopsy

- Definition: fresh tissue sent for rapid histological assessment during the course of an operation, to allow rapid therapeutic decisions to be made at surgery
- The tissue is frozen in liquid nitrogen
- Limitations
  - Destruction of small specimen by ice-crystal artefact
  - May not be diagnostic
  - May be misleading as a result of the destruction
  - Expensive

Interpretation of fine-needle aspiration cytology

- C_1: insufficient material
- C_2: benign tumour
- C_3: atypical cells
- C_4: suspicious of malignancy
- C_5: malignant

Principles of surgery for malignant disease

Role

- Diagnosis and staging
- Therapeutic
  - Curative
  - Palliative

Selection of surgical procedure

- The selection of the surgical procedure depends on:
- The extent of the disease
- Aggression of the tumour
- Availability and effectiveness of alternative and adjunctive therapy
- General health and understanding of the patient
- Acceptance by the patient of the need to undergo surgery

Pre-operative preparation

- Assessment of disease
  - Physical findings
  - Endoscopy
  - Tumour markers
  - Imaging
- Co-existing diseases detected and controlled
- Nutritional support
- Prophylactic antibiotic cover if necessary

Operative findings

- Tumour may be fixed
- Tumour may be unresectable
- Tumour may be resectable but there are unsuspected metastases
- Synchronous tumours may be present

Types of surgery

- Curative surgery for primary tumour
  - Removal of whole tissue containing the tumour plus an intact covering of normal tissue
- Curative surgery for secondaries
  - Block dissection for melanoma in the absence of detectable distant metastases
  - Local recurrence and hepatic metastases for colorectal carcinoma
- Reconstructive surgery
  - Stomach for resected oesophagus, on right gastric or gastro-epiploic arteries
  - Rectus abdominis myocutaneous flap after mastectomy on inferior epigastric artery
  - Latissimus dorsi flap on thoracodorsal vessels
  - Free flaps using microvascular techniques
  - Tissue expansion
- Palliative surgery
  - Palliative resection, bypass or external stoma for obstruction
  - Stenting for oesophageal or biliary obstruction
  - Palliative resection for bleeding gastrointestinal tumours
  - Coeliac axis block for pain

Radiotherapy

Definition

- Therapeutic use of ionising radiation for the treatment of malignant disease

Action

- Causes DNA damage by ionisation, which makes the cell incapable of division
- Therefore, slow-growing tumours are less radiosensitive than rapidly dividing tumours
- Normal tissues respond by accelerated re-population, which is not possible for tumour cells

Fractionation

- Dividing the total dose of radiotherapy into parts spread over several weeks to enable normal cells to re-populate
- Large tumours need large fractions and a large total dose of radiotherapy
- Squamous cell carcinoma and adenocarcinoma are the most radiosensitive tumours
- Normal vital tissues have to be protected, and this may limit radiation dosage

Radiotherapy planning

- Assessment of gross tumour volume (GTV): determined by CT scan
- Clinical target volume (CTV): 0.5–1 cm around the GTV
- Planning target volume (PTV): 0.5 cm around the CTV

Relationship between gross tumour volume, clinical target volume and planning target volume in radiotherapy planning

Planning target volume — Gross tumour volume — Clinical target volume

Radiotherapy as primary therapy

- Sites such as the skin, lung, oesophagus, anal canal and cervix
- Radiosensitive tumours
  - Testicular carcinoma (seminoma)
  - Early Hodgkin's lymphoma
- Inoperable tumours
- Where operations carry high morbidity, high mortality or high disfigurement
- Patients unfit for surgery

Radiotherapy as adjuvant therapy

- To control microscopic spread beyond the resection margin
- To control tumour cells spilled at operation
- For lymph nodal metastases, e.g. from breast cancer, CNS tumours, pancreatic tumours, rectal cancer, parotid gland tumours
- Post-operatively, to the tumour bed
- Pre-operative, to downstage the tumour, e.g. bladder cancer, rectal cancer, sarcoma

Palliative radiotherapy

- To advanced lung carcinoma, for symptom control
- To bone metastases, for pain control
- To spinal cord compression, to prevent motor, sensory and sphincter disturbances
- To brain metastases, to prevent morbidity
- For superior vena cava obstruction

Treatment of systemic disease

- For leukaemias and lymphomas with bone marrow rescue
- Iodine-131 for differentiated cancer of the thyroid

Complications

- Nausea, vomiting and loss of appetite
- Skin changes: hair loss, redness, thinning and spider naevi
- Mouth and jaw: dental abscess, osteoradionecrosis of mandible
- Lungs: radiation pneumonitis, fibrosis
- Heart: pericarditis, fibrosis
- Spinal cord: paralysis

- Abdomen: radiation enteritis, causing chronic ulcer, scarring, stricture and perforation
- Gonads: amenorrhoea, infertility
- Kidneys: renal failure, with anaemia and hypertension
- Muscles: atrophy, calcification, malignancy
- Thyroid: cancer

Immunotherapy

- Treatment of cancers using recombinant cytokines that have immunomodulator activity and anti-tumour activity, e.g. interleukin (IL)-2 and interferon (IFN)-alpha

IL-2

- T-cell growth factor that is central to T-cell-mediated immune response
- Used for treatment of renal cell carcinoma and malignant melanoma

Colony stimulating factors (CSFs)

- Exert effect on haemopoiesis and immune functions
- Reduce chemotherapy-induced haematological toxicity and are useful adjuvants in high-dose chemotherapy and bone marrow transplants, e.g. erythropoietin and granulocyte-CSF

IFN-alpha

- Acts against many solid and haematological malignancies, e.g. hairy cell leukaemia, chronic myeloid leukaemia, Kaposi's sarcoma and malignant melanoma

Hormonal therapy

- Used for patients with breast, prostate and endometrial cancer
- Breast cancer
  - For oestrogen receptor (ER)-positive tumours and progesterone receptor (PR)-positive tumours

- Agents used in pre-menopausal patients
  - Oophorectomy
  - Luteinising hormone releasing hormone (LHRH) agonists
  - Tamoxifen
- Agents used in post-menopausal patients
  - Tamoxifen
  - Anastrazole
  - Megestrol acetate
- Prostate cancer
  - LHRH agonists
  - Orchidectomy
  - Non-steroidal anti-androgens
    - Flutamide
    - Bicalutamide
  - Diethyl stilbestrol

Chemotherapy

Types

- Palliative chemotherapy
- Curative chemotherapy
- Adjuvant chemotherapy
- Neo-adjuvant chemotherapy

Palliative chemotherapy

- To improve symptoms
- To improve quality of life
- Sometimes to improve survival (in some cancer types)

Curative chemotherapy

- For chemosensitive tumours
  - Testicular cancer
  - Acute leukaemias
  - Lymphomas
  - Some paediatric tumours

Adjuvant chemotherapy

- To kill micrometastases after surgery or radiotherapy, e.g. in breast cancer

Neo-adjuvant chemotherapy

- To treat micrometastases that are not visible on imaging

- To reduce the size of the tumour before surgery
- Examples
  - In breast cancer, permitting wide local excision instead of mastectomy
  - In oesophageal cancer
  - In sarcoma

Complications

- Local toxicity: tissue destruction if the chemotherapy agent is extravasated
- Bone marrow toxicity
  - Leukopenia, leading to infections
  - Thrombocytopenia, leading to bleeding
  - Anaemia
- Gastrointestinal toxicity
  - Nausea and vomiting
  - Treated with metoclopramide and lorazepam
- Alopecia, which is temporary
- Carcinogenesis, which is directly related to dosage
- Gonadal damage
  - Sperm banking for males
  - Fertilisation and freezing of ova for females
  - Hormone replacement therapy

Paraneoplastic syndrome

Definition

- Group of symptoms that occur in the presence of neoplasia but that are not directly caused by the tumour itself or its metastases or by associated cachexia

Importance

- Signs and symptoms may be the earliest clinical manifestation of a tumour
- Can lead to morbidity and death
- Can mimic other diseases
- Can mimic metastases, leading to upstaging

Classification

- Humoral: mediated by a secreted tumour product
- Immunological: tumour-associated autoimmune phenomena
- Hematological
- Uncertain cause (idiopathic)

Examples

- Paraneoplastic Cushing's syndrome in bronchogenic carcinoma, due to ACTH (humoral)
- Syndrome of inappropriate ADH (SIADH) in bronchogenic carcinoma, due to ADH (humoral)
- Carcinoid syndrome in liver metastases from carcinoid, due to 5-hydroxy-tryptamine (humoral)
- Acanthosis nigricans in pancreatic carcinoma, due to epidermal growth factors
- Hypertrophic pulmonary osteoarthropathy in bronchogenic carcinoma; cause unknown (idiopathic)
- Hypercalcaemia in epithelial tumours, due to parathyroid hormone-related peptide (humoral)
- Eaton–Lambert syndrome (a myasthenia-like picture) in bronchogenic carcinoma (immunological)

- Dermatomyositis and membranous glomerulonephritis in various cancers (immunological)
- Haematological manifestations
  - Polycythemia
  - Disseminated intravascular coagulation
  - Thrombocythaemia
  - Thrombophlebitis migrans
  - Non-infective thrombotic endocarditis
- Dermatological and soft tissue manifestations
  - Acanthosis nigricans
  - Dermatomyositis
  - Erythrodermia
  - Finger clubbing
- Neuromuscular manifestations
  - Polymyositis
  - Myositis
  - Cerebellar degeneration
  - Demyelinating disorders

Neoplasms associated with paraneoplastic syndrome

- Bronchial carcinoma (small cell and squamous cell carcinomas)
- Breast carcinoma
- Renal cell carcinoma
- Pancreatic adenocarcinoma

Surgically important micro-organisms

Classification

- Conventional pathogens: those that cause infection in a previously healthy person
  - *Staphylococcus aureus:* wound infections
  - *Haemophilus influenzae:* chest infections
  - *Neisseria gonorrhoeae:* gonorrhoea
- Conditional pathogens: those that cause infection in patients who have a predisposition to infection
  - *Pseudomonas aeruginosa:* wound infections
  - *Klebsiella species:* urinary tract infections
- Opportunistic pathogens: those that are usually of low virulence but cause infection in immunocompromised patients
  - *Pneumocystis carinii:* chest infections
  - *Candida albicans:* oesophagitis
  - *Aspergillus fumigates:* aspergillosis

Gram-positive cocci

- Staphylococci
  - Coagulase-positive staphylococci: *S. aureus*
    - Superficial infections
    - Deep infections
    - Food poisoning
    - Toxic shock syndrome
  - Coagulase-negative staphylococci: *Staphylococcus epidermidis*
    - Infection in foreign bodies, e.g. prosthetic valves
  - Antibiotics
    - Penicillin, flucloxacillin
    - Erythromycin, clindamycin
    - Cephalosporins, vancomycin
  - Methicillin-resistant *S. aureus* (MRSA), a major threat to surgical patients
- Streptococci:
  - Beta-haemolytic streptococci
    - Lancefield group A streptococci: ENT infections
    - Lancefield group D streptococci: enterococci (*Streptococcus faecalis*)
  - *Streptococcus viridians:*
    - Alpha-haemolytic *Streptococcus* species
    - Upper respiratory tract commensals
  - *S. pneumoniae* (the pneumococcus)
    - Encapsulated
    - Septicaemia in post-splenectomy patients

Gram-positive rods (bacilli)

- Produce a powerful exotoxin
- Examples
  - *Clostridium perfringens:* gas gangrene
  - *Clostridium tetani:* tetanus
  - *Clostridium botulinum:* botulism
  - *Clostridium difficile:* diarrhoea in antibiotic-associated colitis

Gram-negative cocci

- Intracellular diplococci
  - *N. gonorrhoeae*
  - *Neisseria meningitidis*
- *Moraxella catarrhalis*

Gram-negative rods (bacilli)

- Facultative anaerobes
  - *Escherichia coli:* sepsis, diarrhoea
  - *Klebsiella* species: urinary tract infections
  - *Proteus* species: urinary tract infections
  - *Salmonella* species
    - *Salmonella typhi*
    - *Salmonella paratyphi*
  - *Shigella* species: dysentery
  - *Yersinia* species: mesenteric adenitis
- Aerobes
  - *Pseudomonas* species: affects immunocompromised patients
- Miscellaneous
  - *Campylobacter* species: bacterial food poisoning
  - *H. influenzae:* respiratory tract infections
  - *Pasteurella multocida:* following animal bites

Commensal organisms

Definition

- Normal flora in the body, which can cause infection if there is a breach of body defence or if the commensal organism gains access to another site

Examples of normal flora

- Skin
  - Coagulase-negative staphylococci
  - Diphtheroids
- Upper respiratory tract
  - *S. viridans*
  - Diphtheroids
  - Anaerobes
  - Commensal *Neisseria* species
- Lower gastrointestinal tract
  - Coliforms
    - *E. coli*
    - *Klebsiella* species
  - Faecal streptococci
  - *Pseudomonas* species
  - Anaerobes
    - *Bacteroides* species
    - Clostridia
- Anterior urethra
  - Skin flora
  - Faecal flora

Alteration of commensals

- Broad spectrum antibiotics cause overgrowth of resistant organisms, which in turn causes serious infections

Replacement flora

- Organisms that colonise at various sites when the patient is treated with antimicrobial agents
- An example is *Klebsiella* species in the upper respiratory tract of intubated and/or ventilated patients

Exotoxins and endotoxins

Definition

Substances produced by organisms to cause tissue damage

Actions of exotoxins

- Activation of immune system

Comparison of the features of exotoxins and endoxins	
Exotoxins	**Endotoxins**
Simple protein in nature	Lipopolysaccharide in nature
Heat labile (60°C)	Heat stable (60°C)
Produced by Gram-positive bacteria (e.g. diphtheria, cholera, *Shigella,* tetanus)	An integral part of the cell wall of Gram-negative bacteria
Excreted by living cells, i.e. freely diffusible, specific for each type of organism (toxic organism)	Elaborated after bacterial disintegration, i.e. non-diffusible, non-specific for each type of organism (invasive organism)
Highly antigenic	Weakly antigenic
Strongly toxic	Less toxic
Can be detoxified to toxoid	Cannot be detoxified
Highly specific in action, i.e. has affinity to specific tissue	Less specific in action, i.e. gives generalised effects, e.g. fever, DIC, septic shock

- By direct activation of T cells polyclonally
- By binding to major histocompatibility complex (MHC) antigen-presenting cells

Actions of endotoxins

- Fever: mediated by interleukin (IL)-1
- Shock
- Intravascular coagulation causing disseminated intravascular coagulation, through activation of both coagulation systems
  - Hageman factor activates the intrinsic system
  - Release of monocyte factor activates the extrinsic system
- Disturbance of blood cells
  - Neutropenia
  - Thrombocytopenia
- Disturbance of the immune system
  - Increased B-cell mitosis
  - Increased macrophage activity

Source of surgical infections

Infections in clean wounds (class I wounds)

- Class I wounds are wounds created in surgical procedures during which the respiratory tract, genitourinary tract or gastrointestinal tract has not been entered
- Usual sources of infection
  - Airborne
  - Exogenous bacteria that have entered during surgery
  - In the case of prosthetic implants, patient's own skin flora
- Infection rate is < 2%

Infections in clean contaminated wounds (class II wounds)

- Class II wounds are wounds created in elective surgery during which the respiratory tract, genitourinary tract or gastrointestinal tract has been entered
- Usual source of infection
  - Endogenous flora of the organ that has been surgically resected
- Infection rate is 5%

Infections in contaminated wounds (class III wounds)

- Class III wounds are wounds in which:
  - Acute inflammation was found (not pus)
  - There has been spillage of gastrointestinal contents
- Source of infection is bowel and/or other endogenous flora
- Infection rate is 20–40%

Infections in dirty wounds (class IV wounds)

- Class IV wounds are:
  - Wounds in which pus was found following organ perforation
  - Contaminated traumatic wounds
- Source of infection is organisms from faecal contamination
- Infection rate is 40%

Risk of infection

Clean wounds

- No violation of mucosa
- No inflammation
- No drains
- 2% risk of infection
- No antibiotics are indicated
- Cause of infection: airborne organisms

Clean contaminated wounds

- Incision of mucosa but no spillage
- Clean procedures in immunocompromised patients
- 5–10% risk of infection
- Single pre-operative dose of antibiotic is indicated
- Cause of infection: endogenous flora

Contaminated wounds

- Pre-existing infection
- Spillage of viscus contents
- 20–40% risk of infection
- One pre-operative and two post-operative doses of antibiotic are indicated

Dirty

- Pus found at operation
- Organ perforation
- Contaminated traumatic wounds

- 40% risk of infection
- Full course of antibiotics according to culture is indicated

Principles of asepsis and antisepsis

Definitions

- Asepsis: methods that prevent contamination of wounds and other sites by ensuring that only sterile objects and fluids come into contact with them and that the risks of airborne contamination are minimised
- Antisepsis: use of solutions for disinfection, e.g. chlorhexidine, iodine, alcohol – but does not necessarily imply sterility

Operating theatre clothing

- Gowns
  - Woven cotton clothing is relatively ineffective at preventing the passage of bacteria
  - Disposable, non-woven fabric, Gore-Tex or tightly woven polyester–cotton fabrics are ideal
  - Charnley exhaust gown is used for prosthetic implant surgery
- Masks protect the user's mucous membranes
- Eye protection and visors protect the user's mucous membranes
- Hair and beard must be fully covered by synthetic caps or balaclavas
- Footwear
  - Little role in spread of infection
  - Must protect from sharps injury
- Gloves
  - Sterile: protect patient and user
  - Double gloving: increased protection against blood-borne viruses

Operating theatre air

- The number of people and their movements should be minimised
- Positive-pressure or plenum ventilation system with pressure decreasing from theatre to anaesthetic room to entrance lobby causes organisms to be carried out

- Ultra-clean air system for prosthetic implant surgery: unidirectional or laminar air flow at 300 air changes per hour and re-circulated through high-efficiency particulate air (HEPA) filters

Preparation of the surgeon

- Initial scrub of 3–5 minutes at the start of the list followed by effective hand-washing using an antiseptic in between cases
- Antiseptics used:
  - Chlorhexidine gluconate
  - Hexachlorophene
  - Povidone iodine

Preparation of the patient

- Pre-operative shower using chlorhexidine
- All skin infections identified and pre-treated
- Clippers and/or depilatory cream used as near possible to the time of operation
- Skin preparation: scrubbed first and painted with antiseptic solution
- Drapes

Sterilisation, cleaning and disinfection

- Spillage removed as soon as possible
- Contaminated waste and sharps incinerated

Commonly used antibiotics

Inhibitors of cell wall synthesis

- Beta-lactams
  - Penicillins
    - Penicillin: clostridia
    - Ampicillin, amoxicillin: Gram-negative organisms
    - Piperacillin, carbenicillin: *Pseudomonas* species
    - Cloxacillin, methicillin: staphylococci
  - Cephalosporins
    - First-generation cephalosporins, e.g. cephazolin: staphylococci and streptococci
    - Second-generation cephalosporins, e.g. cefuroxime: *H. influenzae* type B, Gram-negative organisms

- Third-generation cephalosporins, e.g. ceftriaxone: Gram-negative enteric anaerobes
  - Fourth-generation cephalosporins, e.g. ceftazidime: *Pseudomonas* species
  - Carbapenems: broad-spectrum coverage against Gram-positive and Gram-negative organisms and *Pseudomonas* species
  - Aztreonam: a monobactam antibiotic with coverage against Gram-negative organisms and *Pseudomonas* species
- Beta-lactamase inhibitors
  - Clavulanic acid
  - Sulbactam
- Vancomycin
  - Streptococci, including enterococci
  - Staphylococci, including MRSA
  - *C. difficile*

Inhibitors of ribosomal protein synthesis

- Aminoglycosides: Gram-positive rods and Pseudomonas species
- Chloramphenicol: Gram-negative rods and anaerobes
- Clindamycin: anaerobes, staphylococci and streptococci
- Erythromycin: *Legionella species*, *Mycoplasma* species, *Chlamydia* species, staphylococci and streptococci
- Tetracycline: *Neisseria* species, rickettsiae, *Mycoplasma* species, *Chlamydia* species, *Brucella* species, syphilis, staphylococci and streptococci

Inhibitors of folic acid synthesis

- Sulfonamides: Gram-positive and Gram-negative enteric organisms
- Trimethoprim: Gram-negative enteric organisms except *Pseudomonas* species

Inhibitors of DNA synthesis

- Metronidazole
  - Anaerobes, including *Bacteroides* species
  - *C. difficile*
  - *Trichomonas species*
  - Amoebiasis

- Quinolones: Gram-positive and Gram-negative aerobes
- Rifampicin: inhibits DNA-dependent RNA polymerase

Principles of antibiotic prophylaxis

- Used only when contamination of a wound is expected or when surgery on a contaminated site may lead to bacteraemia
- For clean procedures
  - When an implant or a vascular graft is inserted
  - In valvular heart disease, to prevent infective endocarditis
  - During emergency surgery in a patient with pre-existing or recently active infection
  - If an infection would be very severe or have life-threatening consequences
- One dose for clean surgery and three doses for contaminated surgery
- Given parenterally and immediately before surgery; if surgery continues for > 3–4 hours, a further dose is given in the theatre
- Should cover relevant organisms
  - In orthopaedics: staphylococci
  - In bowel surgery: Gram-negative aerobic and anaerobic flora

Antibiotic resistance

- Caused by increasing use of newer antibiotics with increased activity and wider spectrum
- Examples
  - MRSA
    - Resistant to commonly used flucloxacillin
    - Treated with glycopeptides, e.g. vancomycin
    - Of concern in burns, plastic surgery and orthopaedics
  - Vancomycin-resistant *S. aureus* (VRSA)
  - Vancomycin-resistant enterococci (VRE)
    - May cause life-threatening sepsis in patients whose immune defences are already impaired by trauma or poor nutrition
  - Multi-resistant *P. aeruginosa*

Basic principles of control of resistant organisms

- Hand-washing and basic infection-control practices
- Screening at-risk patients to identify those who are colonised
- Isolation of colonised or affected patients
- Control of movements of colonised patients between departments
- Judicious use of antibiotics

Blood-borne viruses

HIV-1 and HIV-2

- RNA virus
- During replication, the viral RNA is reverse transcribed by the enzyme reverse transcriptase into a DNA copy, which is inserted into the chromosome of the infected cell, where it produces new virus particles to infect other cells
- Therefore the patient is infected for life
- Major cellular receptor for HIV is the CD4 antigen, which is present on T-helper lymphocytes
- Gradual depletion of these cells causes opportunistic infections and tumours
- HIV has a lipid envelope and is easily destroyed by heat, disinfectants or detergents, but at ambient temperature it is resistant to drying

Hepatitis B virus

- DNA virus
- Long incubation period (70–180 days)
- Surface coating of the virus particles (HBsAg) is identified by serological testing; its presence implies active infection
- HBeAg, derived from the core particle of the virus, indicates continuing activity and high infectivity
- Long-term carrier state is common
- Transmission
  - Sexual intercourse
  - Blood transfusion
  - HBeAg mother to baby
- Persistent replication leads to:
  - Chronic active hepatitis
  - Cirrhosis
  - Increased risk of hepatocellular carcinoma

Hepatitis C virus

- RNA virus
- Common in injecting drug users and in recipients of unscreened blood or blood products
- Results in a persistent carrier state in > 80% of cases
- Long-term risk of chronic liver disease and hepatocellular carcinoma

Universal precautions

- Body fluids that should be handled with same precautions as blood:
  - Cerebrospinal fluid, semen, vaginal secretions, breast milk, amniotic fluid, peritoneal fluid, and pleural, pericardial and synovial fluids
  - Any other body fluid containing visible blood
  - Unfixed tissues and organs
- Passing of sharp instruments should never be done directly, but rather through the vehicle of a rigid container such as a kidney dish
- Re-sheathing of needles should never be attempted unless a suitable, safe re-sheathing device is available; in its absence, all sharps are discarded directly into approved sharps container
- Suture needles and scalpels should never be left on trays for others to clear
- Cuts and abrasions are covered with water-proof dressings; disposable gloves are worn if there is risk of contamination
- Protective eyewear and mask should be worn if there is likelihood of splashing of blood
- Blood spillage on surfaces are removed by first applying disinfectant, e.g. sodium hypochlorite, and then washing with detergent and water
- All staff likely to be exposed to blood, tissues or other body fluids in the course of their work should be immunised, and antibody levels should be measured (HIV, HBV, HBC)
- Surgical technique
  - Instruments rather than fingers should be used for retraction, holding tissues and tying knots

- Electrocautery, blunt-tipped needles and stapling devices should be used where appropriate
- Double-gloving
- Disposable drapes with self-adhesive film should be used

Immunisation

Classification of induction of immunity

- Active immunisation
  - Natural: following infection
  - Artificial: following vaccination
- Passive immunisation
  - Natural: transplacental transfer of antibodies
  - Artificial: injection of preformed antibodies

Types of vaccines

- Live attenuated organisms
  - Long-lasting immunity
  - Potentially dangerous in immunocompromised patients
  - Examples
    - Bacille Calmette–Guérin (BCG) for tuberculosis
    - Sabine vaccine for polio
    - Measles–mumps–rubella (MMR) vaccine
- Killed organisms
  - Smaller immune response
  - Booster doses are necessary
  - Examples
    - Typhoid
    - Cholera
    - Pertussis (in the diphtheria–pertussis–tetanus, DPT, vaccine)
- Toxoid
  - Does not prevent infection but prevents effects from the toxin that result from infection, e.g. tetanus toxoid
- Other bacterial constituents
  - Polysaccharides, e.g. pneumococcal vaccine
  - Proteins

Passive immunisation (post-exposure)

- For patients exposed to HBsAg-positive blood

- Immunocompromised patients with shingles (varicella-zoster)
- Rarely for botulism and rabies

Management of sharps injuries

- As soon as the patient is stable and can be left to the care of others, wash the site of injury liberally with soap and water
- Avoid scrubbing; encourage bleeding
- Do not use antiseptic preparations
- Wash out splashes to eye or mouth by irrigating with copious volumes of water
- Complete an incident form and contact the occupational health department
- Blood sample must be taken from the injured staff member
- Laboratory testing of the source patient after discussion and informed consent
- If the source patient is a carrier of hepatitis B virus:
  - Those who have never been vaccinated:
    - Hepatitis B immunoglobulin should be given within 48 hours of the exposure
    - Course of hepatitis B vaccination should be started as soon as possible
  - Those who have been vaccinated:
    - If antibody response is > 100/mL in the previous year, no further action is needed
    - If the titre is < 100/mL or blood has not been tested, a booster dose should be given, followed by repeat testing of antibody status
- For hepatitis C virus
  - No prophylaxis
  - Monitoring of liver function tests and hepatitis C virus antibodies
- For HIV
- Post-exposure prophylaxis according to latest local guidelines, e.g. Truvada (tenofovir 245 mg + emtricitabine 200 mg) once daily and Kaletra (lopinavir 400 mg + ritonavir 100 mg) twice daily
  - Treatment should commence as soon as possible, certainly within 1 hour of exposure, and continue for 1 month
  - Negative antibody titre 6 months after exposure indicates absence of infection

Disinfection

Definition

- Process used to reduce the number of viable micro-organisms
- Efficacy depends on:
  - Length of exposure
  - Presence of blood, faeces and organic matter

Examples

- Hypochlorite
  - Antibacterial and antiviral
  - Inactivated by organic matter
- Povidone iodine
  - Antibacterial
  - Used as skin preparation and surgical scrub
- Chlorhexidine
  - Active against Gram-positive bacteria
  - No risk of skin irritation
- Quaternary ammonium salts (cetrimide)
  - Active against Gram-positive bacteria
  - No action against *Pseudomonas* species
- Formaldehyde
  - Antibacterial and antiviral
  - Irritant to eyes, respiratory tract and skin
  - 10% formaldehyde is used to disinfect surfaces
- Glutaraldehyde
  - Antibacterial and antiviral
  - Kills spores slowly
  - May cause hypersensitivity
- Boiling water
  - Kills bacteria, some viruses and some spores
  - Items should be thoroughly cleaned and fully immersed
  - Suitable for proctoscopes and rigid sigmoidoscopes
- Pasteurisation
  - For foodstuffs such as milk
  - Done at 63–66 °C for 30 minutes
  - Non-sporing bacteria are killed

Sterilisation

Definition

- Complete destruction of all micro-organisms, including spores, cysts and viruses

Methods

- Physical sterilisation
  - Moist heat
    - Denaturation of bacterial proteins (DNA and cell membrane)
    - Done at 121 °C with a hold time of 15 minutes or at 134 °C with a hold time of 3 minutes
    - Change of colour of heat-sensitive inks in the sterilisation packs (Bowie–Dick test)
  - Dry heat sterilisation
    - Denaturation of cellular proteins
    - Done at 160 °C with a hold time of 2 hours: kills all micro-organisms
    - Used for objects that can stand high temperatures
  - Irradiation
    - Industrial process
    - Used commercially for catheters, syringes, intravenous lines and so on
  - Filtration
    - For heat-labile solutions, e.g. drugs, intravenous fluids
    - Cellulose acetate filters used for viruses
- Chemical sterilisation
  - Ethylene oxide
    - For vegetative bacteria, spores and viruses
    - Used for electrical equipment, fibre-optic endoscopes and so on
    - Toxic, irritant, mutagenic and may be carcinogenic
  - Glutaraldehyde
    - Used for endoscopes
    - May cause dermatitis

- Steam with formaldehyde
  - Dry saturated steam with formaldehyde for vegetative bacteria, spores and viruses
  - Used for heat-labile instruments, e.g. cystoscopes
  - Done at a low temperature (73 °C) for 2 hours

Nosocomial infections

Definition

- Exogenous infections derived from people or objects in the hospital
- People
  - Medical, nursing, other patients
  - Can be those with infection or subclinical infection, or asymptomatic carriers
- Objects
  - Surgical instruments
  - Anaesthetic equipment
  - Ventilators and humidifiers
  - Parenteral fluids and drugs

Modes of spread

- Contact
- Airborne
- Ingestion

Prevention and control

- Education of staff
  - Hand-washing
  - Correct waste disposal
  - Good nursing care
  - Safe environment
  - Good theatre technique
  - Aseptic surgical technique
- Skin infection and antisepsis
- Sterilisation and disinfection
- Prophylactic antibiotics
- Protective clothing
- Isolation of patients with established infection
- Appropriate design of hospital buildings
- Staff health
  - Immunisation of staff
  - Isolation of infected staff
- Surveillance
  - Infection control
  - Monitoring of infection rates
  - Appropriate policy making

Chapter 8   Principles of surgery

Incisions and wound closure

Principles of incision

- Access
  - To view structures
  - To manipulate tissues
  - To view rear aspect
  - To control other structures that may not lie within minimal exposure
- Avoiding incidental damage to:
  - Nerves and tendons
  - Vascular structures (damage affects healing)
  - Muscles and ligaments around a joint (damage can cause loss of movement)
- Tissue planes: correct anatomy
- Cosmetic aspects
  - Especially in the face, but also in other parts of the body
  - Langer's lines should be taken into account
- Vascular supply
  - Angled incisions heal better than linear ones
  - In an incision made parallel to previous one, intervening tissue is ischaemic
- Bleeding: if not controlled, leads to wound haematoma
- Infection

Principles of closure

- Apposition: tissues on each side of the incision brought together and prevented from separating until the cells have bridged between them
- Tension: relieving incisions and flaps
- Layers: each layer is repaired separately
- Materials: chosen to provide maximum security and minimum tissue reaction

Individual incisions

- Laparotomy
  - Midline vertical incision for exploration
  - Paramedian incision is an alternative (rarely used nowadays)
  - In infants – transverse

- For specific operations, there may be specific placements of incisions, e.g. Kocher's incision
  - Closure
    - Layered
    - Continuous mass closure with suture four times the length of the incision
- Chest surgery
  - Lateral thoracotomy: upper edge of a rib
  - Thoraco-abdominal surgery: along one of the lower ribs and carried through the costal margin into the abdomen
  - Median sternotomy

Skin closure

- Should be cosmetically acceptable
- Inversion of edges must be avoided
- Infection, hypertrophic scars and keloid must be avoided
- Types
  - Continuous closure: subcuticular
  - Interrupted closure
    - Simple
    - Mattress (transverse or vertical)
  - Tapes, clips, steristrips
- Removal of stitches
  - Head and neck: after 3–5 days
  - Inguinal area and upper limb: after 7 days
  - Abdomen and lower limb: after 10 days
  - Dorsal: after 14 days
- Langer's lines should be noted

Peri-operative care

Risk factors adversely influencing peri-operative morbidity

- Age: increased risk in those aged > 60 years or < 1 year
- Cardiovascular disease
  - Recent myocardial infarction (within last 6 months)
  - Hypertension

- Respiratory disease: chronic obstructive or restrictive disease
- Gastrointestinal disease
  - Malnutrition
  - Adhesions
  - Jaundice
- Renal disease: chronic renal failure
- Haematological conditions
  - Anaemia
  - Polycythaemia
  - Thrombocytosis
- Smoking
- Obesity
- Diabetes mellitus
- Drugs
  - Monoamine oxidase inhibitors
  - Oral contraceptives
  - Anticoagulants
- Surgeon, operative severity and emergency surgery

Pre-operative assessment

- Assessment of operative risks: appropriate selection of patients
- Assessment of fitness for anaesthesia and surgery
- Adequate explanation and informed consent
- Correction of nutritional, blood volume and fluid deficiencies and electrolyte disturbances
- Prophylactic measures against common post-operative complications
- Estimation of the amount of blood required
- Assessment of the likely post-operative course and probable need for transfer to a high-dependency or intensive care unit after the operation

How to perform a pre-operative assessment

- History, for risk factors
- Physical examination
- Investigations
  - Routine investigations in all patients
    - Haemoglobin
    - Urea
    - Electrolytes
    - Creatinine
  - Other routine investigations in certain patients

- Liver function tests, in liver disease or alcoholism
- ECG, in those aged > 60 years or with cardiovascular disease
- Chest X-ray, in pulmonary disease and malignancy
- Cervical spine X-ray, in neck problems or rheumatoid arthritis
- Thoracic inlet X-ray, in thyroid enlargement
- Sickle cell screening, in susceptible population
  - Special investigations, when indicated
    - PFT and ABG
    - Cardiac function tests
    - Coagulation screen

Risk scoring systems

- Generic scoring systems
  - Used across a wide range of diseases
  - Examples
    - The American Association of Anesthesiologists (ASA) scoring system (see table)
    - The Acute Physiology and Chronic Health Evaluation (APACHE)
    - The Physiological and Operative Severity Score for enumeration of Morbidity and Mortality (POSSUM)

ASA scoring system

- See table opposite

APACHE

- The sum of acute physiology score (APS), age points and chronic health points
- APS points are based on:
  - Core temperature
  - Mean arterial blood pressure
  - Heart rate
  - Respiratory rate (ventilated or not ventilated)
  - Oxygenation: p_aO_2
  - Arterial pH
  - Serum Na^+
  - Serum K^+
  - Serum creatinine
  - Haematocrit
  - White blood cell count
  - Glasgow coma score (GCS): 15 minus the actual score

Class	Physical status	Mortality
ASA scoring system, showing class based on physical status and mortality associated with each class		
I	Normal healthy individual	0.05%
II	Mild to moderate systemic disease, e.g. diabetes mellitus, hypertension	0.4%
III	Severe systemic disease, not incapacitating, e.g. uncontrolled diabetes mellitus, hypertension	4.5%
IV	Severe incapacitating systemic disease, that is a constant threat to life, e.g. severe persistent angina, hepatic failure	25%
V	Moribund patient, not expected to survive, where surgery is the last resort, e.g. ruptured aortic aneurysm	50%
E – in any class is a patient who requires an emergency operation		

- The points are based on a scale of 0 (for normal range) to 4 (for high or low abnormal) over a 24-hour period
- Age points
- < 44 years scores 0 points
- 45–54 years scores 2 points
- 55–64 years scores 3 points
- 65–74 years scores 4 points
- > 75 years scores 5 points
- Chronic health points
  - Elective post-operative patient scores 2 points
  - Non-operative or emergency post-operative patient scores 5 points
- Original system (APACHE I) had 34 potential acute physiological variables
- Revised system (APACHE II) has 12 acute physiological variables
- Maximum score that can be given is 71; in practice, no patient has exceeded 55
- When the score is > 29, there is a sharp rise in mortality
- If the score is > 35, mortality is > 85%

POSSUM

- For general surgical patients, mainly used in surgical audit
- Highly accurate in predicting both morbidity and mortality
- Scores based on 12 physiological variables and six operative severity variables

Disease-specific scoring systems

Glasgow Coma Scale (GCS)

- Quantitative assessment of the patient's level of consciousness, which is reproducible: see table

Eye opening		Verbal response		Motor response	
Glasgow Coma Scale, based on scores relating to eye opening, verbal response and motor response					
Spontaneous	4	Oriented	5	Obeys	6
To speech	3	Confused conversation	4	Localises pain	5
To pain	2	Inappropriate words	3	Withdraws	4
None	1	Incomprehensive sounds	2	Flexion	3
		None	1	Extension	2
				None	1

- GCS in head injury
  - Severe head injury: < 8
  - Moderate head injury: 9–12
  - Mild head injury: 13–15

New York Heart Association (NYHA) score for cardiac function

- Class I
  - Cardiac disease without limitation of physical activity
  - No symptoms of fatigue, palpitation, dyspnoea or angina pain with ordinary physical activity
- Class II
  - Cardiac disease with slight limitation of physical activity
  - Comfortable at rest
  - Ordinary physical activity leads to symptoms
- Class III
  - Cardiac disease with marked limitation of physical activity
  - Comfortable at rest
  - Less than ordinary physical activity leads to symptoms
- Class IV
  - Cardiac disease with inability to carry on any physical activity without discomfort
  - Symptoms may be present at rest
  - If any physical activity is undertaken, discomfort is increased

Child–Pugh grading of liver disease

- See table

Assessment of severity of pancreatitis

- The presence of three or more criteria using either Ranson's criteria or the Glasgow criteria indicates acute, severe pancreatitis
- Ranson's criteria
  - At admission
    - Age > 55 years
    - White blood cell count > 16×10^9/L
    - Glucose >10 mmol/L
    - AST > 250 u/L
    - LDH > 350 U/L
  - At 48 hours
    - Haematocrit fall > 10%
    - BUN rise > 5 mg/dL
    - Calcium > 2 mmol/L
    - p_aO_2 < 60 mmHg
    - Base deficit > 4 mEq
    - Estimated fluid sequestration > 6 L
  - Glasgow criteria (within 48 hours)
    - Age > 55 years
    - White blood cell count > 15×10^9/L
    - Glucose > 10 mmol/L
    - Albumin < 32 g/L
    - Urea > 16 mmol/L
    - LDH > 600 U/L
    - AST and ALT > 100 U/L
    - p_aO_2 < 60 mmHg
    - Ca^{2+} < 2 mmol/L

Injury scoring systems

- Injury severity score (ISS) – depends on the type and severity of injury

Child–Pugh grading of liver disease: grade A, B or C based on clinical and laboratory parameters

Parameter	Grade A	Grade B	Grade C
Albumin (g/dl)	>3.5	3–3.5	<3
Bilirubin (mmol/L)	<25	25–40	>40
Prothrombin time (S > normal)	<4	4–6	>6
Prothrombin level (%)	>64	40–64	<40
Ascites	None	Controlled	Refractory
Encephalopathy	None	Minimal	Advanced

Injury severity score calculation			
Body region	**Description of injury**	**Abbreviated injury scale**	**Square top three**
Head, neck	Cerebral contusion	3	9
Face	No injury	0	
Chest	Flail chest	4	16
Abdomen	Minor contusion of liver	2	25
	Complex rupture of spleen	5	
Extremities (including pelvis)	Fractured femur	3	
External	No injury	0	
Injury severity score:			**50**

- Anatomical scoring system that provides an overall score for patients with multiple injuries
- Each injury is assigned an abbreviated injury scale (AIS) score and allocated to one of six body regions (see table)
- Only the highest AIS score in each region is use
- The scores of the thee most severely injured body regions are each squared and then added together to produce the ISS score.
- An example of the ISS calculation is shown in the table
- The ISS score ranges from 0 to 75
- If an injury is assigned an AIS of 6 (unsurvivable injury), the ISS score is automatically assigned as 75
- The ISS score is virtually the only anatomical scoring system in use and correlates linearly with mortality, morbidity, hospital stay and other measures of severity

Diabetic ulcer grading

- Wagner's grades
  - Grade 0: pre-ulcerative or post-ulcerative
  - Grade 1: superficial ulcer, partial or full thickness
  - Grade 2: deep ulcer extending to fascia, ligament, tendon or capsule
  - Grade 3: deep ulcer with abscess or osteomyelitis
  - Grade 4: partial forefoot gangrene
  - Grade 5: whole foot gangrene
  - Prognosis depends on presence of three criteria (one point each)
    - Foot ulcer for longer than 2 months
    - Ulcer > 2 cm in diameter
    - Wagner's grade 3 or higher
- University of Texas (UT) grading
  - Grade 0: pre-ulcerative or post-ulcerative
  - Grade 1: superficial ulcer, partial or full thickness
  - Grade 2: deep ulcer extending to fascia, ligament, tendon or capsule
  - Grade 3: penetrating bone or joint
  - For each grade:
    - A: no infection or ischaemia
    - B: infection
    - C: ischaemia
    - D: both infection and ischaemia
- Pressure ulcer scoring system
  - Based on depth of wound and clinical appearance (see table overleaf)

Prognostic scoring systems for cancer

- TNM (tumour, nodes, metastases)
- Pathological grading
- Nottingham prognostic index for breast cancer

Pressure ulcer scoring system		
Stage	Depth of wound	Clinical appearance
I	Limited to epidermis	Non-blanchable erythema
II	Partial thickness skin loss	Abrasion, blister, shallow ulcer
III	Full thickness skin loss with subcutaneous tissue damage	Deep ulcer, eschar, necrosis, infection
IV	Full thickness skin loss with extension through fascia, to muscle, tendon, capsule, bone	Deep ulcer with skin necrosis, infection and exposure of deeper structures

Colorectal carcinoma: Dukes' staging

- See table opposite

Malignant melanoma

- Clarke's levels
  - Level I: involving only the epidermis (*in situ*)
  - Level II: involving the papillary dermis
  - Level III: invading the papillary dermis up to the interface
  - Level IV: involving the reticular dermis
  - Level V: invading the reticular dermis up to the subcutaneous fat
- Breslow's thickness
  - Stage I: < 0.75 mm
  - Stage II: 0.76–1.5 mm
  - Stage III: 1.5–4.0 mm
  - Stage IV: > 4 mm

Non-Hodgkin's lymphoma: Ann-Arbor staging

- Stage I: single lymph node region
- Stage II: more than two lymph node regions on the same side of the diaphragm
- Stage III: lymph node regions on both sides of diaphragm, with or without involvement of the spleen
- Stage IV: disseminated extralymphatic spread
- For each stage:
  - A: no systemic symptoms
  - B: systemic symptoms present (fever, night sweats or weight loss)

Laboratory testing

- Aims
  - Confirm of the diagnosis
  - Exclusion of alternate diagnoses
  - Assessment of fitness for surgery
  - Assessment of risk to others, e.g. hepatitis B virus infection, HIV status, methicillin-resistant *Staphylococcus aureus* (MRSA)
  - Medicolegal coverage, e.g. skull X-ray for head injuries
  - Post-operative assessment, to screen for persistence or recurrence of disease
- Selection of tests
  - Sensitivity, e.g. colonoscopy may be more sensitive than barium enema for colonic polyps
  - Simplicity, e.g. plain X-ray rather than MRI or bone scan
  - Safety, e.g. endoscopy rather than barium studies in perforation; e.g. fine needle aspiration is safer than Tru-Cut, but Tru-Cut gives a better histopathological diagnosis
  - Cost, e.g. ultrasound rather than CT
  - Acceptability to the patient, e.g. barium meal rather than an upper gastrointestinal endoscopy
  - Availability, e.g. CT may be more readily available than MRI
- Limitations of investigations
  - May not correlate with clinical judgement

Duke's staging for colorectal carcinoma (Astler–Collins modification)		
Stage	Depth of penetration and lymph node involvement	5-year survival
A	Limited to mucosa	85%
B_1	Into muscularis propria	
B_2	Through muscularis propria	67%
C_1	Regional lymph node involvement	
C_2	Highest lymph node involvement (at pedicle)	37%
D	Distant metastases	-

- – Wrong report may result from:
  - • Incorrect performance
  - • Incorrect interpretation
  - • Limited sensitivity
- – Complications, e.g. from carotid angiography
- – Financial implications
- • Sequence and timing
  - – Logical sequence of testing should be used, depending on the condition of the patient and the progress of the disease

Imaging methods

Ultrasound

- • Physics
  - – Ultrasound waves are created in a transducer by applying a momentary electric field to a piezo-electric crystal, which vibrates
  - – The transmitted waves interact with soft tissue interfaces and are reflected back, deflected or absorbed
  - – Sound waves that are reflected are used to make the image
  - – The greater the difference in density between two adjacent tissue planes, the greater the amount of reflected sound waves
- • Uses
  - – To visualise soft tissues
  - – To visualise fluid collections in the subcutaneous tissue and within body cavities
  - – Investigation of choice in gallstone diseases

- • Advantages
  - – Real-time image
  - – Safe in pregnancy
  - – Useful for guided procedures
- • Disadvantages
  - – Cannot be used for the brain
  - – Bowel gas prevents adequate visualisation
  - – Retroperitoneum cannot be assessed
  - – Operator-dependent

Computed tomography (CT)

- • Physics
  - – Computer integration of multiple exposures as an X-ray tube travels in a circle around the patient
  - – The circular track is called the gantry
  - – A fan-shaped beam is produced by the tubes and picked up by detectors aligned directly opposite
  - – Computer constructs the image by dividing the gantry into a grid
  - – Each box in the grid is called a voxel and each voxel is given a value in Hounsfield units (HU), depending on the density of tissue in the box
    - • Water: 0 HU
    - • Air: 1000 HU
    - • Abdominal organs: 30–80 HU
    - • Compact bone: > 250 HU
    - • Lung: 80–100 HU

Magnetic resonance imaging (MRI)

- • When a body is placed in a magnetic field, the protons line up along the direction of that field

- Images are generated by the energy released from the protons when they re-align with the magnetic field after application of radiofrequency energy
- Electromagnetic energy is received and converted to images by a computer
- Classified as T_1- and T_2-weighted images
- T1-weighted images
  - Fat appears bright
  - Water appears dark
- T2-weighted images
  - Fat appears dark
  - Water appears bright
- Advantages
  - Unparalleled soft tissue resolution
  - No radiation
  - Multiplanar capabilities
  - Great sensitivity to flow phenomena and temperature changes
- Disadvantages
  - Expensive
  - Not available everywhere
  - Those with implanted metallic objects cannot be scanned
  - Unsuitable for claustrophobic patients

Nuclear scans

- Radionuclide is administered into the body and subsequently undergoes radioactive decay, giving off gamma radiation
- Commonly used radionuclide is technetium
  - Pure gamma-ray emitter
  - Low-dose ionising radiation is delivered to the patient
- The gamma-rays are detected by a gamma-scintillation camera, and the image is formed from the rays

Nutrition

Nutritional assessment

- Biochemical assessment
  - Serum albumin
  - Transferrin
  - Retinol binding protein
- Anthropometric assessment
  - Triceps skin-fold thickness
  - Mid-arm muscle circumference

- Immunological assessment
  - Lymphocyte count
  - Delayed hypersensitivity to skin testing
- Dynamometric assessment
  - Hand grip dynamometry

Body mass index (BMI)

- Calculate by the weight (in kilograms) divided by the height in metres squared
- Interpretation
  - < 16: malnourished
  - 16–19: underweight
  - 19–25: normal
  - 25–30: overweight
  - 30–40: obese
  - > 40: morbidly obese

Nutritional requirements

- Hospitalised patients
  - Protein: 1.5 g/kg/day
  - Energy: 40 kcal/kg/day
    - 30% fat
    - 70% carbohydrate
  - Nitrogen: 14–16 g/day
    - Those with increased energy needs require an additional 0.4 g/kg/day

Purpose of nitrogen administration

- Minimises net losses without wasting administered nitrogen
- Permits maintenance of patient's lean body mass
- Allows adequate supply of nitrogen for repair
- Allows active repletion of lean body mass in a previously compromised patient

Measurement of nitrogen balance

- 24-hour urinary and faecal nitrogen
- 24-hour urinary urea (accounts for 80% of loss) plus 2–3 g for other routes

Enteral nutrition

- Routes
  - Oral
  - Fine-bore nasogastric tube
  - Nasoenteric route
    - Nasoduodenal tube
    - Nasojejunal tube

- Pharyngostomy (rarely used)
- Oesophagostomy (rarely used)
- Percutaneous endoscopic gastrostomy
- Needle catheter jejunostomy
- Advantages
  - Cheaper and more physiological than parenteral nutrition
  - Improves anti-bacterial host defences
  - Blunts hypermetabolic response to trauma
  - Maintains gut mucosal mass
  - Maintains gut barrier function
  - Prevents disruption of gut flora
- Complications
  - Tube-related complications
    - Malpositioning of the tube
    - Removal of the tube
    - Blockage of the tube
  - Diet-related complications
    - Diarrhoea, abdominal bloating and cramps
    - Nausea, regurgitation and aspiration
    - Vitamin and mineral deficiencies
    - Drug interactions
  - Metabolic and biochemical complications
  - Infective complications, resulting from:
    - The diet itself
    - The reservoir
    - Giving sets

Parenteral nutrition

- Categories of patients suitable for total parenteral nutrition (TPN)
  - Medical indications
    - Inflammatory bowel disease
    - Hepatic failure
    - Renal failure
    - Respiratory failure
  - Surgical indications
    - Pre-operative and post-operative care
    - Fistula, burns or sepsis
    - Pancreatitis
  - Orthopaedic indication
    - Polytrauma
  - Miscellaneous indications
    - Patients in intensive care unit
    - Cancer
    - Short bowel syndrome
    - HIV-infection

- Absolute contraindication for TPN is a functioning bowel
- Complications of TPN
  - Catheter problems
    - Pneumothorax
    - Air embolism
    - Haematoma
    - Hydrothorax
    - Haemothorax
    - Hydromediastinum
    - Haemomediastinum
    - Catheter fracture with embolisation of the tip
  - Thrombophlebitis
    - Superior mediastinal syndrome in superior vena cava thrombosis
    - Treated with anticoagulants and urokinase
  - Infection
    - Coagulase-negative staphylococci
    - *Staphylococcus aureus*
    - Coliforms
  - Metabolic complications
    - Osmotic diuresis
    - Acute hyperosmolar syndrome
    - Hyponatraemia
    - Zinc and folate deficiencies
    - Hypophosphataemia
    - Sensitivity reactions
    - Abnormal liver function tests (increased enzymes)
    - Acalculous cholecystitis
    - Cholestasis
    - Hypoglycaemia or hyperglycaemia

Associated medical conditions in a surgical patient

- Medical diagnoses associated with increased surgical morbidity and mortality
  - Ischaemic heart disease
  - Congestive heart failure
  - Arterial hypertension
  - Chronic respiratory disease
  - Diabetes mellitus
  - Cardiac arrhythmias
  - Anaemia
  - Obesity

Aims of management

- Diagnosis of pre-existing medical disease and accurate assessment of degree of problem
- Ensuring that the management of the medical condition is optimised pre-operatively
- Ensuring that specialised post-operative care is available if required

Cardiovascular disease

- Coronary artery disease: myocardial ischaemia will occur whenever the balance between myocardial O_2 supply and demand is disturbed such that demand exceeds supply
  - Blood pressure control
  - Pain management
  - Supplemental O_2
- Arterial hypertension should be stabilised pre-operatively before elective surgery
- Heart failure
  - Inadequacy of heart muscle secondary to ischaemic disease or overloading
  - Treated with digitalis, angiotensin-converting enzyme (ACE) inhibitors, diuretics and/or vasodilators
  - Peri- and intra-operative haemodynamic monitoring and pulmonary capillary wedge pressure monitoring
- Valvular heart disease
  - Antibiotics
  - Avoid peri-operative hypotension
  - Invasive monitoring
- Cardiomyopathies
  - Diuretics
  - Vasodilators
  - Anti-arrhythmics
- Disturbances of rhythm
  - Atrial fibrillation can be caused by:
    - Cardiac disease
    - Thyrotoxicosis
    - Pulmonary embolism
    - Bronchial carcinoma
  - Atrial flutter
- Heart block
  - Atrioventricular heart block
  - Intraventricular conduction defects

- Drugs that further decrease nodal conduction should be avoided
  - Halothane
  - Beta blockers
- Temporary pacemaker may be needed

Respiratory disease

- Asthma
  - Peri-operative nebulisation
  - Pre-medication
  - Post-operative pain management
  - Intermittent positive-pressure ventilation (IPPV) if p_aO_2 is < 6.7 kPa (50 mmHg) or p_aCO_2 is > 6.7 kPa (50 mmHg)
- Chronic bronchitis and emphysema
  - For major surgery: elective tracheostomy and post-operative ventilation
- Smoking
  - Six times higher incidence of post-operative respiratory complications in smokers
  - Carbon monoxide shifts O_2 dissociation curve to the left and has negative inotropic effect, resulting in a decreased O_2 supply
  - Nicotine increases heart rate and systemic blood pressure, leading to increased myocardial demand for O_2

Endocrine dysfunction

- Thyroid disease
  - Bring patient to euthyroid state pre-operatively
  - Avoid disturbances of cardiac rhythm, and hypoxia and hypothermia
- Pituitary disease
  - In hypopituitarism, there is an increased peri-operative risk of hypoglycaemia, hypothermia, water intoxication and respiratory failure: oral hydrocortisone should be given
  - In acromegaly, intubation can be difficult
  - In diabetes insipidus, intravenous vasopressin should be given
- Adrenal disease
  - Addison's disease: peri-operative steroids should be given

- Phaeochromocytoma: alpha-blockers, e.g. phenoxybenzamine, should be given
- Pancreatic disease
  - Diabetes mellitus is controlled with pre-operative and peri-operative insulin

Obesity

- BMI
  - 19–25: normal
  - 25–30: overweight
  - 30–40: obese
  - > 40: morbidly obese
- Pre-operative reduction in BMI for elective cases
- Obese patients are more prone to post operative deep venous thrombosis

Blood disorders

- Anaemia
  - If haemoglobin < 10 g/L, it should be treated pre-operatively
  - Tissue oxygenation is maximal at a haemoglobin of 11 g/L
  - Therefore, over-correction is to be avoided
- Platelet disorders are treated with platelet transfusion
- Haemophilia
  - Cryoprecipitate
  - Fresh frozen plasma
  - Factor IX concentrate

Renal diseases

- Chronic renal failure
  - Glomerular filtration rate < 30 mL/minute
  - May need dialysis
  - Nephrotoxic drugs should be avoided
- Nephrotic syndrome: albumin infusion pre-operatively

Liver disease

- Patients are screened for hepatitis B
- Hepatic and renal support to bring hepatic and renal functions to normal, to avoid peri-operative hepatorenal syndrome
- Ascitic fluid drainage may be needed
- Sepsis should be watched for
- Coagulation problems should be corrected

Alcoholism and drug abuse

- Maintain normal doses of addict's usual drug in the immediate pre-operative and post-operative period

AIDS

- Universal precautions

Patients with transplanted organs

- Continue immunosuppressants
- Look for usual infections, and for tumours and lymphomas

Elderly patients

- Look for decreased cardiorespiratory function

Issues related to medications

- Drugs for which pre-operative dose modification is necessary
  - Oral contraceptives
    - Maintain for minor or peripheral procedures and institute prophylaxis against deep venous thrombosis
    - Stop 1 month before abdominal or pelvic surgery
  - Anticoagulants
    - Stop oral agents at least 1 week before surgery
    - Substitute heparin if continued anticoagulation is necessary
    - Heparin can be rapidly reversed with protamine if necessary
  - Anti-diabetes agents
    - If on diet control: no specific precautions
    - If on oral drugs: omit on morning of surgery and give glucose–K$^+$–insulin sliding scale regimen
    - If controlled by insulin: glucose–K$^+$–insulin sliding scale regimen
  - L-dopa: omit pre-operatively
  - Monoamine oxidase inhibitors carry a significant potential for drug interactions causing serious physiological disturbance

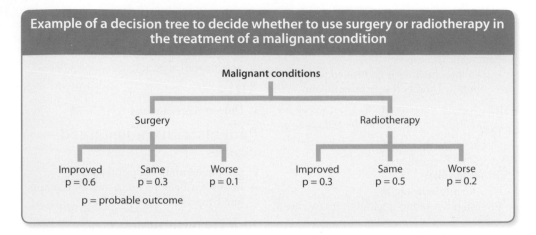

Example of a decision tree to decide whether to use surgery or radiotherapy in the treatment of a malignant condition

Malignant conditions

Surgery

Radiotherapy

Improved
p = 0.6

Same
p = 0.3

Worse
p = 0.1

Improved
p = 0.3

Same
p = 0.5

Worse
p = 0.2

p = probable outcome

- Corticosteroids: give hydrocortisone 100 mg intravenously pre-operatively and every 3 hours peri-operatively
- All other medications need to be taken until the morning of surgery and resumed post-operatively

Decision-making in surgery

- Good surgery requires 75% decision-making and 25% dexterity

Processing information

- Personal and acquired information
  - The validity of a research report must be judged on:
    - Clarity and logic of the investigation
    - Soundness of the interpretation
- Incomplete data
  - It is not always possible to have complete information before making decisions
- Discriminating features
  - Never use too much information
- Oversimplification
  - Tends to brush important factors aside
- Pressures
  - Rank in the order of priority (use triage)

Steps in decision-making

- Algorithm
  - Step-by-step method for progressing through a fairly straightforward clinical decision

- Protocol
  - Set of rules or uniform method of approaching a problem
  - Flow chart
- Guidelines
  - Approval given by an authoritative person or body
- Decision tree (see figure)
  - To allow comparisons of differing treatments, e.g. in malignant conditions
- Deferment
  - When a solution is not forthcoming, put aside if time permits and reconsider later
- Ask advice

Acting on a decision

- Preparation
  - Safe and acceptable routines must be practised
- Anticipation
  - Effects anticipated, recognised and corrected if necessary
- Provisional decisions
  - Subject to change

Personal audit

- Look back on successes and failures

Statistics

Definition

- Mathematical method of demonstrating the probability of a relationship

Components

- Standard deviation: measure of spread of observations around the most common observation
- Mode: the most common observation
- Mean: the average
- Median: the observation with the same numbers of observations higher and lower than itself, i.e. the central observation

Clinical trials

Definition

- Scientific methods of detecting difference in outcomes between treatments

Randomisation

- Ensures that each patient has an equal chance of receiving either treatment

Blinding

- Done in order to limit bias
- If both doctor and patient are kept unaware of which treatment the patient is receiving: double-blinding
- If the doctor is aware but the patient is not aware: single-blinding
- Single-blinding is more prone to bias
- Involvement of an independent agency is necessary to double-blind surgical procedures

Ethics

- Patients should not be denied effective treatment
- Any new treatment should be safe
- Informed consent should be obtained

Phases

- Phase I trials
  - To assess toxicology, clinical pharmacology and appropriate dosage
  - To assess route of administration
- Phase II trials
  - Evaluation of initial efficacy
  - If not effective, the trial is abandoned at phase II
- Phase III trials
  - Both efficacy and safety of the drug are assessed

- If the drug is found to be both effective and safe, it is licensed for use
- Phase IV trials
  - Post-marketing surveillance
  - Continued safety monitoring and assessment of new clinical applications

Audit

Definition

- Systematic critical analysis of the quality of medical care, including the procedures used for diagnosis and treatment, the use of resources, and the resulting outcome and quality of life for the patient

Medical audit

- Assessment by peer review of the medical care provided by the medical profession to the patient

Clinical audit

- Assessment of the total care of the patient by nurses and professions allied to medicine as well as by the doctors

Purpose of audit

- Systematic approach to the review of clinical care to highlight opportunities for improvements and to provide a mechanism for bringing them about
- Gives necessary reassurance to patients, clinicians and managers that an agreed quality of service is being given with available resources

Clinical effectiveness

- Clinically effective interventions maintain and improve health and secure the greatest possible health gain from the available resources

The audit cycle

- Observation of existing practice
- Comparison with standard
- Implementation of change
- Observation of implemented practice

Educational benefits

- Critical review of current practice and comparisons against pre-defined

standards encourages the acquisition and updating of knowledge
- Identification of particular areas where knowledge could be improved or is deficient, suggesting the need for research

Clinical audit committee

- Co-ordinates the audit process

Techniques of audit

- Structure: quality and type of resources available
- Process: what is done to the patient
- Outcome: result of clinical outcome
  - Basic clinical audit: analysis of case type, morbidity and mortality
  - Incident review: strategies to be adopted under certain clinical scenarios
  - Clinical record review: member of another firm invited to review notes
  - Criterion audit: retrospective analysis of clinical records against chosen criteria
  - Adverse occurrence screening
    - Infection
    - Re-admission
  - Comparative audit, with peers
  - Outcome audit: measure of spectrum of skill

Consent

Definition

- Ability of the patients to make a considered choice about what is in their personal interests, after receiving sufficient information about their illness, the proposed treatment and the prognosis

Pre-requisites

- Proposed procedure, its practical applications and probable prognosis
- Probability of specific associated risks or complications
- Probability of risks of other aspects related to the procedure, e.g. anaesthetics, intravenous line, bed rest, catheter
- Other surgical or medical alternatives, including non-treatment, with advantages and disadvantages

To determine whether patient has understood

- Ask patient to repeat what has been said
- Ask patient at various times if they have any questions

Ethical issues in specific situations

- Unconscious patients
  - May proceed without consent
  - Relatives should not be asked to sign
- Children
  - For elective surgery, consent is gained from parent
  - If the parent does not consent, the parent may be over-ridden by court order if life is at stake
  - Legal age for consent is 16 years; under 16 years, consent may be obtained if child is competent
- Patients with mental handicap or psychiatric illness
  - Attempts must be made to obtain consent even if communication is difficult
  - In life-threatening situations, surgery may be done if surgeon and psychiatrist agree (especially in the case of psychosurgery for schizophrenia)
  - In mentally handicapped patients, a surgeon in consultation with the principal carers and close family members can take decision about surgery, e.g. in Alzheimer's disease

Premedication

Definition

- Drugs prescribed by the anaesthetist to be administered pre-operatively to allay anxiety, to relieve pain, to dry saliva and to maintain the dosage of intercurrent medication

Anxiolytics

- Benzodiazepines
  - Diazepam, 0.05–0.3 mg/kg
  - Lorazepam, 0.015–0.06 mg/kg
  - Midazolam, 0.07–0.08 mg/kg

- Phenothiazines
  - Promethazine, 0.2–0.5 mg/kg
  - Uses
    - To calm the patient
    - To help to reduce time spent dwelling on fears
- Opioids
  - Used if analgesia is required

Drying secretions

- Atropine, 0.02 mg/kg
- Hyoscine, 0.008 mg/kg
- Glycopyrrolate, 0.01 mg/kg
- Uses
  - Prior to dental surgery or bronchoscopy
  - Surgery on the lung
  - Paediatric patients
  - Also to prevent bradycardia

Analgesics

- Morphine, 0.1–0.2 mg/kg
- Papaveretum, 0.2–0.4 mg/kg
- Pethidine, 1–1.5 mg/kg
- Uses
  - Continuous background of analgesia to aid the anaesthetic and to extend analgesia into the post-operative period
  - To reduce post-operative analgesic requirement
- Side effects
  - Respiratory and cardiovascular depression
  - Therefore used with caution in a moribund patient

General anaesthesia

Definition

- Reversible, drug-induced state of unresponsiveness to outside stimuli, characterised by non-awareness, analgesia and relaxation of striated muscle

Phases

- Three phases: induction, maintenance and relaxation

Induction phase

- Hypnosis at induction:
  - Thiopentone
    - Side effect: myocardial depression
  - Propofol
    - Short half-life
    - Used in day cases
  - Ketamine
    - Used in patients with shock
    - Stimulates sympathetic nervous system
    - Prevents decrease in cardiac output
- Dissociative anaesthesia with profound analgesia
  - Fentanyl
    - In high doses (10 µg/kg) for induction for cardiac anaesthesia
- Relaxation at induction
  - Suxamethonium
    - For crash induction
    - Side effects: histamine release, bradycardia, hyperkalaemia, persistent neuromuscular block and malignant hyperthermia
- Crash induction
  - Rapid-sequence intravenous induction, cricoid pressure and tracheal intubation
  - Aim is to prevent regurgitation and aspiration of stomach contents for non-fasted patients, patients with hiatus hernia and emergency trauma patients

Maintenance phase

- Hypnosis
  - Halothane
    - Side effects: arrhythmia, hepatic dysfunction
  - Enflurane: less arrhythmogenic than halothane
  - Isoflurane: a calcium antagonist
  - N_2O: background anaesthetic given with 70% O_2 (Entonox)
- Relaxation
  - Suxamethonium: a depolarising agent
  - Curare
    - D-tubocurare: causes hypotension
    - Alcuronium: causes hypotension
    - Vecuronium: causes bradycardia
    - Atracurium: causes histamine release
- Analgesia
  - From premedication
  - Anaesthetic opioid supplementation
  - Analgesia from N_2O

- Consequences of inadequate analgesic depth
  - Catecholamine release following surgical stimulation leading to cardiovascular instability
  - Patient movements during surgery
  - Patient awareness during surgery (rare)

Recovery phase

- Neostigmine
  - Reverses relaxation
  - Side effects
    - Sweating
    - Bradycardia
  - Given with atropine
  - Full reversal confirmed by patient being able to maintain head lifting

Local and regional anaesthesia

Definition

- Reversible blockade of nerve conduction by regionally applied agents for the purpose of sensory ablation, either of traumatised tissue, or to enable minor surgery

Areas of block

- As the pain fibres enter the spinal cord
  - Epidural block
  - Spinal block
  - Paravertebral block
- Along the route of the pain fibres in the neurovascular bundle
  - Field block
  - Specific nerve block
- At the nerve endings
  - Local infiltration around the required site (skin and subcutaneous)

Classification of nerve fibres according to their size and speed of conduction

- A fibres
  - A-alpha fibres
    - Motor and proprioception fibres
    - Fastest conduction

  - A-beta fibres
    - Touch and pressure fibres
    - Slower than A-alpha fibres
  - A-gamma fibres
    - Motor fibres
    - Slower than A-beta fibres
  - A-delta fibres
    - Pain, temperature and touch fibres
    - Slower than A-gamma fibres
- B fibres
  - Pre-ganglionic autonomic fibres
- C fibres
  - Slowest conduction
  - Dorsal root: pain and reflexes
  - Sympathetic: post-ganglionic

Sensitivity to local anaesthesia

- The smaller the fibre, more sensitive it is
- C fibres are the most sensitive

Local anaesthetics

- Action: inducing blockage of nerve conduction in peripheral nerve impulses from destruction of Na^+ channels in the axon membrane
- Types
  - Lignocaine
    - Dose: 3 mg/kg; 5 mg/kg when given with adrenaline
    - Maximum dose: 300 mg
    - Side effect: CNS toxicity
  - Bupivacaine
    - Dose: 1.75 mg/kg; 2.25 mg/kg when given with adrenaline
    - Maximum dose: 175 mg
    - Side effect: cardiovascular toxicity
  - Prilocaine
    - Maximum dose: 600 mg
    - Least toxic of these agents

Clinical applications

- Local infiltration of anaesthetic
  - Alone or with adrenaline
  - Eutectic Mixture of Local Anaesthetics (EMLA) cream: mixture of lignocaine and bupivacaine
- Field blocks and nerve blocks
  - For inguinal hernia
  - Brachial plexus
  - Femoral or sciatic nerve block

- Spinal, epidural or paravertebral block
  - Pain of childbirth and labour
  - Epidural catheter for continuous analgesia
  - Side effects
    - Hypotension resulting from sympathetic block
    - Urinary retention resulting from parasympathetic block

Monitoring of anaesthetised patient

Components

- Anaesthetic and respiratory monitoring
- Cardiovascular monitoring

Anaesthetic and respiratory monitoring

- Basic monitoring (settings of the machine)
  - Supply pressure gauge
  - Flow meters
  - Reservoir bag tension
  - Anaesthetic breathing connection
- Reservoir bag excursions
  - Chest wall movement
  - Respiratory pattern
- O_2 failure alarm
- F_iO_2 analyser and alarm
- Pulse oximetry
- Airway pressure alarm
- Capnography (end tidal CO_2)
- Exhaled gas spirometry

Cardiovascular monitoring

- Basic
  - Skin colour
  - Peripheral perfusion
  - Pulse rate and pulse volume
  - Blood pressure
  - ECG
  - Temperature
  - Central venous pressure
- Urine output
- Arterial cannulation
- Balloon floatation catheter
- Cerebral function monitoring when the circulation to the brain is at risk

Nerve injuries during anaesthesia

Causes

- From faulty positioning of the patient
- Occurs because of compression or traction of nerve trunks

Predisposing positions

- Trendelenburg tilt
- Left or right thoracic position
- Hyperabduction of the arm: brachial plexus injury
- Lithotomy position: common peroneal nerve injury

Nerves most commonly injured

- Popliteal nerve
- Brachial plexus
- Radial nerve
- Ulnar nerve

Safeguards

- Adequate positioning
- Strapping of the patient
- Use of padding for protection

Post-operative monitoring

Immediate recovery phase

- Advantages of recovery ward
  - Close observation and monitoring
  - Immediate availability of staff and equipment
  - Immediate access to operating theatre in the event of a complication
- Patient is nursed in lateral position with jaw held forward
- Patient must not be left unattended until capable of:
  - Protecting own airway
  - Responding to commands
- Causes of airway obstruction
  - Decreased muscle tone of pharyngeal muscles, leading to supraglottic flaccidity

- Remedied by chin lift and jaw thrust or by an oropharyngeal or nasopharyngeal airway
  - Laryngeal oedema
    - Caused by C1 esterase inhibitor deficiency
    - May require tracheostomy

Other monitoring

- Level of consciousness
- ECG
- Central venous pressure
- Blood pressure
- Pulse rate
- Temperature
- Pulse oximetry
- Urine output and output from any drains
- Pain control

Causes of post-operative hypoxia

- Decreased tone of muscles of chest wall
- Changes in bronchomotor and vascular tone
- Diaphragmatic splinting as a result of:
  - Pain
  - Abdominal distension
  - Retained bronchial secretions
    - Decreased functional residual capacity and collapse of dependent segments
    - Increased shunting and ventilation–perfusion mismatch

Oxygen therapy

- Variable performance mask
  - Hudson mask: 5 L/minute
  - Catheter: 4 L/minute
- Fixed performance mask (Venturi mask) is used in patients with chronic lung disease
- Humidification of inspired air is needed to avoid drying and encrustation of bronchial secretions

Diathermy

Principles of diathermy

- Passage of high-frequency alternating current through body tissue

- Where current is locally concentrated, heat is produced, up to 1000 °C

Effects

- Low frequency alternating current (mains frequency – 50 Hz) causes stimulation of neuromuscular tissue
- Severity depends on current (amps) and its pathway
  - 5–10 mA produces a painful muscular contraction
  - 80–100 mA through the heart causes ventricular fibrillation
- If frequency is increased to > 50,000 Hz (50 kHz), there is no response
- Surgical diathermy is 400 kHz to 10 MHz, and high current up to 500 mA can be safely passed through the patient to produce local heat

Monopolar diathermy

- High-frequency current from a generator
- Passes to active electrode held by the surgeon
- Causes local heating
- Current spreads through body tissue
- Returns to generator via patient plate electrode
- Patient plate
  - Should have good contact with the patient
  - Contact area should be at least 70 cm^2
- For cutting
  - Continuous output with temperature up to 1000 °C
  - Causes an arc between the active electrode and the tissue
  - Cell water is vaporised, with tissue disruption
- For coagulation
  - Pulsed output, causing desiccation and sealing of blood vessels

Bipolar diathermy

- Current passes down one limb of the forceps
- It then passes through a small piece of the tissue held by the forceps to be coagulated
- It then passes back to generator via the other limb of the forceps
- Disadvantage: cannot be used for cutting

Safety

- General safety
  - Required safety standards
  - Proper training of staff
- Responsibility rests with the surgeon to check alarm wiring and patient plate
- Alarms activated when circuit continuity is disturbed
- Patient plate
  - Close to the site of operation
  - Away from ECG and other devices
  - Avoid bony prominences, scar tissue and hairy skin
  - Good skin contact is essential
  - No fluid should seep under it
- Patient
  - Avoid skin contact with earthed metal objects, e.g. drip stands, operating table
- Technique
  - Check dial settings before use
  - Spirit-based skin preparations should have evaporated before use
  - Surgeon should activate the machine
  - Replace electrode in insulated quiver after use
  - Should not be used inside the gut
  - Monopolar diathermy should not be used on appendages, e.g. the salpinx, the penis, or on isolated tissue, e.g. the testis, owing to the chance of current density persisting beyond the operative site

Diathermy burns

- Record should include the site of the patient plate
- Site should be inspected for a possible burn at the end of the procedure
- If discovered, the electromedical safety officer is summoned
- All electrical equipment is then examined, including the patient plate lead
- The patient should be informed
- Clinically, a diathermy burn is a full-thickness burn that requires excision

Concurrent pacemakers

- Diathermy may interfere with the pacemaker circuit, causing serious arrhythmias or even cardiac arrest

- If the diathermy is close to pacemaker box, current travels down the pacemaker wire and may cause a myocardial burn, leading to cardiac arrest
- Safe diathermy use with a pacemaker
  - Inform cardiologist and obtain information regarding:
    - Type of pacemaker
    - Indication for insertion
    - Underlying rhythm
  - Avoid diathermy or use bipolar diathermy
  - Patient plate should be placed away from the pacemaker
  - Use only short bursts of diathermy
  - Stop diathermy if arrhythmias occur

Diathermy during laparoscopy

- Dangers
  - Inadvertent contact between the instrument and the bowel
  - Inadvertent contact between the electrode and another instrument that is touching the bowel
- To avoid problems:
  - Insulation of instruments should be complete
  - Adequate view of pneumoperitoneum is needed
  - Technique
    - Avoid excessive diathermy
    - Tent structures before current is applied
    - Bipolar or lower voltage currents are safer

Lasers

Definition

- An acronym for 'light amplification by stimulated emission of radiation'
- Device for producing a highly directional beam of coherent (monochromatic) electromagnetic radiation

Lasing medium

- Commonly gaseous, e.g. argon, CO_2
- May be crystalline, e.g. Nd:YAG (neodymium: yttrium–aluminium–garnet)

Delivery system

- With argon and Nd:YAG, the laser beams are transmitted down fibre-optics to a slit lamp
- With CO_2, the laser beams are transmitted via a series of mirrors through an articulated arm to a micromanipulator

Types

- Nd:YAG laser
  - Penetrates to 3–5 mm
  - Wavelength of 1.06 micrometres
  - Coagulates larger tissue volume
  - Leaves behind eschar of damaged tissue
- CO_2 laser
  - Wavelength of 10.6 micrometres
  - Very little tissue penetration
  - Useful for vaporising surface of tissue
  - Healing is rapid, with minimal scarring
- Argon laser
  - Wavelengths of 0.49 micrometres and 0.51 micrometres
  - Used in ophthalmology and dermatology

Clinical applications

- Gastrointestinal tract (Nd:YAG)
  - Vaporising and debulking recurrent or untreated advanced oesophageal carcinoma
  - Superior to intubation in short malignant oesophageal strictures
  - Controlling haemorrhage from the stomach, oesophagus and duodenum
  - Destruction of small ampullary tumours in the duodenum
  - Palliative resection of advanced rectal carcinoma
  - In laparoscopic surgery – risk of CO_2 embolism
- Urology (Nd:YAG)
  - Low-grade, low-stage transitional cell lesions in the bladder under local anaesthesia
  - If photosensitising agent like haematoporphyrin is used in conjunction with Nd:YAG tissues are sensitised and more easily destroyed

- Ophthalmology
  - ND:YAG to destroy an opaque posterior capsule during extracapsular cataract extraction
  - Argon for trabeculoplasty and in open-angle glaucoma, to reduce intraocular pressure
  - Photocoagulation in diabetic retinopathy to prevent retinal detachment
- ENT
  - CO_2 for haemostasis and for removal of benign tumours, and in premalignant conditions
  - Argon for middle ear surgery
- Vascular surgery
  - CO_2, ND:YAG and argon for angioplasty to vaporise atheromatous plaques
  - A potential complication is perforation of the vessel wall
- Plastic surgery
  - Pulsed ruby lasers to remove tattoos
  - Argon for port wine stain
  - CO_2 to resect atretic bony plates in choanal atresia
- Gynecology
  - CO_2 for cervical and vulval precancerous lesions

Classification according to degree of hazard

- Class I
  - Low-risk, low-power
  - Maximum permissible exposure cannot be exceeded
- Class II
  - Low-risk, low-power, visible radiation
  - Maximum power of 1 mW
  - Safety by natural aversion responses, e.g. blink reflex
- Class IIIa
  - Low-risk, visible radiation
  - Maximum power of 5 mW
  - Eye protection by natural aversion
  - Hazard if the system is focused to a point
- Class IIIb
  - Medium-risk
  - Maximum power is 0.5 W
  - Direct viewing is dangerous

- Class IV
  - High-risk, high-power devices
  - Diffusely reflected beam is dangerous
  - Potential fire hazard
  - Its use requires caution
  - Medical lasers are in this class

Hazards

- Patient hazard
  - Burning of normal tissue
  - Perforation of hollow viscus, e.g. the oesophagus
  - Damage to trachea or lungs during ENT procedures
- Operator hazard
  - Usually to eyes or skin
  - Eye
    - Beams penetrate and are focused on the retina
    - Corneal burns
    - Cataract

Safety measures

- Laser protection adviser should formulate the rules
- Laser safety officer has custody of the laser equipment
- Staff trained in safety precautions
- List of nominated users should be available
- Separate laser control area, with restricted entry
- Adequate eye protection
- Labelling of laser according to its class
- Reflective surfaces should be avoided in the laser control area
- Adequate ventilation in the laser control area with an extract system to vent the fumes

Sutures and ligature materials

Ideal suture

- Small diameter and great tensile strength
- Low tissue reactivity
- Good knot-holding capability to hold knots securely
- Minimal effect on the resistance of the wound to infection

Types of sutures

- Absorbable
  - Plain catgut: natural monofilament
  - Chromic catgut: natural monofilament
  - Polyglycolic acid: synthetic monofilament (Dacron, Dexon)
  - Polyglactin: synthetic braided (Vicryl)
  - Polydioxanone: synthetic monofilament (Maxon/PDS)
- Non-absorbable
  - Silk: natural, braided
  - Linen: natural, braided
  - Stainless steel wire, silver wire: monofilament / braided
  - Iron alloy wire: monofilament (Flexon)
  - Nylon: synthetic, monofilament (Ethilon, Dermalon)
  - Polyester: synthetic, braided (Ticron, Mersilene, Ethibond)
  - Polypropylene: synthetic, monofilament (Prolene)
  - Polytetrafluoroethylene (PTFE): synthetic, expanded monofilament (Gore-Tex)

Factors for selecting a suture or ligature

- Whether material is to be absorbed
- Tensile strength
- Thickness
- Handling and knotting properties
- Intensity of the body's inflammatory reaction to the material

Choice

- Gastrointestinal anastomosis: fine absorbable
  - Synthetic monofilament PDS
  - Coated Vicryl: polyglactin 910
- Abdominal wound closure and vascular anastomosis: longer lasting tensile strength
  - Polyamide (nylon)
  - Polypropylene (prolene)
  - Polytetrafluoroethylene (PTFE – Gore-Tex)
- Metal (titanium) clips can be used:
  - Where access is difficult
  - To demarcate an area for subsequent radiotherapy

- To assess radiologically the response of neoplasm to radiotherapy or chemotherapy

Needles

- Shape
  - Straight: infrequently used
  - Curved: held with needle holder
- Tip
  - For skin or tough fibrous tissue: cutting
  - For breast tissue: round-bodied

Indications for using staples

- When the procedure can be carried out with greater safety with staples, e.g. repair of an anastomotic leak
- When the operative time is significantly reduced and this is considered important
- When the incidence of late complications like stenosis is low, for example in a low anterior resection of the rectum or in an oesophagogastric anastomosis high in the chest

Tourniquets

Indications

- Prevention of bleeding, to ensure accurate operation in a bloodless field
- Prevention of systemic toxicity in isolated limb perfusion
  - With chemotherapeutic drugs in treatment of localised cancers, e.g. melanoma, sarcoma
  - Local anaesthetic drugs (prilocaine) in regional intravenous anaesthesia (Bier's block)

Contraindications

- Elderly patients
- Peripheral vascular disease
- High risk of venous thromboembolism
- To arrest bleeding
- Local anaesthesia

Procedure

- Before application of the tourniquet
  - Check the monitor and the cuff and the adequacy of the cuff breadth
  - Ensure the correct limb has the tourniquet applied
  - Intravenous antibiotics (if indicated) should be given 5 minutes before the cuff is inflated
  - An intravenous cannula should be in position
  - Limb exsanguination is by elevation of the limb for 5 minutes (with the arm at 90° or the leg at 45°) and the use of an Esmarch bandage
  - Appropriate soft padding is needed under the tourniquet
  - Avoid vital structures, e.g. the testis
- After application of the tourniquet
  - Inflation, ideally to the minimal effective pressure for the minimum time required
  - Inflation pressure
    - 250–350 mmHg for the lower limb (nearly 100 mmHg above the systolic blood pressure)
    - 200 mmHg for the upper limb (nearly 50 mmHg above the systolic blood pressure)
  - Inflation time should be noted by the anaesthetist and the theatre staff
  - Skin preparation
  - Deflation at regular intervals to allow reperfusion
    - Every 90 minutes for the upper limb
    - Every 120 minutes for the lower limb
  - Anaesthetist should be warned before total release
  - Total tourniquet time should be recorded in the operative notes
  - Application site should be checked after removal of the tourniquet

Complications and risks

- At the tourniquet site
  - Skin
    - Friction burns, due to movement of a poorly applied tourniquet
    - Chemical burn, due to skin preparation solution getting under the tourniquet
    - Pressure necrosis, due to over-inflation, insufficient padding or inadequate cuff breadth
  - Nerves
    - Neuropraxia, due to over-inflation pressure

- The radial nerve is the most commonly affected; other nerves include the ulnar nerve, median nerve and sciatic nerve
- Distal to the tourniquet site
  - Vascular complications
    - Thrombosis
    - Ischaemia
  - Muscular complications
    - Ischaemia reperfusion toxic injury, which leads to stiffness and weakness without paralysis, which in turn leads to compartment syndrome
- Systemic complications
  - Haemodynamic changes at the time of inflation and deflation
  - Systemic reperfusion injury, due to rhabdomyolysis after deflation
  - Hypercoagulability
  - Pulmonary embolism
  - Haemorrhage after release of the tourniquet

Wound healing

Definition

- Process by which a damaged tissue is restored, as closely as possible to its normal state

Steps

- Haemostasis
  - Formation of clot
  - Proliferation of vessels (granulation tissue)
- Inflammation
  - Influx of plasma constituents from damaged vessels , as a result of the action of mediators
- Regeneration
  - Collagen network laid down by fibroblasts
  - Wound contraction is caused by fibroblasts
  - Connective tissue formation unites the main body of the wound
  - Post-operative strength of the wound is dependent on this step

- Repair
  - Re-epithelialisation from residual adnexal structures

Factors with a deleterious effect on wound healing

- Local factors
  - Infection
  - Ischaemia
  - Foreign body
  - Haematoma
  - Malignancy
  - Denervation
- Systemic factors
  - Poor nutrition
  - Deficiency of vitamin A or vitamin C
  - Protein deficiency
  - Zinc and manganese deficiency
  - Diabetes mellitus
  - Uraemia
  - Jaundice
  - Steroid use
  - Immunosuppressive agents
  - Chemotherapeutic agents
  - Malignant disease
  - Irradiation
  - Advanced age

Types of wound healing

- By primary intention
  - Closure of surgical incision
  - Healing occurs by epithelialisation and connective tissue formation
- By secondary intention
  - When an open wound is allowed to close naturally
  - Healing occurs by wound contraction, connective tissue formation and epithelialisation
  - Heals from the bottom by abundant vascular connective tissue that has a granular appearance
- By tertiary intention
  - Delayed primary closure or secondary suture after healing is established and granulation tissue has formed

Wound strength recovery

- 50–70% of recovery of strength is achieved by the end of 6 months
- Total recovery is rarely achieved

Comparison of hypertrophic scar with keloid	
Hypertrophic scar	**Keloid**
Scars crossing Langer's lines and infection or excessive tension makes them more prone to hypertrophy	Colored races, women are more prone. Familial tendency
Limited to original wound	Spreads beyond
No claw-like processes	Claw-like processes present
No itching	Itching present
No signs/symptoms of increased vascularity	Increased vascularity present
May regress after 6 months	No regression
Does not recur after excision if causative factors are eliminated	Recurs after excision

Wound fibrosis

- Abnormally contracting tissue in a scar occurring as a late consequence of injury
  - Adhesions in the peritoneum
  - Oesophageal stricture
  - Hepatic cirrhosis
- Skin wound fibrosis can lead to:
  - Hypertrophic scars (see table)
  - Keloids (see table)

Treatment of wound complications

- Anti-fibrotic agents (D-penicillamines)
- Compression
- Excision
- Corticosteroids (triamcinolone)

Principles of wound management

Pre-operative management

- Correction of anaemia and renal failure
- Correction of nutritional disorders
- Correction of jaundice, coagulation defects
- Optimal management of diabetes mellitus
- Anticipation of wound failure and corrective measures in immunosuppressed patients and in patients with malignancy

Operative management

- Good irrigation of contaminated wounds
- Removal of foreign bodies
- Debridement down to healthy tissues
- Appropriate positioning of incisions
- Gentle handling of tissues
- Correct selection of suitable suture materials
- Suturing without tension
- Anatomical closure of layers
- Local haemostasis

Post-operative management

- Sterile dressings
- Frequent inspection of wound
- Any discharge should be sent for culture and sensitivities, and appropriate antibiotic therapy instigated
- Prevention of hypoxia (with O_2 therapy)
- Nutritional supplements

Fracture healing

Cells involved in healing

- Osteoblasts
  - Lay down new bone (osteoid)
- Osteoclasts
  - Macrophage lineage cell
  - Reabsorb and remodel new bone

Stages

- Haemorrhage
  - Gap filled with blood clot and plasma-derived proteins
- Acute inflammatory reaction
  - Loosening of periosteum and filling at fracture site
  - Bone necrosis, depending on extent of the injury
- Invasion of macrophages, leading to granulation tissue formation and differentiation into connective tissue stem cells (soft callus)
- Provisional callus formation (woven bone plus cartilage), which unites the fracture ends; origin of callus is the periosteum and medullary cavity
- Ossification of callus: consolidation (hard callus)
- Remodelling and restoration to normal
  - Resorption of cortical bone
  - Removal of excess medullary new bone
  - Woven bone replaced by lamellar bone

Complications

- Fibrous union, caused by improper immobilisation
- Non-union, caused by interposition of soft tissue
- Delayed union, caused by sepsis, foreign body or ischaemia
- Malunion, leading to osteoarthritis

Healing of nervous tissue

CNS

- Most neurones cannot be replaced
- Limited regeneration in the hypothalamic neurohypophyseal system
- In the rest of the CNS:
  - Necrosis elicits proliferation of glial cells and in-growth of capillaries
  - Physical barrier to regeneration of neuronal fibres

Peripheral nervous system

- Severed axon causes nerve cell chromatolysis
  - Swelling
  - Disappearance of Nissl granules

- Breaking up of myelin sheath surrounding the axon
- New neurofibrils sprout from proximal end of a severed axon and invaginate Schwann cells (at a rate of 1 mm/day)
- May or may not reach the end-organ or the distal cut end
- If not, there is a tangle of new nerve fibres embedded in a mass of scar tissue: the traumatic (or stump) neuroma
- Tinel's sign is tenderness at the site of the traumatic neuroma on percussion

Day-care surgery

Definition

- Surgery for a patient who is admitted for investigation or operation on a planned non-residential basis but who requires facilities to recover
- Outpatient surgery: no facilities required for recovery (those done under local anaesthesia)
- Ambulatory surgery: 23 hours' stay

Benefits

- Releases resources and increases total number of patients treated
- Cost containment without jeopardising clinical outcome

Day-care unit

- Self-contained unit with its own admission and reception office, staff rooms, stores, ward, theatre suites and recovery ward
- Closed at nights and at weekends
- Beds are booked in advance and never blocked by emergencies

Selection of patients

- Ideal for patients undergoing operations that require a relatively short general anaesthetic and that do not carry a risk of post-operative complications
- Unsuitable criteria
  - Obesity (BMI > 30)
  - Advanced age (> 65–75 years)
  - ASA score > 2
  - Home conditions
    - Living alone
    - No home telephone
    - > 1 hour journey from the hospital

Examples of day care operations

- General surgery
  - Minor operations on skin and subcutaneous tissues
  - Hernia repair
  - Anal fissure repair and sphincterotomy
  - Lymph node biopsy
  - Rectal polypectomy
- Orthopedic procedures
  - Joint manipulations
  - Ganglion excision
  - Carpal tunnel decompression
  - Excision of palmar fascia for Dupuytren's contracture
- Urology
  - Diagnostic urethrocystoscopy
  - Biopsy of bladder mucosa
  - Circumcision
  - Vasectomy
  - Excision of scrotal lesions

Operational policy

- Efficient booking, with reminder and confirmation protocols is needed
- Pre-admission and discharge policy

Pain management

- Local infiltration anaesthesia
- Opioids with shortest half life, e.g. fentanyl, to avoid post-operative nausea and vomiting
- Non-steroidal anti-inflammatory drugs or cyclo-oxygenase-2 inhibitors

Endoscopic surgery and laparoscopy

Definition

- Surgery through an approach that reduces the trauma of access without compromising exposure

Techniques

- Laparoscopy
- Thoracoscopy
- Endoluminal endoscopy
  - Gastrointestinal

- Urinary
- Respiratory
- Vascular
- Perivesical endoscopy
- Arthroscopy and intra-articular joint surgery
- Combined approaches

Morbidity of open surgical wounds

- Pain leads to decreased mobility, with an increased risk of pulmonary collapse, chest infection and deep venous thrombosis
- Wound infection
- Wound dehiscence
- Bleeding
- Herniation
- Nerve entrapment
- Post-operative pain due to retraction
- Exposure, causing fluid loss by evaporation
- Adynamic ileus

Advantages of minimal access surgery

- Trauma of access and exposure is reduced
- Visualisation is magnified and improved
- Closed environment
  - Decreased exposure and drying
  - Decreased external contamination
- Decreased depression of immune system
- Decreased wound-related complications and adhesion formation
- Decreased hospital stay and post-operative morbidity, and early return to employment

Disadvantages of minimal access surgery

- Difficulties in hand–eye co-ordination, due to:
  - Two-dimensional imaging
  - Lack of navigational cues to judge depth
- Lack of tactile feedback
- Difficulties in dissection and haemostasis in more advanced procedures
- May require separate incision to deliver specimens in excisional surgery
- Possible local biological factors leading to increased chances of wound recurrence

Stereoscopic imaging for laparoscopic surgery

- For critical procedures, knot tying and dissection of closely underlying tissues
- Drawbacks
  - Decreased brightness
  - Necessity to wear glasses
- Image-processing techniques: allow visualisation of any view of the operative region in any orientation

Laparoscopic ultrasound

- A substitute for sense of touch
- Allows visualisation through fluid-filled solid organs as well as vascular structures
- Permits differentiation of solid and cystic masses
- Evaluation of wall layers of hollow viscera
- Enables assessment of the dimensions, infiltration and dissemination of tumours
- Avoids unnecessary tissue dissection
- Aids guided biopsy

Training

- Can be done by simulators

Equipment

- Image systems
  - Light source
    - Xenon: provides natural white light
    - Halogen: white balancing by camera
    - Fibre-optic camera
  - Rigid viewing telescopes
    - 0°, for forward viewing
    - 30°, for angled viewing
  - Flexible telescopes
    - For endoscopies
  - Image display systems
    - One or two television monitors mounted on trolleys that also house the light source, camera control unit and insufflator
- Devices
  - CO_2 insufflator
    - Does not support combustion
    - Soluble
    - Cheap
  - Cardiovascular side effects include decreased cardiac output, increased systemic vascular resistance, increased preload, increased peripheral vascular resistance, and decreased hepatic splanchnic flow
  - Neuroendocrine side effects include release of renin and aldosterone
- Abdominal wall lift gasless systems
  - Rubber tube sling device
  - Planar intraperitoneal device
  - Extraperitoneal device
- Hand-assisted laparoscopic surgery for:
  - Anti-reflux surgery
  - Splenectomy
  - Colonic surgery
- Master–slave manipulators (robot surgery)
  - Under the immediate and constant control of the operator
  - Copies and translates hand movements made by surgeon
  - Especially useful in coronary bypass surgeries

Conversion

- Elective: e.g. planned conversion following decision that continuing laparoscopy is impossible because of dense adhesions or difficult anatomy
- Enforced: e.g. unplanned conversion because of excessive uncontrollable bleeding, injury to bowel, bile duct or other vital structures; e.g. unplanned conversion due to equipment failure

Complications

- General
  - Pneumothorax
  - CO_2 embolism
  - Necrotising infections of port site
  - Thromboembolism
- Iatrogenic injuries
  - Major retroperitoneal vascular injuries
  - Bowel injuries
  - Bile duct injuries
  - Ureteric injuries

Endoluminal minimal access surgery

- Trans-anal endoscopic microsurgery, for rectal tumours up to the peritoneal reflection
- Laparo-endoluminal gastric approach, for lesions in the posterior wall of the stomach, fundus and gastro-oesophageal junction

Interventional flexible endoscopy

Indications

- Retrieval of swallowed or inhaled foreign body
  - Those with sharp edges
  - Those that are corrosive
  - Those that cause acute obstruction
  - Those that remain in the stomach for > 72 hours
  - Bezoars
- Dilatation of benign strictures
  - Solid tapered dilators
  - Balloon dilators
- Percutaneous endoscopic gastrostomy
- Control of gastrointestinal bleeding
  - Thermal therapy
    - Monopolar or bipolar coagulation
    - Argon plasma coagulation
    - Laser probe coagulation
    - Laser photocoagulation
    - Microwave energy
  - Injection therapy
    - Sclerosants
    - Vasoconstrictors
    - Fibrin, thrombin glue and so on
  - Vascular occlusive devices
    - Bands
    - Metal clips
- Treatment of gastrointestinal polyps and early mucosal cancers
  - Laser ablation of mucosal cancer or severe dysplasia
  - Excision of polyps
  - Ablation of premalignant mucosa, e.g. Barrett's oesophagitis
  - Submucosal resection of early gastric cancer
- For palliation of incurable bronchial, gastrointestinal, biliary, pancreatic and colorectal malignancies by:
  - Dilatation
  - Stenting, with expandable metallic stents
  - Recanalisation laser
    - Nd:YAG
    - Photodynamic ablation
- For treatment of ductal stones, cholangitis and pancreatitis
  - Sphincterotomy plus Dormia basket or balloon catheter
  - Pigtail stent for a retained stone
  - Nasobiliary drain for cholangitis
  - Pseudocystogastrostomy
  - Extraction of pancreatic calculi and stenting in chronic pancreatitis

Part 2

System-specific surgery

Cerebral blood flow

- Grey matter: 50 mL/100 g/minute
- White matter: 20 mL/100 g/minute
- Brain receives 17% of cardiac output
- Utilizes 20% of body's O_2
- Cerebral blood flow (CBF) is directly proportional to cerebral perfusion pressure (CPP) and inversely proportional to cerebral vascular resistance (CVR)
- CBF = CPP / CVR

Autoregulation of CBF

- Decreased mean arterial pressure (MAP) results in decreased CVR, maintaining CBF
- If MAP < 50 mmHg, this mechanism is exhausted, leading to decreased CBF
- Reverse is true when MAP increases
- This is exhausted at MAP > 160 mmHg

Mechanisms of autoregulation

- Myogenic response
- Reflex vasodilatation and vasoconstriction responses to relaxation and stretch of the vessel wall caused by changes in perfusion pressure
- Metabolic regulation: vasodilatation in response to accumulation of local metabolites at lower perfusion pressures
- Vasodilator metabolites:
  - CO_2
    - Causes cerebral vasodilatation, i.e. relaxation of smooth muscle in response to decreased pH in the surrounding cerebrospinal fluid (CSF)
    - Hypocapnia leads to cerebral vasoconstriction, decreased CBF and decreased intracranial pressure
    - Lineal relationship of cerebral blood flow and p_aCO_2 is 3–9 kPa
  - O_2
    - Hypoxia increases cerebral blood flow
    - Acts only when p_aO_2 is < 50 mmHg (6.9 kPa)

Interventions that optimize CBF

- Head tilt to 30°
- Neutral positioning of the neck, thereby avoiding venous obstruction
- Blood pressure and oxygenation
  - Avoidance of hypoxia and hypotension
  - Maintenance of MAP at > 90 mmHg and p_aO_2 at > 13.5 kPa
  - Respiratory interventions
    - Hypoxia avoided
    - p_aCO_2 maintained at 4.5–5 kPa
    - Mild hyperventilation may be used in refractory cases
- Pain control, to avoid hypertensive response associated with pain
- Corticosteroids
  - Dexamethasone reduces vasogenic oedema and increased intracranial pressure associated with neoplasms
  - Used cautiously in head trauma
- Reduction of cerebral metabolism
  - Control of temperature and seizures
  - Sedation
  - Induced hypothermia may be useful: it is still under trial
- Osmotherapy
  - Mannitol decreases intracranial pressure and increases CBF
  - Mechanisms
    - Osmotic diuretic effects
    - Increased blood volume with decreased viscosity and improved blood flow characteristics
    - Free radical scavenging effects
    - Decreased CSF production
  - Hypertonic saline also may be used

Assessment of CBF

- Positron emission tomography (PET)
- Single-photon emission CT (SPECT)
- Xenon CT
- CT and MRI perfusion scans
  - Jugular venous saturation ($sJvO_2$) measures brain oxygenation

- Brain tissue oxygen (P_bO_2)
- Cerebral microdialysis (evolving research tool)
  - Can measure glucose, glycerol and glutamate assays
  - Lactate pyruvate ratio to mark anaerobic metabolism
- Regional CBF: thermistor-based CBF monitoring

Intracranial pressure

- Normal intracranial pressure: 5.8–13 mmHg (12–18 cmH$_2$O) in the horizontal position

Munro–Kelly doctrine

- Normal contents of the cranium
  - The brain
  - The CSF
  - The blood and blood vessels
- Any increase in the volume of one component should be accompanied by a decrease in either or both of the other components in order to maintain intracranial pressure

Consequences of head trauma

- Mass lesions
- Increased microvascular permeability, leading to interstitial oedema
- Hypoxia, which causes further cerebral swelling
- Hypercarbia, which causes vasodilatation of blood vessels in the injured parts of the brain

Results of head trauma

- Tentorial herniation
  - Cranial nerve III compression, causing ipsilateral pupillary dilatation
  - Corticospinal tract compression, causing contralateral motor weakness
- Coning, with Cushing's response
  - Decreased respiratory rate
  - Decreased heart rate
  - Increased systolic blood pressure
  - Increased pulse pressure

Raised intracranial pressure

Effects

- Hydrocephalus, due to a space-occupying lesion of the posterior cranial fossa
- Cerebral ischaemia, due to increased intracranial pressure compromising the vascular component
- Brain shift and herniation, which can be trans-tentorial or tonsillar
- Trans-tentorial herniation
  - Caused by a supra-tentorial mass
  - The uncus is pushed over the tentorium cerebelli
  - Results in compression of:
    - Cranial nerve III, with ipsilateral pupillary dilatation
    - Cerebral peduncle, with contralateral hemiparesis and ipsilateral hemiparesis

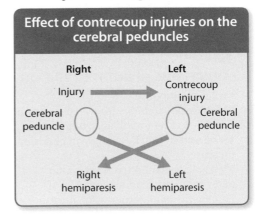

Effect of contrecoup injuries on the cerebral peduncles

Right — Injury → Left — Contrecoup injury

Cerebral peduncle — Cerebral peduncle

Right hemiparesis — Left hemiparesis

- Aqueduct, with headache and vomiting
- Posterior cerebral artery, with cortical blindness
- Brainstem, with coma, decerebrate rigidity and death
- Tonsillar herniation:
  - Cerebellar tonsils move into the foramen magnum
  - Results in respiratory failure and death

Systemic effects

- Caused by autonomic imbalance as a result of compression of the hypothalamus

- Hypertension
- Bradycardia
- Respiratory slowing
- Pulmonary oedema
- Gastrointestinal ulceration

Clinical features

- Headache
- Nausea and vomiting
- Papilloedema
- Decreased level of consciousness

Hydrocephalus

Definition: abnormal accumulation of CSF in the ventricular system of the brain
- Normal values
  - CSF volume: 150 mL
  - Rate of production: 500 mL/day (0.35 mL/minute)
- CSF circulation
  - Produced from the choroid plexus and the ependymal lining of ventricles
  - Passes to third and fourth ventricles the through foramina of Luschka and Magendie
  - Absorbed into the venous system via:
    - The arachnoid villi and granulations
    - Small herniations of the subarachnoid space into the superior sagittal sinus

Classification

- Obstructive hydrocephalus (obstruction within the ventricular system)
  - Congenital hydrocephalus
    - Stenosis of the aqueduct of Sylvius
    - Dandy–Walker syndrome
  - Acquired hydrocephalus
    - Multiple supratentorial tumors e.g. craniopharyngioma
    - Cysts, e.g. colloid cyst
    - Posterior fossa tumors
- Communicating hydrocephalus (obstruction outside the ventricular system)
  - Congenital hydrocephalus
    - Arnold–Chiari malformation (myelomeningocoele)
    - Meningocoele
    - Encephalocoele
    - Venous hypertension

- Achondroplasia
- Cranio-facial syndromes
- Acquired hydrocephalus
  - Subarachnoid haemorrhage
  - Meningeal carcinomatosis
  - Post-meningitis

Clinical features

- Infants (before fusion of the cranial sutures)
  - Increasing head circumference
  - Tense fontanelle
  - Separation of the cranial sutures
    - Episodic apnoea and bradycardia
    - Irritability
- Older children and adults (after fusion of the cranial sutures):
  - Headache
  - Vomiting
  - Altered level of consciousness
  - Visual obscurations
  - Papilloedema
  - Cognitive impairment
  - Poor concentration
  - Gait disturbance

Investigations

- Cranial ultrasound in infants
- CT, MRI
- Intracranial pressure monitoring
- CSF infusion test

Treatment

- External ventricular drainage
- Ventricular shunts
  - Early complications (within first few months of surgery)
    - Infection
    - Malposition
    - Blockage
    - Intracranial bleeding
    - Viscus perforation
    - Overdrainage leading to extra-axial fluid collection
  - Late complications
    - Blockage
    - Disconnection
    - Migration or fracture
    - Overdrainage leading to slit ventricle syndrome
    - Shunt ascites
    - Abdominal pseudocyst

- Endoscopic third ventriculostomy
  - Alternative to ventriculoperitoneal shunting
  - Endoscope passed into the lateral ventricle via a burr hole in the frontal region
  - The tip of the scope is passed through the foramen of Munro, into the third ventricle, the floor of which is perforated and enlarged with a balloon catheter
  - This creates an artificial opening in the basal subarachnoid space
  - Suitable for obstructive hydrocephalus where the obstruction is between the third ventricle and the outflow of the fourth ventricle, e.g. aqueductal stenosis or posterior fossa tumour

Glasgow Coma Scale (GCS)

Function

- Quantitative assessment of the patient's level of consciousness

Components

- Eye opening
  - Spontaneous: 4 points
  - To speech: 3 points
  - To pain: 2 points
  - None: 1 point
- Verbal response
  - Oriented: 5 points
  - Confused: 4 points
  - Inappropriate: 3 points
  - Incomprehensible: 2 points
  - None: 1 point
- Motor response
  - Obeys commands: 6 points
  - Localises pain: 5 points
  - Withdrawal response: 4 points
  - Abnormal flexion: 3 points
  - Abnormal extension: 2 points
  - None: 1 point

Assessment

- Mild derangement: GCS of 13–15 points
- Moderate derangement: GCS of 9–12 points
- Severe derangement: GCS < 8 points

- Associated with:
  - Pupillary dysfunction
  - Lateralised extremity weakness

Epilepsy

- Only one third of cases are in children aged < 15 years
- One fifth of cases cannot be controlled medically
- Surgery is aimed at excising a focal lesion

Surgery for epilepsy

- There should have been an adequate trial of medical treatment before surgery is contemplated
- Hippocampal sclerosis is associated with prolonged febrile convulsions in infancy
- Focal signs may assist in localisation
- Established psychosis is a contraindication for surgery
- MRI is very useful for localising abnormal tissue

Types of surgery

- Partial resection of the temporal lobe: indicated for lesions in the amygdala or hippocampus
- Local anaesthesia may be used if lesions are close to an eloquent area
- Hemi-decortication gives 80% relief from seizures if there is an extensive abnormality
- Resection of the corpus callosum improves seizures, but does not eradicate them

Meningitis

Routes of infection

- Direct spread from middle ear, mastoid, paranasal sinus, or osteomyelitis of vertebrae or skull
- Blood-borne, from septicaemia
- Penetrating wounds to the brain
- Iatrogenic
  - Lumbar puncture
  - Spinal anaesthesia

Common pathogens

- Haemolytic streptococci
- *Staphylococcus aureus*

- *Neisseria meningitidis*
- *Listeria monocytogenes*

Complications

- Cerebral infarction
- Cerebral abscess
- Subdural abscess
- Hydrocephalus
- Epilepsy

Cerebral abscess

Causes

- Routes of infection (direct spread, septicaemia and penetrating wounds to the brain, iatrogenic) and common causative pathogens are the same as for meningitis

Sites

- Temporal lobe or cerebellum, from otitis media
- Frontal lobe, from paranasal sinuses
- Parietal lobe, from haematogenous spread

Complications

- Meningitis
- Intracranial herniation
- Focal neurological deficit
- Epilepsy

Intracranial mass

- Causes increased intracranial pressure, which leads to various clinical presentations

Clinical presentations

- Hydrocephalus: 'sunset appearance'
- Cerebral ischaemia: drowsiness and coma
- Brain shift and herniation
  - Ipsilateral pupillary dilatation
  - Contralateral hemiparesis
- Systemic effects
  - Cushing's response
    - Hypertension
    - Bradycardia
    - Bradypnoea
  - Haemorrhagic pulmonary oedema
  - Gastrointestinal ulceration (Cushing's ulcer)

- Miscellaneous presentation
  - Headache, due to distortion and compression of pain receptors within the dura and around cerebral blood vessels
  - Nausea and vomiting, due to pressure on the vomiting center in the pons and medulla
  - Papilloedema, due to venous obstruction
  - Decreased level of consciousness, leading to coma

Intracranial haemorrhage

Intracerebral haemorrhage

Causes

- Micro-aneurysms
- Vascular tumour

Extracerebral haemorrhage

- Can be extradural, subdural or subarachnoid

Extradural haemorrhage

- Causes
  - Skull fracture at the pterion, with arterial tearing
  - Middle meningeal artery tear as a result of fracture of the temporal bone
- Clinical picture
  - Lucid interval followed by increased intracranial pressure, leading to coma
  - Transtentorial herniation

Subdural haemorrhage

- Causes
  - From small bridging veins
  - Acute haemorrhage as a result of trauma
  - Chronic haemorrhage in the elderly as a result of brain shrinkage
- Clinical picture
  - Personality change
  - Memory loss
  - Confusion
  - Fluctuating level of consciousness

Subarachnoid haemorrhage

- Causes
  - Trauma in association with head injury

- Rupture of a berry aneurysm
- Rupture of a vascular malformation
- Hypertensive haemorrhage
- Coagulation disorder
- Rupture of an intracerebral haematoma
- Tumours
- Vasculitis
- Clinical picture
  - Sudden severe headache

Classification of cerebral tumours

Primary tumours

- Glial tumours
  - Astrocytoma
  - Medulloblastoma
  - Ependymoma
  - Oligodendroglioma
- Non-glial tumours
  - Meningioma
  - Acoustic neuroma
  - Pituitary tumours

Secondary tumours

- Lung cancer
- Breast cancer
- Kidney cancer
- Melanoma

Brainstem death

Definition

- Functioning of the heart and lung without cerebral activity

Prerequisites for diagnosis

- Irreversible brain damage of known aetiology
- Apnoeic coma dependent on artificial ventilation
- Exclusion criteria
  - Reversible drug effects
  - Hypothermia
  - Circulatory, metabolic and endocrine disturbances

Tests for brainstem reflexes

- Pupillary reflexes, which test cranial nerves II and III
- Corneal reflexes, which test cranial nerves V and VII
- Absence of response to supra-orbital pressure
- Gag and cough reflexes, which test cranial nerves IX and X
- Vestibulo-ocular reflexes (elicited by putting 50 mL of ice-cold water into the ear), which test cranial nerves VIII, III and VI
- Absence of spontaneous respiration despite provoking stimuli, which are:
  - Pre-oxygenation with 100% O_2 for 10 minutes
  - Disconnection of the ventilator
  - p_aCO_2 being allowed to rise to 6.6 kPa
  - O_2 given via endotracheal tube at 6L/minute

Jugular venous pulse waves

- High jugular venous pressure
  - Superior vena cava obstruction
  - Tricuspid stenosis
  - Pleural effusion
  - Tension pneumothorax
  - Over-filling
  - Right heart failure
  - Cardiac tamponade
  - Constrictive pericarditis

- Abnormal jugular venous pulse wave
  - Absent 'a': atrial fibrillation
  - Canon 'a': complete heart block
  - Large 'a' and slow 'y': tricuspid stenosis
  - Large 'v': tricuspid incompetence
- Kussmaul's sign
  - Paradoxical increased jugular venous pressure on inspiration, seen in constrictive pericarditis and cardiac tamponade

Representation of the jugular venous pulse wave

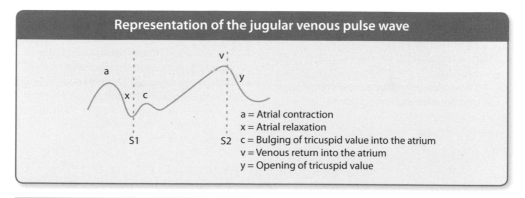

a = Atrial contraction
x = Atrial relaxation
c = Bulging of tricuspid value into the atrium
v = Venous return into the atrium
y = Opening of tricuspid value

Cardiac cycle

Phases and events

Phases and events of the cardiac cycle

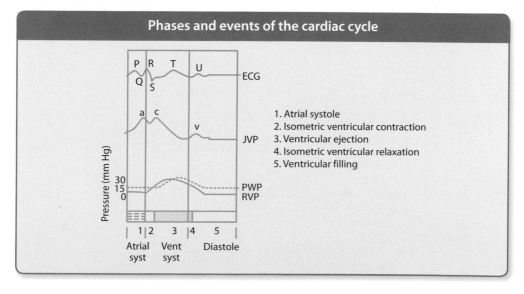

1. Atrial systole
2. Isometric ventricular contraction
3. Ventricular ejection
4. Isometric ventricular relaxation
5. Ventricular filling

Cardiopulmonary bypass

Indications

- Cardiac and supra-diaphragmatic aortic surgeries
- Cardiac and pulmonary support
- Hypothermia

Technique

- Patient is anticoagulated with heparin (300 IU/kg)
- Blood is drained from the right atrium and passed through an oxygenator
- Oxygenated blood is then returned to the ascending aorta

Complications

- Trauma to red blood cells
  - Haemoglobinaemia
  - Haemoglobinuria
- Hypercoagulability
  - Bleeding
  - Disseminated intravascular coagulation
- Systemic inflammatory response syndrome (SIRS), multiple organ dysfunction syndrome (MODS) and acute respiratory distress syndrome (ARDS)
- Air embolism

Fetal circulation

- Oxygenated blood from the placenta passes through the ductus venosus to the right atrium
- From the right atrium, it passes through the foramen ovale to the left heart
- It then passes through the ascending aorta to the brain
- Remaining blood from the right heart and blood from superior vena cava passes to the pulmonary artery
- It then passes through the ductus arteriosus to the descending aorta and supplies the rest of the body
- Venous blood passes back through the umbilical arteries to the placenta
- Thus, more oxygenated blood goes to brain than to the rest of the body

Soft tissue injuries

Definition

- Injuries that involve damage to ligaments, tendon and muscles

Types

- Sprains
- Strains
- Contusions
- Tendonitis
- Bursitis

Sprains

- Complete or partial tears of the ligament from over extension of a joint
- Grade I sprains
  - Minimal pain and swelling
  - No loss of function
- Grade II sprains
  - Incomplete tear with bruising, pain and swelling
  - Difficulty in weight-bearing
- Grade III sprains
  - Severe pain and swelling
  - Inability to weight bear

Strains

- Injury to muscle or tendon caused by twist, pull or overuse
- Can be partial or complete
- Usual site is the hamstring
- Occurs with sporting injuries
- Occurs with recurrent trauma, e.g. lifting weights
- Occurs with chronic strain due to overuse, e.g. tennis elbow

Contusions

- Bruise to soft tissue as a result of direct trauma
- Subcutaneous blood leads to haematoma, discoloration, swelling and pain

Tendonitis

- Inflammation of tendon sheath and/or tendon

Bursitis

- Inflammation of the bursa, due to direct injury, excessive traumatic exercise or overuse

Treatment

- Acronym: RICE
  - R: rest
  - I: ice packs. 24–48 hours
  - C: compression
  - E: elevation
- Grade III sprains should be immobilised in a splint
- Purpose of immobilisation
  - Protection of and support for unstable muscles or tendons
  - Restriction of range of movement
  - Limitation of re-injury to the area
  - Return the area to normal function as soon as possible

Pathophysiology of fractures

- Normal bone fracture: when bone is stressed beyond the load
- Stress fracture: when the fracture is caused by cyclical loading of low magnitude
- Pathological fracture: when a fracture occurs as a result of a force that is within the physiological tolerance, owing to a pre-existing abnormality of the bone

Types of fracture

- Greenstick fracture (occurs in children)
- In adults:
  - Complete or incomplete fractures
  - Displaced or undisplaced fractures
  - Simple or comminuted fractures
  - Open or closed fractures
- Classification according to the direction of force
  - Transverse fractures
  - Oblique fractures
  - Spiral fractures

Complications of fractures

General complications

- Hypovolaemic shock
- Acute respiratory distress syndrome (ARDS)
- Systemic infection and systemic inflammatory response syndrome (SIRS)
- Fat embolism

Early local complications

- Infection
- Nerve injury
- Vascular injury
- Visceral injury
- Compartment syndrome
- Local joint injury and infection

Late local complications

- Complications of healing
  - Delayed union
  - Malunion
  - Non-union
- Joint stiffness and myositis ossificans
- Ischaemic contractures
- Sudeck's atrophy, from disuse
- Avascular necrosis of bone
- Growth disturbance
- Osteoarthritis

Fracture healing

Stages

- Recruitment of bone-forming cell precursors (osteoprogenitors)
- Induction and activation into different cartilage and bone-forming cells (osteo-induction)
- Presence of osteo-conductive surface on which new bone can be produced (callus)

Histological stages

- Haematoma
- Blood clot organised to form granulation tissue
- Callus formation
  - Primary cellular callus
  - External bridging callus
  - Late medullary callus
- Conversion of callus to woven bone by endochondral ossification
- Consolidation and remodelling of woven bone to lamellar bone
- Reconstitution of medullary canal and recovery of bone shape

Factors affecting fracture healing

- General factors
  - Age: healing is faster in children
  - Nutrition and general health
  - Infection, which slows healing
  - Pre-existing abnormal bone, which slows healing
- Local factors
  - Site: upper limb fractures heal faster than lower limb fractures
  - Blood supply, which is dependent on soft tissue attachments
  - Proximity of the bone ends
    - Bone loss
    - Soft tissue interposition
  - Intra-articular fracture, which heal more slowly
  - Nerve supply

Principles of fracture management

- Early treatment
  - 'ABC' of advanced advanced trauma life support (ATLS)
  - Assessment of neurovascular status of the limb
- Reduction
- Holding until the fracture unites
- Rehabilitation to ensure as independent a life as possible

Stages of management

- Reduction of the fracture
  - Only if displaced and malunion will compromise function
- Holding the fracture
  - For comfort
  - To prevent repeat displacement
  - To allow early return to function
- Rehabilitation
  - To build muscle power
  - To reduce stiffness
  - To rebuild proprioception

Indications for leaving a fracture unreduced

- In children, in whom remodelling will correct the position
- In elderly patients, in whom function is more important than cosmetic effect

Types of reduction

- Closed reduction
  - Minimises damage to blood supply
  - Relies on soft tissue attachments to maintain reduction
  - Rarely adequate for intra-articular fractures
  - Difficult to perform in babies when bones cannot be seen on x-rays
- Open reduction
  - Needs careful planning and preparation of the patient (not an emergency procedure)
  - Indications
    - Open fracture
    - Fractures that cannot be reduced closed
    - Displaced intra-articular fracture
    - Grossly unstable fracture
    - Displaced intra-articular fracture in a child
  - Non-rigid: stimulates rapid callus formation

Types of implants

- Plates and screws
- Wires
- Intra-medullary nails

Complications of internal fixation

- Damage to soft tissues and blood supply
- Risk of introducing infection
- Callus formation is inhibited

Femoral neck fractures

Aetiology

- Elderly females: osteoporosis
- Younger patients: chronic alcoholism and chronic medical conditions

Classification

- Intracapsular fractures
  - Displaced high cervical fractures
  - Undisplaced high cervical fractures
  - Basi-cervical fractures
- Extracapsular fractures
  - Two-part intertrochantric fractures
  - Multifragment intertrochanteric fractures
  - Subtrochanteric fractures

Blood supply to the femoral head

- Artery within ligamentum teres, via the joint space
- Lateral and medial circumflex arteries: retrograde entry from capsular attachments

Intracapsular fractures

- Clinical features
  - Undisplaced fractures
    - Pain and tenderness
  - Displaced fractures
    - Shortened and externally rotated limb
- Investigations
  - X-ray
  - Bone scan
  - MRI
- Treatment options
  - Undisplaced fracture (patient of any age)
    - Sliding hip screw
    - Multiple screws
  - Displaced fracture (patient aged > 80 years)
    - Hemiarthroplasty
  - Displaced (patient aged < 80 years)
    - Reduction and sliding hip screw
    - Bipolar hemiarthroplasty
    - Total hip replacement
  - Displaced fracture (younger patient)
    - Reduction and dynamic nail and screw
    - Total hip replacement

Extracapsular fractures

- All patients need sliding a hip screw and plate or an intramedullary device unless unfit for general anaesthesia
- Complication: wound infection

Subtrochanteric fractures

- High-energy fractures with marked displacement
- Extensive blood loss
- Treatment: fixed by intramedullary nail or extramedullary sliding screw and plate
- Complication: delayed union or non-union

Treatment options for complications

- For avascular necrosis after an intracapsular fracture: hip replacement
- For instability after an extracapsular fracture: sliding hip screw
- For insecure fixation or delayed union after a subtrochanteric fracture: intramedullary nail, or plate and screw

Bone and joint infections

Osteomyelitis

- Usually pyogenic
- May be granulomatous (caused by tuberculosis or syphilis)
- May follow a penetrating injury
- Organisms
  - Usually *Staphylococcus aureus*
  - *Haemophilus* species and streptococci in children

Septic arthritis

- Usually pyogenic, may be granulomatous
- Caused by haematogenous spread, penetrating injury or surgery
- Common in immunocompromised patients

Management of osteomyelitis and septic arthritis

- Microbiological diagnosis
- Intravenous antibiotics
- Surgical intervention if conservative treatment fails to produce improvement

Knee aspiration

Purpose

- To establish diagnosis
- To relieve discomfort
- To drain effusion or infected fluid
- To instil medication

Indications

- Crystal-induced arthropathy
- Haemarthrosis
- Limiting joint damage resulting from an infectious process
- Symptomatic relief of a large effusion
- Unexplained joint effusion
- Unexplained monoarthritis

Contraindications

- Bacteraemia
- Surgeon unfamiliar with the anatomy
- Joint prosthesis
- Overlying infection in the soft tissue
- Coagulopathy
- Overlying dermatitis
- Unco-operative patient

Technique

- Site: 1 cm above and lateral to the superolateral aspect of the patella (giving the most direct access to the patella)
- Needle is directed distally

Complications

- Severe pain: indicates needle coming into cartilage and that the needle ought to be redirected
- Infection
- Re-accumulation of fluid; elastic wrap after aspiration may help to prevent this complication

Osteoarthritis

Definition

- Manifestation of degenerative disease

Types

- Primary osteoarthritis
  - With age
  - Affects weight-bearing joints

- Secondary osteoarthritis
  - After pre-existing joint damage (from trauma or infection)
  - Affects any joint

Causative lesion

- Failure of cartilage repair in stressed areas of the joint

Pathological features

- Failure of repair, which leads to loss of radiographic joint space
- Subchondral bone sclerosis and cyst
- Proliferation and remodelling of bone in unstressed areas, causing osteophyte formation
- Capsular thickening and fibrosis, leading to joint stiffness

X-ray criteria for diagnosis

- Progressive cartilage destruction
- Subarticular (subchondral) cyst formation
- Sclerosis of surrounding bone
- Osteophyte formation
- Capsular fibrosis

Rheumatoid arthritis

Definition

- Systemic disease characterised by proliferative and destructive inflammation of the synovium
- Extra-articular rheumatoid arthritis can affect the serosa, blood vessels, viscera, subcutaneous tissue and ocular connective tissue

Joints involved

- Small joints of the hands and feet first, followed by:
  - Knee involvement
  - Shoulder involvement
  - Elbow involvement
  - Cervical spine instability

Pathology

- HLA-DR-4 or Dw-4
- Activation of T-helper cells by an unknown microbial pathogen
- T-helper cells produce cytokines, which activate inflammation within the joint

- B cells are activated to produce rheumatoid factor (auto-antibodies against IgG in synovial fluid and serum)
- Immune complexes in the synovial fluid lead to local tissue damage by a type III hypersensitivity reaction

Joint replacement

Definition

- Replacement of painful, arthritic, worn or diseased parts of the joint with artificial surfaces shaped in such a way as to allow joint movement

Types

- Total joint replacement: all joint surfaces replaced
- Hemiarthroplasty: the joint surface of only one bone is replaced
- Unicompartmental arthroplasty in the knee: only the inner or outer sides of both surfaces of the knee are replaced

Replacement material

- Prosthesis or implants made of high-density polyethylene
- Ceramic-bearing surface
- Metal-on-metal
- Bonded to bone by polymethylmethacrylate (PMMA) cement

Technique

- Dislocation of joint after exposure
- Joint surface and bones close to it are removed
- Implantation of prosthetic component and PMMA cement
- Reduction of dislocation
- Repair of muscle and ligaments over the joint where possible

Other techniques

- Cementless fixation
- Resurfacing or more radical removal of bone
- Minimally invasive technique

Indications

- Disabling pain and loss of function
- Benefits must be weighed against the risk of the procedure

Contraindications

- Infection (absolute contraindication)
  - Close to operative area
  - Anywhere in the body
- Other co-morbid conditions (relative contraindications)

Pre-operative work-up

- Complete routine laboratory tests
- X-ray of joint
- Planning of implant design (templating)

Post-operative care

- Early mobilisation to minimise the risk of deep venous thrombosis and pneumonia
- Physiotherapy

Complications

- General complications
  - Myocardial infarction
  - Stroke
  - Deep venous thrombosis
  - Pneumonia
  - Urinary tract infection
- Specific complications
  - Malposition
  - Fracture of adjacent bone
  - Damage to nerves
  - Damage to blood vessels
- Long-term complications
  - Chronic infection
  - Persistent pain and/or weakness
  - Loss of range of motion
  - Loosening of components as a result of fatigue (caused by inflammatory reaction to fragment and wear debris: called osteolysis)
  - Wear on the bearing surface

Prognosis

- Excellent in 95% of cases
- Pain relief is reliable
- Full range of motion is not always accomplished

Compartment syndrome

Definitions

- A progressive condition in which the elevated tissue pressure within the confined myofascial compartment exceeds the capillary pressure and ultimately compromises the circulation to the muscles and nerves
- Can also be defined as a limb- and life-threatening condition observed when the capillary perfusion pressure falls below tissue pressure in a closed anatomic space
- Untreated, compartment syndrome leads to tissue necrosis, permanent functional impairment and if severe, renal failure and death

Sites

- Wherever a compartment is present
  - Hand
  - Forearm
  - Upper arm
  - Abdomen
  - Buttock
  - Entire lower extremity

Cause

- Any injury, including vigorous exercise

Pathophysiology

- If fluid is introduced into a fixed volume, the pressure increases
- The increased pressure leads to extraneous compression and decreased tissue perfusion, and autoregulatory mechanisms are overwhelmed
- Normal cellular metabolism requires an O_2 tension of 5–7 mmHg
- This O_2 tension is easily maintained as a result of the capillary perfusion pressure (CPP) of 25 mmHg and the interstitial pressure (ISP) of 4–6 mmHg
- Normal tissue perfusion pressure is CPP minus ISP
- If ISP increases, tissue perfusion pressure is overwhelmed
- Initially, there is an increase in venous pressure and capillary flow stops, leading to hypoxia and release of vasoactive substances, which increase endothelial permeability and increases ISP further
- Slowing of nerve conduction decreases tissue pH and promotes muscle necrosis and release of myoglobin
- 6 hours is currently accepted as upper limit of viability

Signs and symptoms

- Early
  - Increased pain
  - Pain on passive movement
  - Paraesthesia
- Late
  - Decreased distal sensation
  - Compartment swelling and tension
  - Decreased muscle power
  - Decreased pulse pressure in the distal limb
- Loss of pulse is a very late sign

Diagnosis

- Urine for myoglobin
- Blood for creatine phosphokinase

Treatment

- O_2 inhalation
- Fasciotomy
- Mannitol
- Alkalinisation of urine

Complications

- Peripheral nerve damage
- Contractures
- Limb loss
- Renal failure
- Systemic inflammatory response syndrome (SIRS), multiple organ dysfunction syndrome (MODS) and death

Bone tumours

Primary tumours

- Bone-forming tumours
  - Osteoma
  - Osteosarcoma
- Cartilage-forming tumours
  - Chondroma
  - Chondrosarcoma
- Fibrous tumours
  - Fibroma
  - Fibrosarcoma
- Tumours of uncertain origin
  - Giant cell tumour (osteoclastoma)
  - Ewing's sarcoma

Secondary tumours

- From prostate, lung, breast or kidney
- Usually osteolytic
- Tumours from the prostate may be:
  - Osteoblastic
  - Osteogenic

Haemopoietic tumours

- Leukaemia
- Lymphoma
- Multiple myeloma

Metabolic bone disease

- Disorders of calcium, phosphate and vitamin D metabolism
- May be endocrine, renal or gastrointestinal in origin
- Classification
  - Hypercalcaemia, e.g. hyperparathyroidism
  - Hypocalcaemia
    - Rickets and osteomalacia
    - Renal osteodystrophy
  - Normocalcaemia with decreased bone mass
    - Osteoporosis
    - Scurvy
  - Normocalcaemia with increased bone mass
    - Osteopetrosis
    - Paget's disease

Low back pain and sciatica

- Incidence is 70-90%
- Site: intervertebral disc

Pathology

- Degenerative changes
  - Deterioration of proteoglycans within the disc leads to loss of its hydrophilic properties and the disc becomes dehydrated
  - The disc becomes narrower and therefore narrows the nerve root canals
  - Secondary changes occur in the facet joints, with osteophytes and narrowing

- The annulus is the source of pain
  - Tears of the annulus cause part of the nucleus to herniate through the posterolateral corner, leading compression of the nerve root in the lateral part of the spinal canal
  - Central disc protrusion leads to compression of the cauda equina
- Spinal stenosis, as a result of ageing

Clinical features

- Back pain radiating to the thigh
- Spinal tumour and infection must be ruled out
- Cauda equina syndrome: sudden onset of saddle anaesthesia with altered bladder and bowel function

Treatment

- Conservative
- If severe, decompression

Treatment of simple sciatica

- Epidural corticosteroid injection
- Chemonucleolysis
- Laser discectomy
- Microdiscectomy
- Standard discectomy

Cervical degenerative disease

Types

- Cervical radiculopathy
  - Neck and radicular pain
- Cervical myelopathy
  - Pain and stiffness in the neck
  - Loss of dexterity
  - Unsteadiness of gait
  - Restricted cervical spine movement

Differential diagnosis

- Cervical rib
- Ulnar or median nerve entrapment
- Metastatic cervical spine disease
- Distal brachial plexus involvement resulting from an apical lung tumour (Pancoast's tumour)

Management

- Non-operative
  - Rest
  - Analgesia
  - Cervical collar
- Surgery
  - Anterior discectomy
  - Posterior foraminectomy

Principles of hand trauma

Vascular injuries

- Division injuries
  - Tourniquets should be avoided
  - Vessels should not be clipped blindly
- Compartment syndrome
  - Release of cast
  - Fasciotomy

Metacarpal and phalangeal fractures

- Fifth metacarpal neck (Boxer's fracture): best left untreated
- Spiral fracture of metacarpal may lead to rotator malunion: K wire fixation
- Phalangeal fracture needs early mobilisation to avoid stiffness

Ligament injuries

- Carpal instability caused by scapholunate ligament rupture: early repair and K wire

Tendons

- Mallet finger
  - Caused by forced flexion of the distal interphalangeal joint
  - Rupture of insertion of the long extensor tendon
  - Treated with closed reduction and splintage in full extension (mallet splint)
- Flexor tendon injury
  - Primary repair under magnification
- Extensor tendon injury
  - Primary suture and splintage for 4 weeks

Diseases of the foot

- Congenital
- Talipes equinovarus
- Developmental
  - Planovalgus: decreased lateral arch
  - Pes cavus: increased lateral arch
- Acquired
  - Injury
  - Minor infection
    - Blisters
    - Ingrowing toe nail
  - Major infection
    - Diabetic foot
    - Madura foot
  - Arthritic
    - Rheumatoid arthritis
    - Hallus rigidus
- Ageing
  - Hallus valgus
- Deformities
  - Hammer toe
    - Extension of the metacarpophalangeal joints
    - Flexion of the proximal interphalangeal joints
    - Extension of the distal interphalangeal joints
  - Claw toe associated with pes cavus
  - Mallet toe: only the distal interphalangeal joint is involved
  - Curly toe
  - Metatarsalgia, due to cavus foot
  - Morton's neuritis: entrapment of digital nerves

Trigger finger

- Caused by thickening of the opening of flexor tendon sheath, which snares the tendon
- Causes a small nodule in the flexor tendon
- When proximal interphalangeal joint is flexed, it locks and snaps into extension
- Treatment
  - Corticosteroid injection into the sheath
  - Release of pulley at the level of the metacarpophalangeal joint
  - In rheumatoid arthritis: synovectomy

Ganglion

- Smooth, well-defined, fluctuant and trans-illuminant swelling around the wrist or small joints
- Consists of a compressed collagen sheath filled with mucoid substance
- Treatment
  - Conservative
    - Aspiration
    - Compression
  - Surgery
    - Traced down to source and excised (usually the scapholunate ligament or the scaphoid–trapezo-trapezoid joint)

Carpal tunnel syndrome

- Common in perimenopausal women
- Pain is worst at night and relieved by hanging the hand out of bed
- Causes numbness and/or clumsiness
  - Weakness of the abductor pollicis brevis muscle
  - Altered sensation in lateral three and a half fingers
- Tinel's percussion sign is positive over the carpal tunnel
- Phalen's test (tingling in the hand when wrist is fully flexed) is positive
- Thenar wasting in advanced cases
- Electrophysiology to confirm diagnosis
- Treatment
  - Splinting the wrist in extension at night
  - Injecting corticosteroid into the carpal canal
  - Surgical release of the transverse carpal ligament

Dupuytren's disease

- Autosomal-dominant inheritance
- Associated with:
  - Age
  - Smoking
  - Pulmonary tuberculosis
  - Epilepsy
  - AIDS
  - Alcoholic cirrhosis

- Caused by proliferation of myofibroblasts in the palmar fascia and subsequent contracture of the fascia
- Flexion deformity of metacarpophalangeal and proximal interphalangeal joints
- Surgical release if severe
  - Z plasty
  - Full-thickness graft
- Recurrence is common

Amputations

- Traumatic
- Non-traumatic
  - In 50% of people with diabetes mellitus in India
  - 80% are due to vascular causes in the UK
  - In 20–30% of people with diabetes mellitus in the UK

Types

- Above-knee amputation
- Gritti–Stokes amputation
- Through-knee amputation
- Below-knee amputation
- Symes' amputation
- Trans-tarsal amputation
- Trans-metatarsal amputation

Post-amputation problems

- Patients who have had a below-knee amputation need 63% more energy to walk with a prosthesis than with a normal limb
- Patients who have had an above-knee amputation need needs 117% more energy to walk with a prothesis than with a normal limb

Principles

- Preserve the knee if possible
- Wheelchair-bound patients need disarticulation

Technique

- Tissue handling with care
- Length of the flap needs to be one and a half times the circumference at the amputation level

- Tension-free
- Bone edges are bevelled
- Trimming and correct shape
- Perioperative physiotherapy and occupational therapy

Below-knee amputations

- Ideal length of stump is 12.5–13.5 cm, with retention of the fibular head for stability
- Long posterior flap
- Myoplasty: suturing of agonist and antagonist muscle over bone
- Complications
  - Early complications
    - Haemorrhage
    - Haematoma
    - Infection
    - Phantom pain
    - Urinary retention
  - Late complications
    - Flap breakdown
    - Contractures
    - Causalgia or neuralgia
    - Osteomyelitis
    - Failure to use prosthesis

Ray amputation

- Definition: toe (or finger) and corresponding part of the metatarsal (or metacarpal) is removed

Symes amputation

- Performed in infection
- Removal of malleoli and anchoring heel pad after ankle dislocation

Deciding the level of amputation

- Clinical evaluation
- Duplex scan
- Transcutaneous oximetry
- Trial cuts
- Angiogram

Sympathectomy

- Provides pre-amputation vasodilatation
- Improves skin vascularity

Peripheral vascular disease and limb ischaemia

Aetiology

- Atherosclerosis affecting the macrocirculation and the microcirculation
- Common sites of atherosclerosis in the macrocirculation
  - Coronary system
  - Carotid bifurcation
  - Aorto-iliac system
  - Femoro-distal system
- Effects of atherosclerosis on the microcirculation
  - Decreased perfusion pressure
  - Increased interaction of cellular elements with endothelium

Risk factors

- Smoking
- Hyperlipidaemia
- Hypertension
- Diabetes mellitus

Pathophysiology

Macrocirculation

- Atherosclerosis (focal intimal accumulation of lipids and fibrous tissue beneath the epithelium of large and medium-sized vessels) can be composed of:
  - Fatty streaks
  - Fibrous plaques
  - A combination of both
- Compensatory collateral vessels develop

Microcirculation

- Decreased perfusion pressure results in:
  - Vasodilatation
  - Increased plasma viscosity
  - Activation of platelets
  - Increased vascular permeability

Clinical features

- Intermittent claudication

Differential diagnosis

- Popliteal artery entrapment syndrome
- Persistent sciatic artery
- Fibromuscular dysplasia
- Cystic adventitial disease

Investigations

- Ankle–brachial pressure index (ABPI):
  - > 1: normal
  - < 0.9: mild PVD
  - < 0.7: moderate P VD
  - < 0.5: severe PVD
  - Unreliable in calcified arteries
- Exercise tests in patients who are asymptomatic at rest
- Full blood count, cholesterol, glucose, urea and electrolytes
- Transcutaneous O_2 tension
- Duplex ultrasound
- Arteriography (digital subtraction angiography) can provide a 'road map'
  - Shows site, size, number and extent of lesions and distal run-off

Management

- Risk factor modification
  - Stopping smoking
  - Control of diabetes mellitus and hypertension
  - Weight reduction
  - Decrease lipid levels
  - Decrease homocystine levels
- Exercise programmes
- Drugs
  - Pentoxyfilline: decreases red blood cell deformability
  - Anti-platelet drugs
  - Prostaglandins
  - Calcium channel blockers
- Endovascular interventions
  - Percutaneous transluminal angioplasty (PTA)
  - Stenting
  - Endarterectomy
- Surgery
  - Aorto-bifemoral bypass
  - Femoro-popliteal bypass
  - Femoro-distal bypass
    - Anterior tibial artery
    - Posterior tibial artery
    - Venous graft only
  - Lumbar sympathectomy (of doubtful value)

Signs and symptoms of lower limb arterial occlusion

General signs and symptoms

- Intermittent claudication
  - Reproducible, ischaemic, lower limb muscular pain that is brought on by activity, forcing the patient to stop, and relieved by rest
  - Causes
    - Anoxia
    - Acidosis
    - Accumulation of metabolites
- Rest pain
- Coldness, numbness and paraesthesia
- Colour changes in the skin, brittle nails and loss of hair
  - Blanching on elevation
  - Purple on dependency
- Ulceration and gangrene
- Temperature: cold
- Decreased sensation and/or decreased movement
- Pulsation
  - Decreased or absent
  - Disappearing pulse
- Systolic bruit, conducted distally
- Venous refilling
- Erectile dysfunction (Leriche's syndrome)

Clinical features according to level of arterial occlusion

- Aorto-iliac artery
  - Claudication of buttocks, thighs and calves
  - Femoral and distal pulses absent
  - Bruit over aorto-iliac region
  - Erectile dysfunction
- Iliac artery
  - Unilateral claudication of thigh, buttocks and calf
  - Bruit over iliac region
  - Unilateral absence of femoral and distal pulses
- Femoro-popliteal artery
  - Unilateral claudication of the calf
  - Femoral pulses palpable
  - Unilateral absence of distal pulses

- Distal arteries
  - Femoral and popliteal pulses palpable
  - Ankle pulses absent
  - Claudication of calf and/or foot

Occlusive carotid artery disease

Definition of stroke

- Focal (or occasionally global) loss of cerebral function that lasts for > 24 hours and that, after investigation, is found to have a vascular cause
- Transient ischemic attack (TIA): same but lasting < 24 hours

Main risk factors for a stroke

- Hypertension
- Ischaemic heart disease
- Smoking
- Hyperlipidaemia
- History of TIA
- Diabetes
- Hyperfibrinogenaemia

Most common site

- The origin of the internal carotid artery

Clinical features

- May be asymptomatic
- History of TIA
- Amaurosis fugax (transient monocular loss of vision)

Investigations

- Carotid angiography or magnetic resonance angiography
- Duplex ultrasound
- CT scanning: to differentiate haemorrhage from infarction

Management

- Optimal medical therapy
  - Treatment of ischaemic heart disease
  - Control of blood pressure
  - Change of lifestyle
- Carotid endarterectomy
  - Indicated if there is > 70% stenosis
  - Indicated if severely symptomatic even if < 70% stenosis

- Under general or local anaesthesia
- Shunt or patch
- Carotid angioplasty

Renovascular disease

Types

- Fibromuscular dysplasia
  - Non-inflammatory
  - Non-atheromatous
  - Segmental arteriopathy
- Atheromatous
  - Risk factors are same as for generalised atherosclerosis

Clinical presentation

- Incidental and non-significant
- Significant with normal serum creatinine
- Ischaemic renal disease

Investigations

- For incidental findings and those with normal creatinine
  - Renal scintigraphy
  - Renal duplex scan
- For those with renal disease
  - Intra-arterial digital subtraction angiography

Treatment

- PTA
- Endovascular stenting
- Surgery
  - Aorto-renal bypass
  - Endarterectomy
- Medical therapy
  - Anti-hypertensives (avoid angiotensin converting enzyme inhibitors)
  - Aspirin

Arterial embolism and acute limb ischaemia

Aetiology

- Underlying peripheral vascular disease is the most common cause

Risk factors

- The same as for peripheral vascular disease

Clinical features

- Mnemonic: '6 Ps'
  - Pain
  - Pallor
  - Pulselessness
  - Paralysis
  - Paraesthesia
  - Perishing cold
- Venous guttering
- Doppler signals: absence of Doppler-detectable venous flow indicates a poor prognosis

Investigations

- Routine baseline tests
- If time permits – digital subtraction angiography plus interventional thrombolysis; if not, on-table digital subtraction angiography
- Duplex ultrasound
  - For aortic and popliteal aneurysms
  - To assess run-off vessels

Management options

- Heparin
- Thrombolysis
  - Agents
    - Streptokinase
    - Tissue plasminogen activator (TPA)
    - Urokinase
  - Techniques
    - High-dose bolus
    - Pulse spray
    - Low-dose infusions
- Surgery
  - Fogarty's embolectomy
  - Intra-operative thrombolysis
  - Intra-operative angioplasty
  - Atherectomy
  - Reconstruction and/or fasciotomy
- Amputation

Aneurysms

Definition

- Abnormal localised dilatation of an artery or chamber of heart due to weakening of the wall

Classification

- According to structure

- True aneurysm: wall formed by layers of affected vessel
- False aneurysm: wall formed by connective tissue
- According to shape
  - Fusiform aneurysm: dilatation of segment of whole circumference
  - Saccular aneurysm: dilatation of only part of the circumference

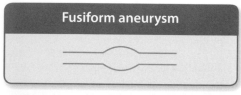

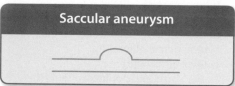

- According to cause
  - Berry aneurysm: congenital defect in the media at the junction of vessels around circle of Willis; may lead to subarachnoid haemorrhage
  - Atheromatous aneurysm: most common in the abdominal aorta
  - Mycotic aneurysm: associated with subacute infective endocarditis
  - Syphilitic aneurysm: common in the thoracic aorta
  - Dissection
    - In the thoracic aorta, caused by medial necrosis
    - Marfan's syndrome
    - Hypertension

False aneurysms

- Otherwise called pulsating haematomas
- Due to an injury causing a small defect
- Repaired by controlling the defect

Arteriovenous aneurysms

- Otherwise called aneurysmal varices
- Follows trauma or an arteriovenous fistula
- Causes
  - Distal increase in venous pressure
  - Distal ischaemia resulting from steal syndrome

Aortic dissection

Definition

- Entry and propagation of blood into the layers of the aortic wall as the result of an intimal tear

Plane of cleavage

- Initially an intimal tear
- Propagation phase: between the inner two thirds and the outer one third of the media

Classification

- Stanford's classification
  - Type A: involving only the ascending aorta
  - Type B: involving the descending aorta, with or without the ascending aorta
- DeBakey's classification
  - Type I: involving the ascending aorta, the arch and the descending aorta
  - Type II: confined to the ascending aorta
  - Type III: confined to the descending aorta beyond the origin of the subclavian artery

Pathology

- Myxoid degeneration: loss of elastic fibres, which are replaced by a proteoglycan-rich matrix
- Cystic medial necrosis, as a result of injury or occlusion of the vasa vasora

Predisposing factors

- Inherited defects of collagen
  - Marfan's syndrome
  - Ehlers–Danlos syndrome
  - Pseudoxanthoma elasticum
- Hypertension, which causes shearing forces across the intima
- Pregnancy, in which microscopic changes occur in the media
- Bicuspid aortic valve
- Traumatic aortic injury
- Iatrogenic
  - Cardiac catheterisation
  - Aortic cannulation for cardiac surgery
  - Aortic valve replacement

Outcomes

- Propagation

- Into the abdominal aorta
  - Gut ischaemia
  - Renal failure
- Into the intercostal or lumbar vessels
  - Spinal cord ischaemia (arteria radicularis magna)
- Into the carotid arteries
  - Stroke
- Into the coronary arteries
  - Angina or myocardial infarction
- Involvement of the aortic valve ring
  - – Acute aortic regurgitation
- Rupture
  - Into the pericardium
    - Cardiac tamponade
  - Into the pleura
    - Haemothorax
  - Into the abdomen
    - Retroperitoneal haemorrhage
- Compression of surrounding structures
  - Trachea
  - Oesophagus
  - Superior vena cava
- Re-entry through another intimal tear, resulting in a 'double-barrelled aorta'

Clinical features

- Cardiogenic or hypovolaemic shock
- New diastolic murmur from aortic regurgitation
- Cardiac tamponade (Beck's triad)
  - Muffled heart sounds
  - Increased central venous pressure (congested neck veins)
  - Decreased blood pressure
- Pulsus paradoxus
- Asymmetric pulse and/or blood pressure
- Stroke or spinal cord involvement

Investigations

- Aims
  - To make a definitive diagnosis
  - To discover:
    - Extent of the dissection
    - Presence of complications
    - Presence of any other co-morbidity
- ECG: to establish presence of myocardial infarction
- Chest X-ray, which (in 80% of cases) shows:
  - Widened mediastinum
  - Displacement of the aortic knuckle

- Depression of the left main bronchus
- Haemothorax
- Angiography ('gold-standard' investigation)
  - To determine extent of dissection
  - To assess coronary anatomy
  - To allow visualisation of ventricular and valve function
  - Disadvantages
    - Invasive
    - Contrast worsens renal function
- CT and MRI
  - 85–90% sensitivity and specificity
  - Disadvantage: no information on cardiac function
- Trans-oesophageal echocardiography
  - 95% sensitivity and specificity
  - Advantages
    - Used at bedside
    - Assesses cardiac and valve functions

Management

- 'ABC'
- Fluid resuscitation and control of blood pressure
  - Two wide-bored intravenous cannulae are inserted, and blood samples are taken for:
    - Baseline investigations
    - Cross match of 10 units of blood
  - Adequate intravenous fluids, ensuring a urine output of 30–40 mL/hour
  - Central venous line for monitoring
  - Labetalol for control of
    - Velocity of ejection fraction
    - Blood pressure
- Surgery
  - Replacement of diseased segment with a prosthetic graft
  - If aortic root is involved:
    - Re-implantation of coronary arteries in the graft
    - Aortic valve replacement or re-suspension
  - If arch is involved:
    - Deep hypothermic circulatory arrest, which is required for pressure control
  - Stenting in some instances
- For Stanford's type B aneurysms
  - Conservative management
  - Surgery confers no added benefits

Arterial trauma

Types

- Direct penetrating trauma
  - Stab wounds
  - Gunshot wounds
- Blunt trauma
  - Road traffic accidents
  - Violence
    - Laceration
    - Transection
    - Contusion
    - Spasm

Results

- Thrombosis
- Haematoma
- Pseudoaneurysm
- Traumatic arteriovenous fistula
- Partial transection results in more blood loss than complete transection, owing to loss of retraction of the vessel

Management

- 'ABC' of advanced trauma life support
- Prioritisation of other accompanying life-threatening injuries
- Brink's classification of severity of injury
  - Category I: patient in shock from ongoing haemorrhage
  - Category II: haemodynamically stable patient with potential for significant morbidity
  - Category III: clinically suspected injury in a stable patient
- Local clinical signs
  - History of persistent arterial bleeding
  - Large or expanding haematoma
  - Major haemorrhage with hypotension
  - Decreased or absent distal pulse
  - Injury to anatomically related nerves
  - Bruit at or distal to the suspected injury site
  - '5Ps' of distal ischaemia
    - Pain
    - Pallor
    - Pulselessness
    - Paralysis
    - Paraesthesia
- Timing of treatment should be ideally within 4–6 hours

- Biplanar angiography or digital subtraction angiography
- Interventional radiology
  - Vascular stents in intimal injuries
  - Graft-covered stents in full-thickness injuries
- Brink's category I trauma requires immediate operative intervention
- Brink's category II and category III trauma requires thorough and rapid evaluation including angiography

General operative principles

- Prepare and drape in anticipation of a vein graft
- Incision parallel to the injured vessel
- Balloon catheter thrombectomy prior to vascular repair
- Systemic heparinisation (50–75 units/kg) or local heparinisation if systemic is contraindicated
- Arterial repair
  - Simple lateral arteriorrhaphy
  - < 2 cm loss: resection and primary anastomosis
  - > 2 cm loss: autogenous vein or prosthetic material interposition; polytetrafluoroethylene (PTFE) is the most infection-resistant)
  - Accompanying venous injuries repaired

Varicosities

Definition

- Tortuous and dilated veins associated with valvular incompetence

Pathogenesis

- Poor support of venous wall
  - Familial
  - Obesity
  - Prolonged dependency
- Increased pressure within the lumen
  - Venous thrombosis
  - Pregnancy
  - Tumour compressing the vein

Clinical features

- Sapheno-femoral incompetence
- Sapheno-popliteal incompetence
- Perforator incompetence

Complications

- Superficial thrombophlebitis
- Venous eczema
- Lipodermatosclerosis
- Venous pigmentation, due to haemosiderin deposition
- Haemorrhage
- Stasis ulcer, which may become malignant (Marjolin's ulcer)

Lipodermatosclerosis

- Occurs in the skin of the gaiter area
- Clinical features
  - Pigmentation
  - Induration
  - Tenderness
  - Inflammation
- Pathogenesis
  - Persistent increased venous pressure in surface veins
  - Distension of the capillary bed
  - Fibrin deposition around capillaries
  - Prevents diffusion of O_2 and nutrients to tissues
  - Necrosis of subcutaneous fat
  - Tissues become fibrosed (sclerosis)

Varicose veins

Definition

- Permanently elongated, dilated and tortuous veins of the superficial venous system, usually affecting the lower limb

Assembly

- Superficial veins
  - Long saphenous vein
  - Short saphenous vein
- Deep vein
- Venous junctions
  - Sapheno-femoral junction
  - Sapheno-popliteal junction
- Perforators
  - Cockett's perforators: mid-thigh level
  - Boyd's perforators: below the knee
  - Dodd's perforators: above the ankle
- Muscle pump

Clinical features

- Feeling of heaviness in the legs
- Oedematous, restless legs
- Aches
- Muscle cramps
- Poor cosmesis

Complications

- Corona phlebectatica (ankle flare)
- Lipodermatosclerosis
- Atrophie blanche
- Oedema
- Haemorrhage
- Eczema
- Acute thrombophlebitis

Differential diagnosis

- For pain
  - Rheumatological disorders
  - Neurological disorders
  - Orthopaedic disorders
  - Lymphatic disorders
  - Arterial disorders
- For oedema
  - Lymphoedema

Clinical tests

- Schwartz tap test: for superficial valves
- Morrissey cough test: for saphena varix
- Trendelenburg test: for junctional incompetence
  - Sapheno-femoral junction
  - Sapheno-popliteal junction
- Modified Perthes test: for deep venous thrombosis (DVT)
- Fegan's test: for locating incompetent perforators

Investigations

- Hand-held Doppler
  - For all uncomplicated varicose veins
  - For sapheno-femoral junction incompetence: calf compression and release causes gurgle of > 0.5 seconds (enhanced by the Valsalva manoeuvre)
  - Less accurate for sapheno-popliteal incompetence
- Duplex ultrasound
  - For deep system (secondary varicose veins)

- For sapheno-popliteal junction
- For recurrent varicose veins
- For atypical varicose veins
- Other investigations
  - Plethysmography
  - Varicography
  - Ovarian phlebography

Treatment

- Reassurance, in asymptomatic patients
- Compression stockings
  - Advantages
    - Relieves symptoms
    - Conceals veins
    - Prevents deterioration of skin lesions
    - Decreases recurrence after surgery
    - Helps in differential diagnosis if signs and symptoms are not typical
  - Disadvantages
    - Poor compliance
    - Expensive
  - Classes of graduated compression stockings
    - Class I: < 25 mmHg of pressure, for heaviness and fatigue
    - Class II: 30–40 mmHg of pressure, for moderate oedema and post-sclerotherapy veins
    - Class III: 40–50 mmHg of pressure, for post-phlebitic limbs
    - Class IV: > 50 mmHg of pressure, for severe chronic venous insufficiency and lymphoedema
  - Pressures given by compression stockings
    - 100% at the ankle
    - 70% at the calf
    - 50% at the thigh
- Sclerotherapy
  - For residual non-stem veins
  - Agents
    - Sodium tetradecyl sulphate (STS), 0.1%, 0.2% or 0.3%
    - Polidocanol, 3%
    - Hypertonic saline
  - Empty vein completely before injecting and bandage for 6–8 weeks
  - Complications
    - Anaphylaxis

- Allergy
- Ulceration
- Arterial injury
- Pigmentation
- DVT
- Surgery
  - Only in symptomatic patients
  - Sapheno-femoral junction ligation
    - Groin crease incision
    - Ligate and divide all tributaries beyond secondary branching
    - Long saphenous vein flush ligated with femoral vein junction
    - Perforate invagination stripper (PIN stripper) is used, since this causes less haematoma and pain
    - Strip always from above downwards, but only to 4 cm below the knee, since below that, the saphenous nerve is likely to be injured
    - Feel the stripper in its entire course before stripping
  - Sapheno-popliteal junction ligation
    - Ligate deep to deep fascia
    - Close deep fascia
    - No stripping
    - The nerve likely to be injured is the common peroneal nerve
  - Subfascial endoscopic perforator surgery (SEPS)
    - Avoids incision through diseased skin
    - Post-operative compression bandage for 1 week

Complications of surgery

- Bruising
- Nerve injury
- Major vessel injury (from the stripper being in the wrong vein)
- Arterial injury
- DVT
- Wound problems

Recurrence

- 20% of cases
- Types
  - True recurrence: neovascularisation
  - False recurrence: technique failure

Venous ulcers

Differential diagnosis for leg ulcers

- Superficial venous incompetence
  - Primary
  - Secondary
- Ischaemic disease
  - Arterial obstructive disease
  - Pressure sores
- Trauma, burns
- Vasculitis
  - Rheumatoid arthritis
  - Scleroderma
- Neoplasia
  - Basal cell carcinoma
  - Squamous cell carcinoma
  - Kaposi's sarcoma
  - Melanoma
  - Epithelioma
- Neuropathic problems
  - Diabetes mellitus
  - Syringomyelia
  - Alcoholism
  - Paralysis
- Syphilis
- Tuberculosis
- Pyoderma gangrenosum
- Necrobiotic lipoidica
- Arteriovenous fistula or malformation
- Blood dyscrasia
  - Sickle cell disease
  - Leukaemia
  - Haemolytic jaundice
- Artefactual damage
- Marjolin's ulcer
- Tropical ulcer
- Primary skin disease

Distinguishing features of arterial and venous ulcers

Clinical features	Arterial	Venous
Age	>60 years	40–60 years
Risk factors	Smoking, diabetes mellitus, hyperlipidaemia hypertension	Previous DVT, thrombophilia, varicose veins
Past history	Peripheral, coronary and cerebrovascular disease	Overt or occult DVT (leg swelling after pregnancy, fracture, etc.)
Symptoms	Severe pain unless there is neuropathy, relieved by dependency	Not very severe pain, relieved by elevation
Site	Pressure areas	Medial 70% (gaiter area) Lateral 20% Both 10%
Edge	Regular, punched out, indolent	Irregular with neoepithelium
Base	Deep, sloughy or necrotic with no granulation tissue May comprise major tendon, bone or joint	Pink and granulating. May be covered with yellowish slough
Surrounding skin	Severe limb ischaemia	LDS, eczema, atrophie blanche
Veins	Empty, guttering on elevation	Full, varicose
Swelling	Absent	Present

Investigations

- Hand-held Doppler
- Duplex ultrasound
- Phlebography
  - Ascending
  - Descending
  - Varicography
- CT and magnetic resonance venography
- Ambulatory venous pressure measurement

Aims of dressing for venous ulcers

- To control (absorb) odour, exudate and/or bleeding
- To occlude pathogenic bacteria and to minimise colonisation
- To relieve pain
- To enhance the wound environment and speed up healing
- To protect the wound from further environmental or iatrogenic injury
- To maintain the wound at body temperature
- To reduce excessive scarring and/or recurrence
- To hide the wound from sight
- Dressings and topical agents are not helpful in ulcer healing

Venous dermatitis

- May represent an inflammatory or immunological response to substances that are not usually found in the skin but that are present as a result of venous hypertension
- Contact dermatitis is due to the application of external substances

Treatment

- Pharmacotherapy
  - Veno-active drugs, e.g. flavonoids
  - Antibiotics (if infection is present)
- Physical therapy
  - Elevation and bed rest
  - Exercise for calf muscles
  - Compression bandaging

Healing and recurrence

- 74% healing at 10–12 weeks with compression
- < 30% healing without compression

Surgery

- Debridement is of no value
- Skin grafting
  - If the base is healthy and venous insufficiency is corrected
  - Split skin and pinch grafting

Deep venous thrombosis (DVT)

- Common post-operative complication

Aetiology (Virchow's triad)

- Stasis
- Endothelial injury
- Hypercoagulable blood

Pathophysiology

- Aggregation of platelets in an area of stasis (valve pockets) or at an area of endothelial damage
- Activation of clotting cascade by surgical trauma: the fibrin produced overwhelms the fibrinolytic system

Sequelae

- Post-operative fatal pulmonary embolism at a rate of two in 1000 cases, which increases to five in 1000 for high-risk orthopaedic surgery
- Fatalities occur < 30 minutes after onset of symptoms
- Post-thrombotic syndrome in 60% of cases of proximal DVT and in 30% of cases of calf DVT

Risk factors

- Patient factors
  - Increasing age
  - Immobility (> 4 days)
  - Obesity
  - Malignancy
  - Previous or family history of deep

venous thrombosis or pulmonary embolism
- Previous DVT associated with oral contraceptive use or pregnancy
- Underlying surgical conditions
- Risk categorisation for proposed surgical procedures
  - Low risk (< 1%)
    - Surgeries under local anaesthesia
    - Day surgeries
  - Medium risk (1–10%):
    - Major general, urological, gynaecological or cardiothoracic surgery or neurosurgery
    - Major trauma
    - Minor surgery or trauma in patients with a previous history of venous thromboembolism or thrombophilia
  - High risk (10–60%)
    - Fracture or major surgery to the pelvis, hip or leg
    - Major pelvic or abdominal surgery for cancer
    - Major surgery in patients with a previous history of venous thromboembolism or thrombophilia
    - Critical lower limb ischaemia or amputation

Thromboprophylaxis

- To identify those at medium or high risk and to provide appropriate prophylaxis
- Methods
  - Mechanical
    - Graduated elastic compression stockings
    - Intermittent pneumatic compression devices
  - Pharmacological
    - Unfractionated heparin (5000 units subcutaneously every 8 hours)
    - Low-molecular-weight (LMW) heparin
    - Dose-adjusted warfarin
    - Dextran 70
    - Aspirin
  - In neurosurgery and ophthalmology, mechanical prophylaxis is preferred
  - Advantages of LMW heparin over unfractionated heparin

- Decreased risk of heparin-induced thrombocytopenia
- Monitoring is not necessary
- Once- or twice-daily dosing as against 8-hourly dosing or infusion
- Disadvantage of LMW heparin over unfractionated heparin
  - Less easy to reverse with protamine sulphate
- Duration of thromboprophylaxis
  - For proximal DVT and pulmonary embolism: 6 months
  - For calf DVT: 6 weeks
  - Continued if risk factor persists
- Classes of graduated compression stockings
  - Class I: < 25 mmHg of pressure, for heaviness and fatigue
  - Class II: 30–40 mmHg of pressure, for moderate oedema and post-sclerotherapy veins
  - Class III: 40–50 mmHg of pressure, for post-phlebitic limbs
  - Class IV: > 50 mmHg of pressure, for severe chronic venous insufficiency and lymphoedema
- Pressure given by compression stockings
  - 100% at the ankle
  - 70% at the calf
  - 50% at the thigh
- Mechanisms of action
  - Heparin
    - Increases affinity of antithrombin for thrombin and factor Xa
    - Leads to prolongation of the activated partial thromboplastin time (aPTT)
  - LMW heparin
    - Increases cleavage of factor Xa by antithrombin
    - So no prolongation of the aPTT
  - Warfarin
    - Inhibits vitamin K-dependent epoxide reductase
    - Prevents conversion of vitamin K-dependent factors (factors II, VII, IX and X)
  - Aspirin
    - Irreversibly inhibits cyclo-oxygenase
    - Prevents thromboxane-mediated platelet activation

Pulmonary embolism

- > 90% of pulmonary emboli are from lower limb DVT

Clinical features

- Acute dyspnoea, pleuritic chest pain and haemoptysis
- Low-grade fever, cyanosis, tachycardia, hypotension, tachypnoea and increased jugular venous pressure
- Sudden cardiovascular collapse in massive pulmonary embolism

Investigations

- Chest X-ray
  - To exclude other pathology
  - Pulmonary embolism shows as:
    - Atelectasis
    - Prominent hilar markings
    - Pleural effusion
- ECG
  - Right heart strain
  - Ischaemia
- Arterial blood gases
  - Hypoxia and hypocarbia
- Echocardiography
  - Right ventricular dyskinesia
- Angiography
  - Standard test for pulmonary embolism
  - Done through the pulmonary artery
  - Intraluminal filling defects and abrupt cut-off
- Ventilation–perfusion (V–Q) scanning
- CT angiography (more sensitive than V/Q scanning)

Treatment

- Intravenous thrombolysis
- Venous thrombectomy under intravenous heparinisation
- Pulmonary embolectomy

Lymphoedema
Definition

- Accumulation of tissue fluid caused by lymphatic obstruction or defective lymphatic drainage

Types

- Primary lymphoedema, due to aplasia or hypoplasia of the lymphatics
  - Congenital lymphoedema
    - Milroy's disease
    - Occurs shortly after birth
  - Lymphoedema praecox, which presents at puberty
  - Lymphoedema tarda, which presents at around 30 years of age
- Secondary lymphoedema, caused by damage to the lymphatic channels
  - Aetiology
    - Infection
    - Surgery
    - Radiotherapy
    - Malignant infiltration
    - Trauma
  - Special situations
    - Filarial lymphoedema: elephantiasis of lower limbs and scrotum
    - Small intestinal lymphoedema, due to malignant infiltration; causes decreased absorption of fat soluble vitamins
    - Thoracic duct lymphoedema: chylous effusions of the pleural and peritoneal cavities

Clinical staging

- Latent
  - Increased interstitial fluid
  - No apparent lymphoedema
- Stage I
  - Pitting oedema
  - Disappears on elevation
- Stage II
  - Non-pitting oedema
  - Does not disappear on elevation
- Stage III
  - Oedema associated with irreversible skin changes

Complications

- Infection
- Dermatophytosis and onychomycosis of the skin and nails
- Lymphangiectasia
- Lymphangiosarcoma

Factitious lymphoedema

- Causes
    - Application of tourniquet
    - Hysterical disuse

Investigations

- Laboratory
    - Full blood count
    - Renal function tests
    - Liver function tests
    - Autoimmune serology
    - Midnight sample for microfilariae
- Arterial Doppler scanning to rule out major disease
- Contrast lymphangiography
- Isotope lymphoscintigraphy
- CT and MRI

Treatment

- Elevation
- Reduction procedures
- Bypass procedures, e.g. lymphovenous bypass

Chapter 13   Skin

Soft tissue infections

Cellulitis

- Spreading infection in the subcutaneous tissue occurring after a skin abrasion or minor trauma
- Organisms
  - *Staphylococcus aureus* or beta-haemolytic streptococci
  - Both produce enzymes that degrade tissue and allow spread of infection
- Clinical features
  - Well-demarcated area of inflammation
  - Cardinal signs of acute inflammation, systemic signs, leukocytosis, lymphadenitis and localised skin necrosis
- Predisposing factors
  - Lymphoedema
  - Venous stasis
  - Diabetes mellitus
  - Surgical wounds
- Management
  - Rest and elevation
  - Antibiotics
    - Benzylpenicillin
    - Flucloxacillin

Necrotising soft tissue infections

- Caused by infection with virulent bacteria
- Toxins can cause widespread skin and fascial necrosis
- Infection spreads along fascial planes
- Meleney's synergistic gangrene
  - Around surgical wounds, stomas and cutaneous fistulae
  - Infection with both *S. aureus* and anaerobic streptococci
  - Initially indistinguishable from cellulitis
  - Skin ulceration
  - No systemic toxicity
  - Management
    - Antibiotics
    - Surgical debridement
- Necrotising fasciitis
  - Immunocompromised patients
    - Diabetes mellitus

- Alcoholism
- Intravenous drug abuse
- Sites
  - Limbs
  - Post-operative surgical wounds
  - Perineum (anorectal sepsis)
  - Male genitalia (Fournier's gangrene)
- Organisms
  - Facultative anaerobes
  - Streptococci
  - *Escherichia coli*
  - Anaerobes
- Exotoxins produce severe toxicity
- Clinical features
  - Severe pain
  - Severe toxicity
  - Cutaneous gangrene
  - Haemorrhagic fluid ooze from the wound
- If untreated, may result in multiple organ dysfunction syndrome (MODS), with a 30% mortality
- X-ray shows gas in the subcutaneous tissue
- Management
  - Antibiotics
  - Early debridement
  - Hyperbaric oxygen
- For MODS:
  - Fluids
  - Transfer to a high-dependency unit
  - Organ support

Benign skin lesions

Epidermoid cysts

- Sebaceous cysts
  - Derived from epidermis lining the hair follicle and sebaceous glands
- Unilocular dermal cysts, with punctum
  - Histologically – epidermal cells with keratin layers
- Steatocystoma multiplex: multiple cysts containing only sebum
- Treatment
  - Excision
  - If infected, incision and excision at a later date

Keratoacanthoma

- Rapidly growing nodule with a central crater containing a keratin plug
- Grows over 6 weeks and shrinks leaving a depressed scar
- Differential diagnosis is squamous cell carcinoma
- If it does not regress by 6 weeks, excision biopsy is needed

Molluscum contagiosum

- Caused by a pox virus of low virulence
- Affects children and young adults
- Crop of smooth umbilicated lesions up to 1 cm in diameter
- Treatment
  - Curettage
  - Cryotherapy
  - Topical trichloro-acetic acid

Warts

- Epithelial hyperplasia triggered by human papilloma virus (HPV)
- Commonly occurs on the hands of children and regresses spontaneously
- Treatment
  - Cryotherapy
  - Coagulation
  - Desiccation or surgical excision

Keloids

- Proliferation of fibrous tissue following trauma, surgical incision or burn
- Raised, red, sensitive area that transgresses the original margins of injury
- More common in black skin by a factor of 12:1
- Common areas are the back, neck, ear lobe, presternal skin and the deltoid area
- Histopathology shows an overgrowth of collagen with a disorganised fibrillar structure
- Treatment
  - Surgical excision leads to recurrence
  - Intralesional injection of corticosteroids
  - Specially designed, tight-fitting elastic garments providing continuous firm pressure

Actinic keratosis

- Also known as senile keratosis or solar keratosis

- Common in Caucasians
- Red, scaly patch
- Premalignant
- Excision only if there is an indication of malignant change

Benign pigmented naevus

- Intradermal, junctional and compound varieties
- Excision only when there is a possibility of malignancy

Skin cancer

Aetiology

- Exposure to ultraviolet light
- Genetic predisposition
- Immunosuppression (less recognised)

Classification

Classification according to the cell of origin

- Epidermal
  - Basal cell carcinoma
  - Squamous cell carcinoma
  - Melanoma
  - Merkel cell carcinoma (neuroendocrine)
- Constituents of dermis
  - Atypical fibroxanthoma
  - Dermatofibrosarcoma protuberans
  - Leiomyosarcoma
  - Angiosarcoma
  - Kaposi's sarcoma
- Adnexal
  - Eccrine sweat gland carcinoma
  - Sebaceous gland carcinoma
  - Cutaneous lymphomas
    - From T cells: mycosis fungoides
    - From B cells: marginal zone lymphoma, follicular lymphoma, diffuse large B-cell lymphoma
    - Metastatic cutaneous lymphoma

Malignant melanoma

- Definition: malignant proliferation of melanocytes arising from a pre-existing naevus or normal skin
- Melanocytes are cells of neuro-ectodermal origin and are found distributed along the epidermal basal layers of the skin and mucous membranes

- Incidence of melanoma
  - Higher in females
  - Higher in fair-skinned people
- Types of melanoma
  - Superficial spreading melanoma: 65% of cases
  - Nodular (amelanotic) melanoma: 10% of cases
  - Lentigo maligna (Hutchinson's freckle): 15% of cases
  - Acral lentiginous: melanoma < 5% of cases
  - (Rare: desmoplastic, neurotropic and uveal)
- Risk factors
  - Skin characteristics
    - Multiple benign naevi >100
    - Multiple atypical naevi
    - Giant pigmented hairy naevus: 20 cm diameter or covering > 50% of the body surface area
  - Genetic predisposition if more than three first-degree relatives are affected (caused by a mutation in the *CDKN2A* gene)
  - Previous skin cancer
  - Immunosuppression
  - Fitzpatrick skin type I, i.e. skin that burns without tanning
  - Exposure to sunlight
    - Intense intermittent exposure
    - Significant adult exposure, especially if associated with sunburn before the age of 10 years
    - Geographical location
- Clinical diagnosis
  - 'ABCDE' system
    - Asymmetry
    - Border irregularity
    - Colour variation
    - Diameter > 6 mm
    - Evolving lesion
  - UK 'seven point checklist'
    - Major criteria: change in size, irregular shape, irregular colour
    - Minor criteria: largest diameter > 7 mm, inflammation, oozing, change in sensation
    - If one major or three minor criteria are present, the lesion is suspicious of melanoma until proved otherwise

- Clinical suspicion
  - Increase in pigmentation
  - Increase in size
  - Bleeding
  - Ulceration or crusting
  - Spread of pigmentation
  - Red halo
  - Satellite lesions
  - Pain or itching
- Staging
  - Breslow's thickness
    - Measured as the maximum recordable dimensions (depth) from the granular layer of the epidermis to the base of the tumour (if the lesion is ulcerated, to the base of the ulcer)
    - It is preferred because the skin layers may be distorted by the tumour
    - Stage I: < 0.75 mm (> 95% cure rate)
    - Stage II: 0.76–1.49 mm (90% cure rate)
    - Stage III: 1.5–3.0 mm (50% cure rate)
    - Stage IV: > 3.0 mm (< 40% cure rate)
  - Clarke's levels
    - Measured as the depth of dermal invasion in reference to normal skin layers
    - Stage I: only in the epidermis, above the basement membrane (*in situ*)
    - Stage II: invasion of the basement membrane into the papillary dermis
    - Stage III: invasion of the papillary dermis into the papillary–reticular junction
    - Stage IV: invasion of the reticular dermis
    - Stage V: invasion of the subcutaneous fat
  - TNM staging
    - Tx: tumour cannot be assessed
    - T0: no primary
    - Tis: melanoma *in situ* (equivalent to Clarke's stage I)
    - T1: up to the papillary dermis (equivalent to Clarke's stage II)
    - T2: up to the reticular dermis (equivalent to Clarke's stage III)
    - T3: invading the reticular dermis (equivalent to Clarke's stage IV)
    - T4: up to the subcutaneous fat (equivalent to Clarke's stage V)

- Nx: nodes cannot be assessed
- N0: no nodes
- N1: regional nodes
- N2: Second level nodes
- N3: distant nodes
- Mx: metastases cannot be assessed
- M0: no metastases
- M1: distant metastases with or without in-transit metastases
- B1: with ulceration
- B2: without ulceration
  - American Joint Committee on Cancer (AJCC) staging
    - Stage 0: *in situ* (equivalent to Tis N0 M0)
    - Stage IA: equivalent to Breslow's stage I and to T1 N0 M0
    - Stage IB: equivalent to Breslow's stage II and to T2 N0 M0
    - Stage IIA: equivalent to Breslow's stage III and to T3 N0 M0
    - Stage IIB: equivalent to Breslow's stage IV and to T4 N0 M0
    - Stage IIIA: any size, one to three microscopic lymph nodes, no distant mets (equivalent to T_{ANY} N1 M0)
    - Stage IIIB: any size, with satellites or in-transit metastases, one to three macroscopic lymph nodes (equivalent to T_{ANY} N2 M0)
    - Stage IIIC: with ulceration
    - Stage IV: distant metastases (equivalent to T_{ANY} N_{ANY} M1)

Malignant melanoma: prognostic factors

Factor	Adverse criteria
Nodal involvement	Worse with the number of nodes involved
Thickness	>4 mm
Mitoses	>10/mm^2
Ulceration	Yes
Age	Increasing age
Site	Head > neck > trunk
Sex	Male

Principles of skin cover

Principles of wound management

- Assessment of the patient
  - Nutrition
  - Anaemia (needs to be corrected)
  - Diabetes mellitus
- Assessment of the area
  - Ischaemia (needs to be corrected)
  - Insensate foot (mandates a change of shoes)
  - Sinus over osteomyelitis (needs bone debridement)
- Assessment of the wound
  - Necrotic tissue
  - Debris leads to contamination
    - Irrigation by pulsating jet lavage
    - If > 100,000 organisms/g of tissue are present, the take of grafts and primary healing is poor
    - Needs debridement
    - 'Second-look policy', 24–48 hours later

Closure of acute wounds

- Primary or delayed primary closure
- Secondary closure
- Tertiary closure

Reconstructive ladder

- Conservative management
  - Fingertip injuries in children
  - Acute pressure sores
  - Patient not fit for surgery
  - Uncorrectable local factors
- Direct closure
  - Good approximation of dermis
  - Tension-free
  - Interrupted: only on the face
- Skin grafts
  - Definition
    - Transfer of a segment of skin that has been separated from its blood supply
  - Types
    - Split-thickness grafts
    - Full-thickness grafts: especially in the face
  - Criteria
    - Thinner grafts require less nutrition and are more likely to take

- Vascularised, non-infected wounds, clean granulation tissue or wounds created following tissue excision
- Immobilisation following grafting
- Donor tissue should match recipient skin in colour and texture
- Grafting should not be done on bone without periosteum, on denuded cartilage or on irradiated wounds
- Bacterial load of > 100,000/g of tissue will mean that the graft will not take
- Seromas and haematomas should be avoided by meshing of the graft
  - Protected skin graft blades
    - Dermatome
    - Humby knife
    - Watson and Cobbett modification
- Tissue expansion
  - Principles: tissue's ability to stretch and proliferate under continuous moderate tension
  - Procedure
    - Subdermal insertion of a tissue expander (soft silicone bag)
    - After 6–8 weeks, excess tissue is designed as flap for closure of the defect
- Flaps
  - Definition: skin that retains its blood supply and that is used to cover wounds on an avascular bed that is unlikely to support a skin graft

- Random-pattern flaps
  - No specific blood vessel in the pedicle
  - Nourishment is through dermal plexus
  - Length of the flap should not be > 1.5–2 times the width of its base
- Axial flap
  - Artery and its accompanying venae comitantes are included in the base of the flap
  - Deltopectoral flap, based on perforating vessels of internal mammary
  - Forehead flap based on anterior branch of superficial temporal artery
- Myocutaneous flap
  - Survival of skin overlying a muscle is possible because of the presence of a pedicle of muscle consisting of its dominant vessel
  - Examples of muscles that can be used: latissimus dorsi, pectoralis major and rectus abdominis
- Fascial flaps
  - Based on perforating vessels at the deep fascia
  - For repairing defects in the lower limbs
- Free flaps
  - By microvascular reconstruction

Pathophysiology

Three concentric zones

- Zone of coagulation
- Zone of stasis
- Zone of hyperaemia

Degrees of burns

- First-degree burn
  - Erythema
- Second-degree burn
  - Superficial partial thickness burn but basal layer not destroyed
  - Deep partial thickness burn
    - Basal layer destroyed
    - Will heal under optimal conditions
- Third-degree burn
  - Full-thickness burn
- Fourth-degree burn
  - Injury to the subcutaneous tissues

Pathology

- Microscopic picture
  - Coagulation–necrosis of cells
  - Thrombosis of vessels
  - Accumulation of fluid and infiltrates
- Destruction of tissues (depth depends on heat of causative agent and contact time)
  - Loss of barrier to infection
  - Fluid loss from surface
  - Red blood cell destruction
- Release of mediators
  - Vasoactive amines
  - Prostaglandins
  - Leukotrienes
  - O_2 free radicals
  - Cytokines: interleukin (IL)-1, IL-2, IL-6
- Increased capillary permeability all over the body
  - Greatest in the first 12 hours
  - Oedema
  - Third space sequestration
  - Loss of circulating fluid volume
  - Hypovolaemic shock
- Increased metabolic rate

Consequences of burns

Early consequences

- Hypovolaemia (loss of protein, fluids and electrolytes)
- Metabolic derangements
  - Hyponatraemia leading on to hypernatraemia
  - Hyperkalaemia leading on to hypokalaemia
- Sepsis (local or generalised)
- Haemolysis leading to anaemia
- Hypothermia

Short-term consequences

- Acute tubular necrosis, due to:
  - Hypovolaemia
  - Haemoglobinuria
  - Myoglobinuria
- Respiratory failure, due to:
  - Smoke inhalation
  - Airway obstruction
  - Acute respiratory distress syndrome (ARDS)
- Catabolism, nutritional depletion
- Venous thrombosis
- Cushing's ulcer and/or erosive gastritis

Long-term consequences

- Permanent disfigurement
- Hypertrophic scars and contractures
- Prolonged hospitalisation
- Psychological problems
- Impaired function

Systemic response to burns

Cardiovascular responses

- Decreased cardiac output, due to:
  - Alteration in Starling's forces and oedema
  - Release of myocardial depressant substances
- Fluid loss, which leads to burns shock

- Progressive anaemia, due to:
  - Loss of red blood cells
  - Trapping of red blood cells
  - Microangiopathic haemolytic anaemia

Renal responses

- Hypovolaemia and myoglobinuria, which lead to acute renal failure

Pulmonary responses

- Upper airway oedema and obstruction
- Ventilation–perfusion imbalance
- Pulmonary oedema, leading to ARDS

Gastrointestinal responses

- Reflex ileus and acute gastric dilatation
- Ulceration as a result of mucosal ischaemia

Musculoskeletal responses

- Osteoporosis
- Demineralisation

Neuroendocrine responses

- Catecholamine-mediated hypermetabolism
- Increased corticosteroids, leading to Na$^+$ and water conservation

Metabolic and nutritional responses

- Hypermetabolism

Immune system responses

- Decreased cellular immunity
- Lymphopenia

Psychiatric responses

- Depression
- Psychosis

Initial clinical assessment of burns

- 'ABCD' of acute trauma life support
- Treatment of immediate life-threatening problems
- History and physical examination
- Age: extremes of age have greater mortality and morbidity

- Extent of burn
  - Only partial-thickness and full-thickness
  - Wallace's 'rule of 9' (with modification in children)
- Depth of burn
  - Superficial burns
    - Painful
    - Erythematous
    - Blanching of tissues
    - Blisters
  - Deep burns
    - Thick-walled blisters
    - Non-blanching wound bed
    - Dry, leathery eschar
    - Absent pin-prick sensation
- Location of burn
  - Primary areas
    - Head and neck
    - Hands
    - Feet
    - Perineum
    - Genitalia
- Inhalation injury
  - History of confinement in closed space with heavy smoke
  - Singed nasal vibrissae
  - Conjunctivitis
  - Pharyngeal oedema
  - Hoarseness and stridor
- Co-morbid factors
  - Associated trauma
  - Cardiovascular, renal, respiratory and metabolic diseases
  - Seizures
  - Alcohol and drug addiction
  - Pre-admission hypovolaemia

Clinical categorisation of burns

	Major	Moderate	Minor
Partial thickness	>25%	10-25%	<15%
Full thickness	>10%	2-10%	<2%
Primary area	Yes	No	No
Inhalation	Yes	No	No
Comorbidity	Yes	No	No
Associated injury	Yes	No	No

Management of burns

- 'ABC' of advanced trauma life support
- Tetanus prophylaxis
- Two wide-bore cannulae are inserted and blood is drawn for basic laboratory work
- Fluid resuscitation
  - Crystalloids initially
  - Colloids after 24 hours
  - Blood
- Urinary catheter
- Relief of pain and anxiety
- Local wound management
  - Cold water and saline irrigation
  - Debridement of blisters
  - Absorbent dressing
  - Elevation of extremity
  - Surgical escharotomy if indicated
- Enteral or parenteral nutrition

Parkland's formula for fluid resuscitation

- Volume of fluid: 2–4 mL/kg body weight multiplied by the percentage of total body surface area burnt
- First half of the volume, given in the first 8 hours as lactated Ringer's solution
- Second half of the volume, given in the next 16 hours
- After 24 hours
  - Dextrose and water
  - Colloid to replace remaining plasma volume (0.5 mL/kg multiplied by the percentage of total body surface area burnt

Assessment of adequate resuscitation

- Urine output 30–50 mL/hour in an adult or 1 mL/kg/hour in a child
- Clear, lucid sensorium
- Pulse rate < 120 beats/minute
- Haematocrit < 60%

Monitoring

- Central venous pressure line
- Swan–Ganz catheter

Respiratory management

- O_2 with F_iO_2 of 100%

- Indirect laryngoscopy and intubation, with intermittent positive-pressure ventilation (IPPV) if indicated
- Escharotomy if indicated

Nutritional management

- Nitrogen: 20 g/day/percentage of total body surface area burnt
- 25 kcal/kg/day plus 40 kcal/day/percentage of total body surface area burnt
- Ascorbic acid 1 g, thiamine 50 mg, riboflavin 50 mg, nicotinamide 50 mg, plus vitamins A and D

Burn wound management

- Initial cooling, cleaning and debridement
- Early excision and grafting
- Occlusive or open dressing
- Biological dressings:
  - Allograft skin
  - Xenograft skin
  - Amniotic membrane
- Prevention of contracture
  - Splinting in optimal position
  - Range-of-motion exercises

Complications of burns

- Renal failure
- Inhalation injury: three types
  - Pulmonary complications and death within 45 seconds
  - Oedematous response resulting from noxious gases, with immediate death
  - Progressive hypoxia and hypercarbia: several hours after admission
- Other pulmonary complications
  - Atelectasis
  - Pneumonia
  - Pulmonary emboli
  - Emphysema
  - Pneumothorax
  - Pulmonary oedema
- Hyperglycemia
- Gastroduodenal ulceration with bleeding
- Biliary stasis and acalculous cholecystitis
- Bacterial, viral and fungal infections of the lung and burn wound

Congenital neck lumps

Thyroglossal cyst

- Most common condition arising from persistence of remnants of the thyroglossal tract
- Infection, rupture, drainage of the cyst or incomplete removal leads to sinus formation
- Intimately related to the hyoid bone
- Clinically causes a midline swelling that moves with deglutition
- Diagnosis is confirmed by ultrasound
- Treatment: removal of cyst together with the track and the hyoid bone (Sistrunk's operation)
- May develop papillary carcinoma of thyroid

Branchial apparatus abnormalities

- Fistula
  - Persistence of second pouch and breakdown of epithelium
  - Opens externally in the lower third of the neck anterior to the sternocleidomastoid muscle
  - Infection leads to abscess
  - Should be removed if symptomatic
- Cyst
  - Presents in the third decade
  - 60% are on the left
  - Site: anterior border of the sternocleidomastoid muscle at the junction of the upper one third and the lower two thirds
  - Complications: infection and pressure effects
  - Diagnosed by fine-needle aspiration cytology, CT scanning or MRI
  - Surgical removal
- Carcinoma
  - Derived from ectopic squamous epithelium

Neurogenic tumours

- Derived from neural crest cells
- Classification

- Neurofibromas
  - von Recklinghausen's disease
  - Plexiform tumours
- Schwannomas
- Paragangliomas (chemodectoma)
- Carotid body tumours
- Glomus tumours of the vagus
- Carotid body tumours
  - At the bifurcation of common carotid artery
  - High incidence in population at high altitude
  - Slow-growing
  - Transmitted pulsation
  - Diagnosed by CT scan, MRI or angiograph; check for other paragangliomas
  - Removed if possible

Lymphangiomas

- From sequestration of lymphoid tissue derived from primary lymph sacs
- Classification
  - Simplex: oral cavity tumours
  - Cavernous: oral cavity tumours
  - Cystic hygromas
    - Cervicofacial
    - Infiltrates tissue planes
    - Small: treatment is by excision
    - Large: injection of OK432 after aspiration

Dermoid cysts

- Epidermoid cysts
- Dermoid cysts occur in the midline
- Teratoid cysts
- Excision is the treatment of choice

Laryngocoeles

- Caused by a remnant of the lateral laryngeal sac, which distends to form a laryngocoele
- May have co-existing carcinoma
- If large, cause stridor
- Treatment is by excision

Inflammatory swellings

- Cat-scratch disease
- Toxoplasmosis

- Brucellosis
- Infectious mononucleosis
- Tuberculosis
  - Cold abscess
  - Collar-stud abscess
  - Sinus

Malignant neck swellings

- Levels of neck nodes
  - Level I: submental nodes
  - Level II: upper jugular nodes (skull base to carotid bifurcation)
  - Level III: middle jugular nodes (carotid bifurcation to cricothyroid membrane)
  - Level IV: lower jugular nodes (cricothyroid membrane to clavicle)
  - Level V: posterior triangle nodes
  - Level VI: anterior compartment nodes

Salivary gland disorders

Infections and inflammations

- Mumps
  - More common in children
  - Incubation period: 21 days
  - Diffuse bilateral interstitial parotid inflammation (occasionally unilateral)
  - 20% have submandibular and other gland involvement
  - May lead to epididymo-orchitis or meningo-encephalitis
- Acute bacterial sialadenitis
  - Infection from the oral cavity
  - Predisposing factors
    - Poor dental hygiene
    - Periodontal abscess
    - Hyposecretion of saliva
    - Stones in the duct with obstruction
  - Risk factors
    - Extremes of age: more common in neonates and the elderly
    - Post-surgery
  - Clinical features
    - Fever, trismus and dysphagia
    - Painful enlargement of the salivary gland
  - Organisms
    - *Staphylococcus aureus*
    - *Streptococcus viridans*
    - *Escherichia coli*

- Treatment
  - Broad-spectrum antibiotics
  - Restoration of good oral hygiene
  - Removal of duct stones
  - Drainage of abscess

Tumours

- 80% involve the parotid gland
- 60% are benign
- Pleomorphic adenoma
  - Superficial lobe is commonly affected
  - Slow-growing, painless mass
  - Facial nerve is not involved
  - Histology: epithelial and stromal cells
    - Rich in proteoglycans
    - From myoepithelial cells
  - False capsule of connective tissue and glandular tissue
  - Treatment is by excision, preserving the facial nerve
  - Recurrence if the false capsule is breached
  - Recurred tumour may encapsulate the facial nerve
- Warthin's tumour
  - Adenolymphoma characterised by cystic spaces surrounded by eosinophilic columnar cells
  - Stroma contains lymphoid follicles
  - Malignant transformation is rare
  - Treatment is by surgical removal
- Muco-epidermoid tumour
  - Most common malignant tumour of the parotid
  - Sheets of squamous cells and tumour-containing cells surrounding cystic spaces
  - May metastasise to lymph nodes, brain and lungs
- Adenocystic carcinoma
  - From myoepithelial cells and cells of the intercalated ducts
  - Submandibular and minor glands are affected more frequently than the parotid glands
  - Histology: cribriform appearance
  - Early perineural invasion is common, causing facial palsy
  - Eradication is difficult, owing to the local infiltration

Stones (sialolithiasis)

- Primary calculi
  - More common in the submandibular glands
  - Contain phosphate and carbonate
  - Caused by stasis and changes in the physicochemical characteristics of the saliva
- Secondary calculi
  - Hyperparathyroidism
  - Hyperuricaemia
  - Hypercalcaemia
- Clinical features:
  - Recurrent and progressive glandular swelling, initially associated with meals
  - Stones are felt along the duct on palpation
  - Calculi are radio-opaque
- Treatment
  - Distal: excision and marsupialisation
  - Proximal: excision of gland and duct

Miscellaneous salivary gland conditions

- Sjögren's syndrome
  - Clinical syndrome affecting salivary and lacrimal glands, associated with dry eyes (keratoconjunctivitis sicca) and dry mouth (xerostomia)
  - Associated with rheumatoid arthritis, systemic lupus erythematosus and other systemic autoimmune diseases
  - Painless progressive enlargement of glands
  - Microscopic appearance
    - Glandular atrophy
    - Lymphocyte infiltration
    - Duct proliferation
  - Risk of developing lymphoma

Chapter 16

Respiratory system

Surface anatomy and lung anatomy

Angle of Louis

- Junction of the manubrium and the body of the sternum
- Articulation of second costal cartilage
- Corresponds to:
  - Lower border of T4
  - Bifurcation of the trachea
  - Meeting of the two pleural sacs
  - Start and end of the aortic arch (the highest point of the arch is at the middle of the manubrium in an adult)

Suprasternal notch

- Lower border of T2

Third intercostal space

- Important for internal mammary artery ligation

Oblique fissure

- From the sixth costochondral junction along sixth rib to meet the T3 spinous process

Horizontal fissure

- Only seen on the right side
- From the fourth costochondral junction along the fourth rib to join the oblique fissure at the fifth rib in the midaxillary line

Lobes and segments of the lung

- Right lung
  - Upper lobe
    - Apical segment
    - Anterior segment
    - Posterior segment
  - Middle lobe
    - Lateral segment
    - Medial segment
  - Lower lobe
    - Superior (apical) segment
    - Inferior segment (with lateral, medial, posterior and anterior parts)

- Left lung
  - Upper lobe
    - Apical segment
    - Anterior segment
    - Posterior segment
    - Superior lingular segment
    - Inferior lingular segment
  - Lower lobe: same as the right lower lobe

Dead space

Definition

- The volume of inspired air that is not involved in gas exchange, i.e. ventilated areas without perfusion
- The proportion of tidal volume that does not participate in gas exchange

Types

- Anatomical dead space
  - Formed by gas conducting airways that are not involved in gas exchange
    - Mouth and nasal cavity
    - Larynx and pharynx
    - Trachea and upper bronchial airways, up to the first 16 generations
- Alveolar dead space
  - Formed by the alveoli that are being ventilated but not perfused and so not contributing to gas exchange
  - Occurs mainly at the top of the lung in the erect posture
- Physiologic dead space
  - The sum of the anatomic and alveolar dead spaces
  - Normally it is 2–3 mL/kg of body weight

Importance

- If the dead space is large, it can interfere with breathing, as the body works to ventilate the lungs and the ventilated air does not take part in gas exchange, i.e. a ventilation–perfusion (V–Q) mismatch

Factors increasing anatomical dead space

- Increased size of the subject (obesity)
- Standing posture
- Increased lung volumes, e.g. in chronic obstructive pulmonary disease (COPD), which causes air trapping
- Bronchodilatation

Factors increasing alveolar dead space

- Hypotension and hypoventilation
- Emphysema and pulmonary embolism
- Positive-pressure ventilation

Diaphragm

- Origin
- Anterior: the xiphoid
- Lateral: the lower 6 costal cartilages
- Posterior
  - Medial and lateral lumbocostal arches
  - Median arcuate ligament
  - Bodies of upper three lumbar vertebrae
- Insertion: central tendon

Nerve supply

- Phrenic nerve (from C3, C4 and C5): motor supply plus sensory supply to the central part
- Lower six intercostal nerves: sensory supply to the periphery

Openings

- Aortic opening: centrally at the T12 level
  - Transmits the aorta, the azygos vein and the thoracic duct

- Oesophageal opening: to the left of the midline a the T10 level
  - Transmits the oesophagus, the right and left vagus nerves and the oesophageal branch of left gastric artery
  - The left vagus nerve is anterior to the oesophagus; the right vagus nerve is posterior to the oesophagus
- Inferior vena cava opening: to the right of the midline at the T8 level
  - Transmits the inferior vena cava and the phrenic nerve

Respiration

Definition

- Process of exchange of O_2 and CO_2 within the lungs
- Types
  - External respiration: respiration of the body as a whole
  - Internal respiration: respiration at the cellular level

Components

- Transport of O_2 and CO_2 by the circulation
- Gas exchange across the alveolar capillary membrane
- Mechanics of breathing required to produce an effective inspiration and expiration
- Nervous and chemical control of the respiratory centre (the respiratory drive)

Main respiratory muscles

- Diaphragm
- Intercostal muscles

Accessory muscles

- Muscles of the neck and shoulder girdle
- Abdominal muscles

Diaphragmatic descent

- 1.5 cm in quiet breathing
- Up to 10 cm in deep breathing
- Increases the longitudinal thoracic diameter

Gas exchange

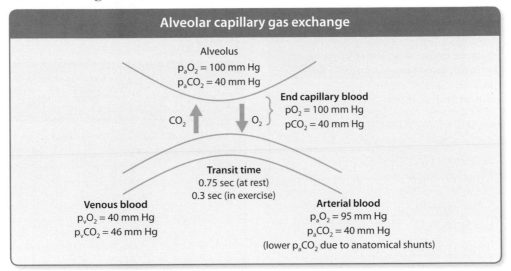

Alveolar capillary gas exchange

Alveolus
$p_aO_2 = 100$ mm Hg
$p_aCO_2 = 40$ mm Hg

End capillary blood
$pO_2 = 100$ mm Hg
$pCO_2 = 40$ mm Hg

CO_2 O_2

Transit time
0.75 sec (at rest)
0.3 sec (in exercise)

Venous blood
$p_vO_2 = 40$ mm Hg
$p_vCO_2 = 46$ mm Hg

Arterial blood
$p_aO_2 = 95$ mm Hg
$p_aCO_2 = 40$ mm Hg
(lower p_aCO_2 due to anatomical shunts)

Intercostal muscles

- Bucket-handle movement
  - Lowers the ribs
  - Increases transverse diameter of the chest
- Pump handle movement
  - Affects the upper two ribs
  - Increases anteroposterior diameter of the chest

Expiratory muscles

- Internal intercostal muscles
  - Contract during forced expiration
- Abdominal muscles
  - Rectus abdominis
  - Internal and external obliques
  - Transversus

Partial pressures

Definition

- Pressure exerted by any one gas in a mixture of gases

Gaseous composition of dry air

- O_2: 20.98%
- CO_2: 0.04%
- NO_2: 78.06%
- Argon and helium (inert): 0.92%

Atmospheric pressure

- Atmospheric pressure at sea level: 760 mmHg (1 atmosphere)
- pO_2 of air: $0.21 \times 760 = 160$ mmHg
- pN_2 of air: $0.79 \times 760 = 600$ mmHg
- pCO_2 of air: $0.0004 \times 760 = 0.3$ mmHg

High altitude

- Composition of the air is the same
- However, the barometric pressure is decreased
- Therefore, pO_2 is decreased
- At 3000 m, alveolar pO_2 is 60 mmHg

Intrapleural pressure

- Normal: 2.5 mmHg
- At the start of inspiration: minus 6 mmHg
- In forced inspiration: down to minus 32 mmHg

Lung volumes and capacities

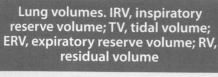

Lung volumes. IRV, inspiratory reserve volume; TV, tidal volume; ERV, expiratory reserve volume; RV, residual volume

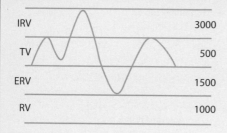

IRV	3000
TV	500
ERV	1500
RV	1000

Lung capacities

- Abbreviations
  - Inspiratory capacity: IC
  - Inspiratory reserve volume: IRV
  - Tidal volume: TV
  - Vital capacity: VC
  - Expiratory reserve volume: ERV
  - Functional residual capacity: FRC
  - Residual volume: RV
  - Total lung capacity: TLC
- IC = IRV + TV = 3000 mL + 500 mL
  = 3500 mL
- VC = IC + ERV = 3500 mL + 1500 mL
  = 5000 mL
- FRC = ERV + RV = 1500 mL + 1000 mL
  = 2500 mL
- TLC = VC + RV = 5000 mL + 1000 mL
  = 6000 mL
- Minute volume = TV × respiratory rate (12 breaths/minutes) = 0.5 L × 12
  = 6 L/minute
- Alveolar ventilation = (500 − 150) mL × 12
  = 4.2 L/min

Measurement of FRC

- Gas dilution method
- N_2 washout

FEV–FEV1 ratio

- Normal: 0.7 (70%)
- Obstructive lung disease: < 70%
- Restrictive lung disease: ≥ 70%

Partial pressures of gases in various parts of the respiratory and circulatory systems (mmHg)

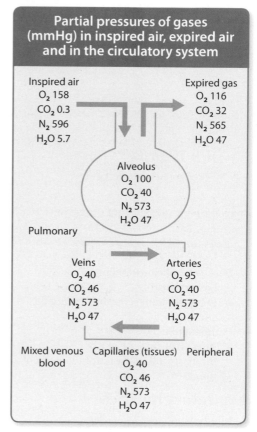

Partial pressures of gases (mmHg) in inspired air, expired air and in the circulatory system

Inspired air
O_2 158
CO_2 0.3
N_2 596
H_2O 5.7

Expired gas
O_2 116
CO_2 32
N_2 565
H_2O 47

Alveolus
O_2 100
CO_2 40
N_2 573
H_2O 47

Pulmonary

Veins
O_2 40
CO_2 46
N_2 573
H_2O 47

Arteries
O_2 95
CO_2 40
N_2 573
H_2O 47

Mixed venous blood   Capillaries (tissues)   Peripheral
O_2 40
CO_2 46
N_2 573
H_2O 47

O_2 partial pressures

- In the atmosphere: 21 kPa
- In the trachea: 19 kPa
- In the alveoli: 14 kPa
- In the arteries: 13.3 kPa

CO_2 partial pressures (kPa)

- In the atmosphere: 0.03 kPa
- In the alveoli: 5.3 kPa
- In the arteries: 5.3 kPa
- In the veins: 6.1 kPa
- In exhaled air: 4 0.03

Pressure difference between the pulmonary capillaries and the oncotic pressure

- Pulmonary capillary pressure: 10 mmHg
- Oncotic pressure: 25 mmHg
- This difference in pressure of 15 mmHg keeps the alveoli free of fluid

Oxyhaemoglobin dissociation curve

- P50
  - 50% haemoglobin saturation
  - p$_a$O$_2$: 26 mmHg
  - Steepest point of the oxyhaemoglobin dissociation curve
  - Most sensitive point for detecting a curve shift
  - Index of O$_2$ affinity
- Causes of right shift (Bohr effect)
  - Anaemia
  - Heat (increased body temperature)
  - Increased CO$_2$
  - Acidosis
  - Increased 2,3-diphosphoglycerate (2,3-DPG)
- Causes of left shift
  - Opposite causes to right shift
  - Carbon monoxide
  - Abnormal haemoglobin
- Advancing age
  - Normal p$_a$O$_2$: 60 mmHg
  - Normal haemoglobin: 90% saturated

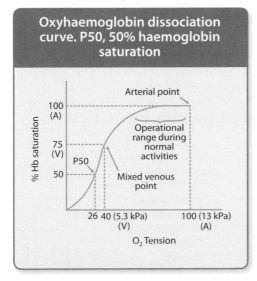

Oxyhaemoglobin dissociation curve. P50, 50% haemoglobin saturation

Quaternary function of haemoglobin

- Each O$_2$ molecule added facilitates the uptake of the next O$_2$ molecule
- This gives rise to the sigmoid shape of the O$_2$ dissociation curve

O$_2$ tension

- Arterial O$_2$ tension: 13 kPa (98 mmHg)
- Venous O$_2$ tension: 5.3 kPa (40 mmHg)
- Tissue O$_2$ tension: 5.3 kPa
- Alveolar gas O$_2$ tension: 13 kPa
- Gradient of 8 kPa between alveolar and venous oxygen tension which facilitates oxygen diffusion from alveolus to venous blood, which then becomes arterial blood
- Gradient of 8 kPa between arterial and tissue oxygen tension which facilitates oxygen diffusion from arterial blood to tissues
- When fully saturated, each gram of normal haemoglobin contains 1.34 mL of O$_2$

O$_2$ cascade

- Definition: incremental drops in pO$_2$ from the atmosphere to the arterial blood
- Atmosphere: 21 kPa
- Trachea: 19.8 kPa
- Alveolar air: 14 kPa
- Arteries: 13.3 kPa
- Relevance
  - Gas diffuses from areas of high pressure to areas of low pressure
  - The cascade facilitates diffusion of O$_2$ from the atmosphere down to the alveoli, and then to arterial blood

CO$_2$ transport

- Arterial pCO$_2$: 40 mmHg (5.3 kPa)
- Venous pCO$_2$: 46 mmHg (6 kPa)
- CO$_2$ is 20 times more soluble than O$_2$
- Therefore, the 6 mmHg difference is sufficient to permit adequate uptake

Steps in CO$_2$ transport

- CO$_2$ enters red blood cells:
  - With haemoglobin, as carbamino-haemoglobin
  - As carbonic acid
- Carbonic acid dissociates into H$^+$ (taken up by reduced haemoglobin) and HCO$_3^-$

- The lower alveolar pCO_2 (40 mmHg) compared with the venous pCO_2 (46 mmHg) favours release

Haldane effect

- Binding of O_2 to haemoglobin reduces its affinity for CO_2
- Therefore, venous blood carries more CO_2 than arterial blood, causing the gradient

Transport of CO_2

- CO_2 is transported as:
  - HCO_3 ions
  - Carbamino compounds
  - Physically, dissolved in solution: $CO_2 + H_2O \rightarrow H_2CO_3 \rightarrow H^+ + HCO_3^-$
- H_2CO_3 generates H^+ within red blood cells
- Carbamino compounds are bound with haemoglobin
- Both these reduce O_2 affinity
- Therefore venous blood has more CO_2 than arterial blood
- HCO_3 diffuses out of red blood cells, causing Cl^- to enter the cells (the 'chloride shift')

Changes in pCO_2 along the respiratory tree

- Venous pCO_2: 6.1 kPa
- Arterial pCO_2: 5.3 kPa
- Alveolar pCO_2: 5.3 kPa
- pCO_2 of exhaled air: 4 kPa
- pCO_2 of atmospheric air: 0.03 kPa

Arterial blood gases

Normal values at a body temperature of 37 °C

- pH: 7.36–7.44 (H^+: 44–36 mmol/L)
- p_aO_2: 75-100 mmHg (10–13.3 kPa)
- p_aCO_2: 35–42 mmHg (4.6-5.6 kPa)
- HCO_3^-: 22–26 mmol/L
- Base excess: ± 2

Interpretation

- pH
  - Increased in acadaemia
  - Decreased in alkalaemia
- p_aCO_2
  - Increased in respiratory acidosis
  - Decreased in respiratory alkalosis

- HCO_3^-
  - Increased in metabolic alkalosis
  - Decreased in metabolic acidosis

Compliance of the lung

Definitions

- Force required to produce a given change in lung volume
- The lower the compliance, the greater the force required
- Also defined as the change in lung volume per unit change in airway pressure
- Normal value: 0.2 L/cmH_2O (200 mL/cmH_2O)

Surfactant

- Lipoprotein produced by type II alveolar cells
- Functions as an agent that lowers surface tension, thus maintaining compliance
- Functions
  - Increases compliance and decreases work of breathing
  - Stabilises smaller alveoli, preventing collapse
  - Decreases transudation of fluid from the interstitium

Factors affecting compliance

- Increased by COPD and old age
- Decreased by fibrosis, pulmonary oedema, acute respiratory distress syndrome (ARDS) and pulmonary congestion

Elastance

- The inverse of compliance, i.e. 1/compliance: a measure of the elastic recoil of lung

Pulmonary blood flow

- Normal: 5.5 L/minute
- Control of pulmonary blood flow
  - Active control
    - Neuronal, via the sympathetic nervous system
    - Humoral
  - Passive control
    - Cardiac output
    - Gravity

Ventilation–perfusion (V–Q) ratio

Normal variation

- From apex to base in the erect posture: more ventilation at the apex, more perfusion at the base
- V–Q ratio is low at the base and high at the apex

Normal value

- Ratio of alveolar ventilation to pulmonary blood flow: 4.2 L/min to 5.5 L/min = 0.8

Factors affecting the V–Q ratio

- If ventilation decreases:
  - pO_2 of the alveoli decreases
  - pCO_2 increases
- If perfusion decreases:
  - pCO_2 decreases
  - pO_2 increases

Control of respiration

Aim

- To keep the p_aO_2, p_aCO_2 and pH within their narrow, normal limits
- Controlled by highly developed negative feedback systems that consist of sensors, controllers and effectors

Sensors

- Relay and sense information, thus detecting changes in:
  - Blood gases: p_aO_2, p_aCO_2
  - pH
  - Movements and muscles
- Chemoreceptors
  - Central chemoreceptors detect changes in p_aCO_2
  - Peripheral chemoreceptors detect changes in p_aO_2, pH
- Receptors within the lungs
  - Chemical receptors
    - Juxta-capillary (J) receptors
    - Irritant receptors
  - Mechanical receptors
    - Pulmonary stretch receptors

- Receptors outside the lungs
  - Chemical receptors
    - Upper respiratory tract (cough)
    - Joints
  - Mechanical receptors
    - Respiratory muscles
    - Baroreceptors

Controllers

- Co-ordinators of information from sensors, tuning automaticity and rhythmicity of respiration and voluntary control
- Respiratory centre (brainstem)
  - Medulla
    - Dorsal: controls inspiration
    - Ventral: controls expiration
  - Pons
    - Apneustic (in the lower pons): prolongs inspiration
    - Pneumotaxic (in the upper pons): inhibits the inspiratory centre
  - Cerebral cortex
    - Exerts voluntary control over automatic brainstem controls so that respiration can be modified by:
    - Speech, eating, drinking and sleeping
    - Sneezing, yawning and vomiting
    - Activity and exercise
    - Pain, fever and hypothermia
    - Fear and anger (through the limbic system in the hypothalamus)

Effectors

- Muscles that produce ventilation
  - Respiratory muscles
    - Diaphragm: the main muscle of respiration
    - Intercostal muscles and chest wall muscles
    - Abdominal wall muscles
  - Accessory muscles
    - Alae nasi
    - Sternocleidomastoid muscle
    - Scalene muscles
    - Pectoral muscles
    - Serratus anterior muscle
    - Latissimus dorsi (for forced expiration)

Central control

- Apneustic centre and pneumotaxic centre in the pons: afferents from vagus nerve
- Afferents from the carotid body via the carotid sinus and the glossopharyngeal nerve
- Afferents from the aortic bodies via the vagus nerve
- Medullary chemoreceptors on the ventral surface of medulla

Quiet breathing

- Inspiratory component of respiratory centre initiates respiration
- Hering–Breuer reflex (carried by vagal afferents) from the distending lung reach the expiratory component of the respiratory centre and inhibit inspiration

Chemical regulation

- Central chemoreceptors
  - Involved in day-to-day respiratory control
  - Chemosensitive areas on the ventral surface of the medulla oblongata, near the floor of the fourth ventricle and the exit of cranial nerves IX and X
  - Very sensitive to the pH changes of the extracellular fluid of the brain, which is most affected by the H^+ ion content of the cerebrospinal fluid (CSF)
  - Because the CSF is separated from the circulation by the blood–brain barrier, there is a slow diffusion of H^+ and HCO_3^-, but CO_2 moves freely, allowing rapid reflection of blood CO_2 in the CSF
  - Because the CSF also has much lower and slower buffering capacity than blood, small changes in p_aCO_2 leads to larger changes in CSF pH than in blood pH
  - Thus, when p_aCO_2 rises, there is a rise in CSF pCO_2, which liberates H^+, which in turn lowers the pH of the extracellular fluid
  - This stimulates central chemoreceptors and the respiratory centre and increases the rate and depth of respiration, which increases the minute volume

- CO_2 is washed off until pCO_2 returns to normal
- The opposite happens when p_aCO_2 falls
- Peripheral chemoreceptors
  - Carotid bodies, which lie at the bifurcation of common carotid artery and the aortic bodies (which lie along the aortic arch)
  - They contain glomus cells with a large dopamine content
  - They have very large blood flow per unit weight because of their location
  - Sensitive to changes in p_aO_2 and arterial pH, and to a lesser extent to changes in p_aCO_2
  - Response to changes in arterial pH is mediated only by carotid bodies, as H^+ cannot readily cross the blood–brain barrier
  - Thus when p_aO_2 decreases, there is decrease in arterial pH and an increase in p_aCO_2
  - This stimulates the respiratory centre and increases the rate and depth of respiration, increases the minute volume and returns the values to normal

Receptors within the lungs

- Mechanical receptors
  - Primary pulmonary stretch receptors within the smooth muscles of the airways
  - Very sensitive to lung distension, discharging impulses via the vagus nerve
  - These impulses decrease the respiratory rate, i.e. slowing of inspiration and increasing of the expiration time (Hering–Breuer inflation reflex)
  - This mechanism is of importance in newborn but is not useful for day-to-day respiratory control
- Chemical receptors
  - J receptors:
    - Located in the alveolar wall, close to the capillaries
    - Thought to stimulate inspiration following an increase in pulmonary blood flow

- Irritant receptors
  - Located in the airway epithelial cells
  - Stimulated by noxious gases, cold air and smoke
  - Discharge impulses via vagus nerve, which increase the respiratory rate and cause bronchospasm

Receptors outside the lungs

- Mechanical receptors
  - Respiratory muscle receptors
    - Relay information on muscle length
    - Stimulated by stretch
    - Help control the force of contraction, i.e. inhibit excessive contraction forces
    - This decreases the rate of respiration, with the sensation of dyspnoea
  - Joint muscle receptors
    - Sensitive to limb movements
    - Utilise gamma stretch receptors and an associated reflex
    - Stimulates of respiration at the start of exercise, which decreases minute ventilation
  - Carotid and aortic sinus baroreceptors
    - Increased blood pressure causes stimulation of these receptors
    - Results in hypoventilation or even apnoea
- Chemical receptors
  - Found in the nose and upper airway
  - Sensitive to chemical stimulation: coughing, sneezing and laryngeal spasm

Arterial O$_2$ saturation

- O$_2$ delivery to tissues depends on
  - Cardiac output
  - Haemoglobin concentration
  - S$_a$O$_2$ (saturation of O$_2$)

Arterial partial pressure of O$_2$ (p$_a$O$_2$)

- Normal p$_a$O$_2$ in a healthy young person at sea level is 100 mmHg (13.3 kPa) and corresponds to an S$_a$O$_2$ of almost 100%
- The p$_a$O$_2$ of mixed venous blood (p$_v$O$_2$) is 40 mmHg (5.3 kPa), which is associated with an S$_a$O$_2$ of 70%

- Normal p$_a$O$_2$ falls with advancing age: 60 mmHg in an 80-year-old
- At a p$_a$O$_2$ of 60 mmHg, haemoglobin is 90% saturated

Arterial saturation of O$_2$ (S$_a$O$_2$)

- Can be measured by pulse oximeter, though this fails in intense vasoconstriction and gives inaccurate figures in methaemoglobinaemia and jaundice
- Normal O$_2$ tension at cellular level: 5–7 mmHg
- Capillary perfusion pressure: 25 mmHg
- Therefore there is a normal tissue perfusion pressure of 20 mmHg
- This facilitates O$_2$ release into the tissues

O$_2$ delivery

- VO$_2$ = total consumption of O$_2$/minute
- DO$_2$ – O$_2$ delivery/minute
- Normal VO$_2$ = 100–160 mL/minute
- Normal DO$_2$ = 500–720 mL/minute
- Therefore, normally only 20–25% of DO$_2$ is being taken up: this is called the O$_2$ extraction ratio
- The O$_2$ extraction ratio increases if DO$_2$ decreases down to 300 mL/minute
- Below this level, VO$_2$ also decreases

Tissue oxygenation

- Tissue oxygenation can be measured by:
  - Gastric tonometry (pH)
  - Mixed venous O$_2$ saturation (pulmonary capillary wedge pressure, PCWP)
  - Micro-electron technology

Other (non-ventilatory) functions of the lung

Defence mechanisms

- Humidification of air
- Immunoglobulin production (IgA) in bronchial epithelium
- Pulmonary alveolar macrophages
- Mechanical defence
  - Hairs in the upper respiratory tract
  - Tonsils and adenoids
  - Ciliary mechanisms

Metabolic and endocrine functions

- Manufacture of surfactant
- Fibrinolytic system
- Synthesis of prostaglandins, histamine and kallikrein
- Conversion of angiotensin I to angiotensin II in the pulmonary circulation (angiotensin converting enzyme is located in the vascular epithelium of pulmonary capillaries)

Valsalva manoeuvre

Definition

- Forced expiration against a closed glottis

Examples

- Coughing
- Straining
  - To lift heavy objects
  - At defaecation

Phases

- Phase I
  - Increase in intrathoracic pressure, leading to pressure on the thoracic aorta and a transient increase in blood pressure
- Phase II
  - Increase in intrathoracic pressure, leading to decreased venous return, decreased stroke volume and decreased cardiac output
  - This in turn leads to decreased mean arterial pressure, causing reflex tachycardia and peripheral vasoconstriction together with the decrease in blood pressure
- Phase III
  - Opening the glottis causes a sudden drop in blood pressure
- Phase IV
  - Decreased intrathoracic pressure leads to improved venous return and increased blood pressure, causing reflex bradycardia (through the vagus nerve)

Uses of the Valsalva manoeuvre

- For testing autonomic functions in neuropathy: there may be no reflex bradycardia through the vagus nerve in autonomic dysfunction
- For termination of paroxysms of ventricular tachycardia, by way of reflex bradycardia through the vagus nerve

Chronic obstructive pulmonary disease (COPD)

Definition

- Reduced expiratory airflow with reduction of respiratory reserve

Causes

- Chronic bronchitis
- Emphysema
- Asthma

Mechanisms

- Increased airway resistance
  - Mucosal swelling
  - Bronchospasm
- Turbulence caused by tortuosity of the airway
- Decreased lung recoil caused by loss of pulmonary elastin

Clinical types

- 'Blue bloaters' (chronic bronchitis)
  - Hypercarbia
  - Polycythaemia
  - Pulmonary hypertension
  - Cor pulmonale
- 'Pink puffers' (emphysema):
  - Constant dyspnoea
  - Less cough and sputum than in chronic bronchitis
  - Blood gases normal because of increased ventilation

Respiratory failure

Definition

- Arterial O_2 tension at sea level of < 8.4 kPa, i.e. hypoxia resulting from inadequate gas exchange within the lung
- 8.4 kPa is the critical point in the O_2 dissociation curve

Types

- Type I: hypoxia plus $p_aCO_2 < 6.6$ kPa (50 mmHg), i.e. normal or low p_aCO_2
- Type II: hypoxia plus $p_aCO_2 > 6.6$ kPa (50 mmHg), i.e. hypercapnia

Causes

- Type I
  - Pulmonary and cardiac causes
  - Alveolar hyperventilation occurs to maintain normal p_aCO_2
- Type II:
  - Disorders of the CNS and peripheral nervous system, and musculoskeletal abnormalities
  - Alveolar hypoventilation

In COPD

- Type I or II due to V–Q imbalance
- Depends on hypoxic drive for respiratory stimulation

Mechanisms of respiratory failure

- Type I
  - V–Q imbalance
    - Present normally
    - Increases in lung disorders
  - Physiological shunting
    - Pneumonia
    - Left ventricular failure
  - Alveolar capillary block
    - Fibrosing alveolitis (with thickening of alveolar membrane)
- Type II
  - Extra-pulmonary ventilator failure (EPVF)
  - Depression of the neurological respiratory drive
  - Increased impedance
    - Morbid obesity
    - Chest trauma
    - Tension pneumothorax
    - Ruptured diaphragm
    - Kyphoscoliosis

Stridor

Definition

- Noisy breathing caused by turbulent airflow through upper respiratory tract
- The cardinal feature of acute upper respiratory tract obstruction

Anatomy and pathophysiology

- Upper airway begins at the nose and mouth and ends at the carina (at the level of the T4–T5 vertebra and the sternal angle)
- Obstruction is likely to occur at the sites of anatomical narrowing
  - At the hypopharynx at the base of the tongue
  - At the false and true vocal cords at the laryngeal opening

Classification

- Supraglottic stridor: above the true vocal cords
- Glottic stridor: involving true vocal cords
- Infraglottic stridor: below the vocal cords and above the carina

Aetiology

- Functional causes
  - CNS depression
    - Head injury
    - Cerebrovascular accident with cardiopulmonary arrest
    - Shock, with hypoxia
    - Metabolic encephalopathies
    - Drug overdose
  - Peripheral nervous system and neuromuscular dysfunction
    - Recurrent laryngeal nerve palsy
    - Post-operative thyroidectomy
    - Inflammation
    - Tumour infiltration
    - Obstructive sleep apnoea
    - Myasthenia gravis
    - Guillain-Barré polyneuritis
    - Laryngospasm
    - Hypocalcemic vocal cord spasm
- Mechanical causes
  - Intrinsic
    - In lumen
    - In wall
  - Extrinsic: outside the wall
  - Foreign body aspiration: most common cause, especially in the elderly and those living in institutions
  - Congenital conditions
    - Choanal atresia (affecting the nose)

- Conditions affecting the oropharynx, e.g. facial malformation (such as Pierre–Robin syndrome and Treacher–Collins syndrome), macroglossia, cystic hygromas, vallecular cyst
- Conditions affecting the larynx, e.g. congenital subglottic stenosis, laryngeal webs, laryngocoeles
- Vascular rings (affecting the trachea)
- Trauma
  - External trauma (blunt or penetrating)
  - Inhalational thermal injury in burns
  - Ingestion of toxic chemicals or caustic agents
- Inflammatory conditions and infections
  - Epiglottitis
  - Retropharyngeal cellulitis or abscess
  - Ludwig's angina
  - Diphtheria
  - Tetanus
  - Bacterial tracheitis
  - Laryngotracheobronchitis (croup)
- Laryngeal oedema
  - Allergic laryngeal oedema
  - Hereditary angioedema
  - Post-intubation oedema
  - Acquired cholinesterase deficiency
  - ACE inhibitor associated antihypertensives
- Neoplastic changes
  - Pharyngeal, laryngeal and tracheobronchial carcinoma
  - Laryngeal papilloma
  - Vocal cord polyposis
- Miscellaneous
  - Cricoarytenoid arthritis (a feature of rheumatoid arthritis)
  - Achalasia
  - Myxoedema
  - Hysterical stridor

Acute respiratory distress syndrome (ARDS)

Definition

- A clinical syndrome characterised by type I respiratory failure, non-cardiogenic pulmonary oedema and hypoxia refractory to O_2 therapy

Causes

- Shock
- Sepsis
- Pancreatitis
- Trauma
- Aspiration
- Near drowning
- See figure opposite

Clinical presentation

- Refractory hypoxaemia ($p_aO_2 < 8$ kPa with $F_iO_2 > 0.04$ or p_aO_2–F_iO_2 ratio < 20 kPa)
- X-ray shows bilateral diffuse pulmonary infiltrates
- Total compliance < 30 mL/cm H_2O
- Pulmonary artery occlusion pressure < 15–18 mmHg with normal oncotic pressures

Phases

- Phase I
  - Occurs in 16–24 hours
  - Tachycardia and tachypnoea
  - Chest X-ray normal
- Phase II
  - Occurs in 48 hours
  - Dyspnoea and cyanosis with inspiratory rhonchi
- Phase III
  - Occurs in 72 hours
  - Marked tachypnoea and dyspnoea
  - High-pitched rhonchi
  - Chest X-ray shows bilateral diffuse pulmonary infiltrates ('white-out')
- Phase IV
  - Occurs after 72 hours
  - Lethargy and restlessness, leading to coma
  - Respiratory and metabolic acidosis
  - Hypoxaemia
  - Hypotension
- Mortality is 50–60%
- Death occurs within 2–4 weeks

Fat embolism

Incidence

- 0.5–3% with single long bone or pelvic fracture
- Up to 30% with multiple injuries

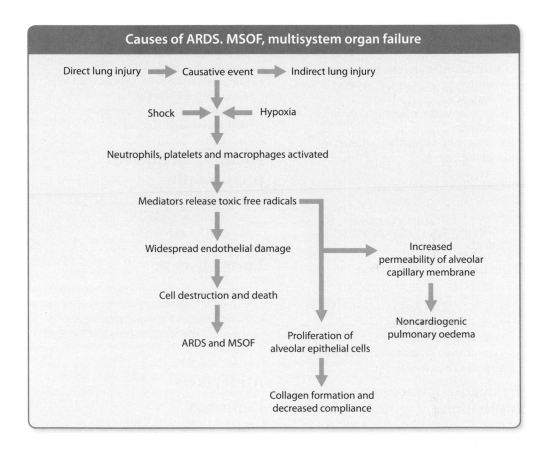

Causes of ARDS. MSOF, multisystem organ failure

Direct lung injury → Causative event → Indirect lung injury

Shock → ← Hypoxia

Neutrophils, platelets and macrophages activated

Mediators release toxic free radicals

Widespread endothelial damage → Increased permeability of alveolar capillary membrane

Cell destruction and death

ARDS and MSOF → Proliferation of alveolar epithelial cells → Noncardiogenic pulmonary oedema

Collagen formation and decreased compliance

Clinical features

- Pulmonary changes
  - V–Q mismatch
  - Decreased alveolar surfactant activity
  - Segmental hypoperfusion
- Neurological dysfunction, due to hypoxia
- Petechial rash
- Arrhythmias
- Renal changes
  - Lipidaemia
  - Tubular damage
  - Ischaemic glomerulotubular dysfunction

Diagnosis

- Fat globules in body fluids
- Diagnostic triad
  - Petechial haemorrhages in the skin
  - Mental confusion
  - Respiratory failure

- Skin biopsy
  - Petechial haemorrhages
  - Fat globules in the blood vessels of the skin

Aspiration syndromes

Causes

- Decreased level of consciousness
  - Anaesthesia
  - Head injury
  - Drug overdose
- Decreased protective reflexes
  - After extubation
  - Myasthenia
  - Neck or pharyngeal injury
- Gastric regurgitation
  - Gastro-oesophageal reflux disease
  - Nasogastric intubation
  - Achalasia

Factors predisposing to post-operative aspiration

- Inadequate pre-operative fasting, e.g. emergency operations in trauma patients
- Pregnancy
- Gastro-oesophageal reflux disease
  - Obesity
  - Pregnancy, and third trimester in particular
  - Hiatus hernia
- Gastric outlet obstruction
- Small bowel obstruction
- Acute abdomen
- Drugs that delay gastric emptying, e.g. opioids

Factors increasing the sensitivity of response to aspiration of gastric contents

- Acidity: pH < 2.5
- Volume: > 4 mL/kg
- Type of aspirate: particles cause more response than fluids

Protective manoeuvres at intubation

- Pharmacological
  - Increase in gastric pH and decrease in volume
    - Histamine-2 receptor blockers, e.g. ranitidine
    - Antacids, e.g. sodium citrate
  - Increased gastric emptying
    - Metoclopramide
    - Cisapride
- Mechanical
  - Pre-oxygenation with 100% O_2
  - Cricoid pressure
  - Rapid sequence intubation

Aspiration of liquids

- Acid
  - Immediate bronchospasm
  - Loss of surfactant
  - ARDS
- Neutral liquids
  - Near drowning
  - Pulmonary dysfunction
- Infected liquids:
  - Hospital-acquired pneumonia

Aspiration of solids

- Upper airway obstruction
- Paradoxical chest wall movements
- Heimlich manoeuvre may be tried to dislodge foreign body
- Smaller objects cause aspiration pneumonia and abscess

Hospital-acquired pneumonia

- Definition: infective consolidation developing > 3 days after admission to hospital for any reason

Lung abscess

- Definition: cavitating lesions produced by pyogenic organisms
- Abscess following aspiration usually occurs in the apical segment of the right lower lobe

Atelectasis

Definition

- Absence of air from all or part of lung

Aetiology

- Bronchial obstruction
  - Sputum
  - Foreign body
  - Tumour
- Alveolar hypoventilation, leading to absorption of air and collapse
- Pleural effusion or pulmonary oedema
- Endobronchial intubation with collapse of the opposite lung

Physiological consequences

- V–Q mismatch
- Decreased lung compliance and increased work of breathing
- Predisposition to infection, owing to retention of secretions

Absorption atelectasis

- When a high F_iO_2 is given, it gets absorbed because of the faster absorption of O_2 compared with nitrogen, and nitrogen splinting of the alveoli is absent, leading to atelectasis

Post-operative atelectasis

- Risk factors
  - Upper abdominal and thoracic surgery: decreased lung expansion from pain and diaphragmatic splinting
  - Body mass index > 27
  - Smoking
  - Age > 60 years
  - COPD
- Management
  - Pre-operative breathing exercises
  - Intra-operative measures
    - Humidification
    - Adequate tidal volume
    - Avoid high F_iO_2
  - Post-operative measures
    - Head-up position
    - Analgesia
    - Early mobilisation
    - Breathing exercises
    - Continuous positive airway pressure (CPAP)
    - Airway suction

Post-operative respiratory insufficiency

Definition

- Insufficiency of the mobility of the lungs to exchange gases sufficiently to meet the physiologic needs in the post-operative period
- More specifically, inadequate oxygenation, impaired CO_2 exhalation, or both
- It is a serious complication, increasing the morbidity and mortality and resulting in extended and expensive hospitalisation

Risk factors

- Pre-operative factors
  - Extremes of age: > 70 years or < 1 year
  - Smoking
  - Obesity
  - Trauma
  - Precipitating disease
    - COPD
    - Neuromuscular disease
- Intra-operative factors

- Anaesthetic factors
  - Anaesthesia: general or spinal
  - Excess fluid administration
  - Blood transfusion
  - Inadequate endotracheal suctioning
  - Insufficient positive end-expiratory pressure (PEEP)
- Operative factors
  - Prolonged procedures (> 3 hours)
  - Oropharyngeal procedures
  - Intra-oral lacerations
  - Gastroscopy
  - Chest wall and lung procedures
  - Upper abdominal procedures
- Patient factors
  - Atelectasis
  - Aspiration
  - Cardiovascular insufficiency
- Post-operative factors
  - Prolonged neuromuscular blockade
  - Prolonged or over-sedation
  - Inadequate tracheal suctioning
  - Cardiovascular instability

Causes

- Caused by one or a combination of:
  - Atelectasis
    - Mucus plug
    - Impaired cough reflex
  - Pulmonary oedema
    - Cardiogenic
    - Non-cardiogenic
  - Aspiration – with or without pneumonia
  - Pulmonary embolism: from deep venous thrombosis
  - Bronchospasm: from reactive airway disease
  - Pneumothorax or haemothorax
    - Trauma
    - Line insertion

Evaluation and management

- Pre-operative management: organised evaluation to identify and correct risk factors
- Post-operative management: early detection of the underlying causes, by:
  - Symptoms and signs, e.g. anxiety, agitation, confusion, dyspnoea, tachypnoea, cyanosis, bradycardia or tachycardia, hypotension or hypertension

- Physical examination of lungs, which may show dullness on percussion, decreased or absent breath sounds or basal crepitations
  - Arterial blood gases
  - Chest X-ray
  - Prevention, by:
    - Early mobilisation
    - Humidification of inspired gases
    - Chest physiotherapy
    - Adequate control of pain

Treatment

- Treatment of pre-existing disease
- Bedside bronchoscopy with lavage
- Corticosteroids and antibiotics, when indicated
- Treatment of thromboembolism

Ventilatory support

Definition

- Respiratory support through endotracheal intubation for a patient who cannot breathe spontaneously

Indications

- General anaesthesia
- Patient's respiratory apparatus fatigued because of acidosis (commonly as a result of medical or surgical sepsis)
- Central ventilatory failure
  - Alcohol
  - Drugs
  - Brain injury
  - Local injury (chest or abdomen)
- Elective ventilation after major upper abdominal operations
- Respiratory arrest or rate of < 8 breaths/minute or > 35 breaths/minute in trauma patients
- Peripheral O_2 saturation < 90% on 60% O_2
- Sweating or fatigue
- Agitation, confusion or refusal of an O_2 mask
- Diminished conscious level (Glasgow Coma Score < 8)
- Airway obstruction or impairment
- Rising p_aCO_2 > 6.6 kPa

Types of ventilators

- Pressure-controlled ventilators
  - PEEP or CPAP
  - Set pressure is pushed into the lung irrespective of volume, to maintain V–Q ratio
  - Given with an endotracheal tube without a cuff
  - Indications
    - Children
    - Large air leak (bronchopleural fistula)
- Volume-controlled ventilators
  - Controlled mechanical ventilation (CMV) or synchronized intermittent mandatory ventilation (SIMV)
  - Given with a cuffed endotracheal tube
  - A fixed tidal volume is delivered
  - In thoracic surgery using one-lung ventilation, half the tidal volume is delivered (250 mL)

Aims of assisted ventilation

- To bring p_aO_2 to > 10 kPa (80 mmHg)
- To bring p_aCO_2 to < 5.5 kPa (40 mmHg)

Benefits of ventilation

- Elimination of CO_2
- Improved oxygenation by
  - Decreased respiratory work and O_2 consumption by respiratory muscles
  - Administration of high F_iO_2
  - Recruitment of collapsed or oedematous alveoli (with PEEP) in hypoxaemic respiratory failure

Modes of ventilation

- CMV
  - Preset tidal volume at a preset rate
  - Tidal volume is 10 mL/kg
  - Barotrauma is more common
- SIMV
  - Preset tidal volume synchronised with patient's respiratory effort
  - Used as a weaning mode
  - If no respiratory effort occurs, the next breath is given after a set time

- Pressure support ventilation
  - When patient's effort is detected, a preset pressure is applied
  - If no effort is detected, there is no ventilation
  - Good for weaning
- Pressure-controlled ventilation
  - Positive airway pressure with fixed rate
  - Patient's effort is not required
  - Used in paediatrics with an uncuffed endotracheal tube
- PEEP
  - To splint the alveoli open in expiration by increasing the FRC
  - Improves matching of the V–Q ratio
  - Ideal pressure: 5–10 cmH$_2$O
- CPAP
  - Spontaneous respiration with continuously increasing airway pressure
  - PEEP without positive pressure ventilation
  - Patient breathes spontaneously, plus there is the benefit of airway splinting
  - Used via an endotracheal tube or a tight-fitting mask
- Pressure-controlled inverse-ratio ventilation
  - Ratio of inspiration to expiration is altered from the normal 1:2 to 2:1
  - Increased mean airway pressure leads to increased recruitment
- Prone ventilation
  - Redistributes the V–Q ratio
- IPPV
  - Up to 20–30 cmH$_2$O to 10 mL/kg body weight
  - Disadvantages
    - Decreased venous return
    - Compression of heart
    - Decreased dead space
    - All of these lead to decreased cardiac output
- Extended mandatory minute volume (EMMV) ventilation
  - Patient breathes spontaneously but is topped up to a preset minute volume

- Triggering
  - Allows patient to take spontaneous breath by decreasing the airway pressure
- Inspiratory-assisted ventilation
  - Patient's respiratory efforts are assisted with positive pressure
- High-frequency ventilation
  - Cycles of > 20/minute with small tidal volumes, to maintain blood gases
  - Useful in management of bronchopleural fistula

Weaning

- When normal O$_2$ saturation can be maintained with an F$_i$O$_2$ < 50%
- Muscle relaxants are stopped
- Sedation is gradually reduced
- Patient is observed for distress

Flail chest

Definition

- Condition that occurs when two or more ribs are fractured in two or more places, producing a segment that is disconnected from the rest of the thoracic cage

Signs and symptoms

- Paradoxical chest wall movement with respiration
- May be absent in the early stages as a result of spasm of the chest wall musculature

Sources of massive haemothorax in flail chest

- Neurovascular bundle under the ribs
- Internal mammary artery
- Large lacerations of the lung surface

Treatment

- PEEP
- Definitive treatment is internal fixation of fracture ribs if thoracotomy is done for any other reason

- Pain management
  - Opioids
  - Intermittent posterior intercostal nerve block
  - Epidural analgesia (the best form of pain management in this condition)

Lung cancer

Associated factors

- Cigarette smoking
- Arsenic
- Asbestos
- Polycyclic aromatic compounds
- Male sex
- Diet: vitamin A has a protective effect

Molecular biological aspects

- Oncogenes
  - *myc*
  - k-*ras*
  - her-2/*neu*
  - *bcl*-2
- Tumour-suppressor genes
  - *p53*
  - *RB*-1

Important pathological types

- Epithelial
  - Squamous cell carcinoma
  - Adenocarcinoma
  - Large cell carcinoma
  - Adenosquamous carcinoma
- Epithelial and neuroendocrine
  - Small cell carcinoma
  - Carcinoid
- Epithelial of salivary gland type
  - Adenoid cystic carcinoma
  - Muco-epidermoid carcinoma

Spread

- Local
  - Central tumours
    - Extrinsic compression of bronchus, which causes distal pneumonia
    - Tumour embolus along pulmonary vein
    - Via the aorta
    - Into the pericardium
    - Superior vena cava syndrome
  - Peripheral tumours

- Into the chest wall
- Pancoast's syndrome
- To the diaphragm
- Dissemination
  - Lymphatic spread to the mediastinal nodes
  - Distant spread
    - Liver
    - Adrenal glands
    - Elsewhere in the lungs
    - Brain
    - Bone
    - Kidney

Clinical features

- Caused by the tumour itself:
  - Cough
  - Haemoptysis
  - Weight loss
- Caused by infiltration of the tumour:
  - Hoarseness
  - Jaundice
  - Bone pain
- Paraneoplastic manifestations
- Gynaecomastia
- Syndrome of inappropriate ADH (SIADH)
- Myasthenia
- Clubbing
- Acanthosis nigricans
- Thrombophlebitis migrans

Diagnosis

- Sputum cytology
- Bronchoscopy
- Needle biopsy
- Thoracoscopy
- Thoracotomy

Staging

- TNM
  - T1: < 3 cm in diameter
  - T2: > 3 cm in diameter or involving the main bronchus
  - T3: involving the chest wall or mediastinum
  - T4: pleural effusion or satellite tumours
  - N0: no nodes
  - N1: peribronchial nodes involved
  - N2: mediastinal nodes involved
  - N3: contralateral nodes involved
  - M0: no distant metastases
  - M1: distant metastases

- Stage I: T1, T2
- Stage II: T3, N1
- Stage III: T4, N3
- Stage IV: M1

Management

- Surgical resection – for T1, T2, N0, N1 lesions
- Radiotherapy and cisplatin chemotherapy for palliation

Pleura

- Normal volume of the pleural fluid: 15 mL

Pleural effusion

- Abnormal amount of fluid within pleural space
- If volume > 100 mL, it can be detected in a chest X-ray
- If volume > 500 mL, it can be detected clinically

Mechanisms

- Increased capillary hydrostatic pressure
- Decreased colloid osmotic pressure
- Increased capillary permeability
- Decreased lymphatic drainage

Empyema

- Infection of the pleural space

Pneumothorax

- Air in the pleural space
  - Classification
    - Traumatic pneumothorax and spontaneous pneumothorax: caused by rupture of apical blebs
    - Closed pneumothorax, open pneumothorax, valvular pneumothorax (tension pneumothorax)

Haemothorax

- Accumulation of blood in the pleural space
- Indications for thoracotomy after insertion of an intercostal drain
  - Initial return of 1000–1500 mL of blood
  - Continued bleeding of 200–300 mL/hour

Empyema thoracis

Definition

- Collection of pus in the pleural cavity

Causes

- Pulmonary infections
  - Lung abscess
  - Pneumonia
  - Bronchiectasis
- Trauma
  - Chest injury
  - Post-thoracotomy
  - Ruptured oesophagus
- Trans-diaphragmatic pathology
  - Subphrenic abscess
  - Hepatic amoebiasis
- Iatrogenic
  - Needle aspiration
- Osteomyelitis of ribs or vertebrae
- Septicaemia with multiple small lung abscesses

Pathogenesis

- Dry pleurisy causes a protein-rich pleural effusion, which becomes purulent and causes compression of the lung and a shift of the mediastinum to the opposite side
- Fibrin is deposited on the pleural surface, causing empyema to get walled off and the space fixed, resulting in anaerobic respiration and a fall in pH within the empyema space
- If not drained, continued formation of fibrin results in restriction of the chest wall and diaphragmatic movement, causing a flattened, immobile hemithorax with overlapping ribs, and scoliosis
- Collar-stud abscess: discharging fistula on the surface (empyemia necessitanes)

Pyopneumothorax

- Pus and air in the pleural space, causing considerable toxaemia

Causes

- Bronchopleural fistula
- Rupture of a lung abscess
- Gas-forming organisms

Clinical features

- Fever, swinging temperature and failure to respond to treatment
- Leukocytosis
- Increased C-reactive protein (> 200)
- Clubbing
- Collar stud abscess
- Chest X-ray shows collapse, fibrosis and scoliosis
- Late empyema acts as a chronic septic focus and causes:
  - Toxaemia
  - Malaise
  - Anorexia
  - Weight loss
  - Chest pain

Treatment

- Early pyopneumothorax
  - Aspiration
  - Irrigation of the empyema space after aspiration
  - Vigorous physiotherapy
  - Chest tube with underwater-seal drain
- Late pyopneumothorax
  - Thoracotomy and decortication if patient is fit
  - If patient not fit, limited aspiration and chest tube placement, and conservative supportive management with antibiotics and respiratory support until patient becomes fit

Pneumothorax

Definition

- Air in the pleural space

Classification

- Spontaneous pneumothorax
  - Simple pneumothorax
  - Tension pneumothorax
- Traumatic pneumothorax
  - Open pneumothorax
  - Tension pneumothorax

Spontaneous pneumothorax

- Rupture of alveolus leads to decreased negative pressure in the chest
- This results in depression of the diaphragm and shift of the mediastinum to the opposite side
- p_aO_2 decreases, owing to V–Q mismatch
- When the source of the pneumothorax is sealed, re-expansion takes place at about 1.25% of the volume of the hemithorax per day
- Classification
  - Primary spontaneous pneumothorax, due to rupture of apical bulla
  - Secondary spontaneous pneumothorax, associated with pulmonary disease
- Signs and symptoms
  - Pleuritic pain on the affected side
  - Dyspnoea
  - Decreased chest movements and resonance to percussion on the affected side
- Treatment
  - Small pneumothorax (occupying < 20% of the hemithorax): no treatment
  - Large or symptomatic pneumothorax: chest tube

Tension pneumothorax

- Valvular type of pneumothorax, in which air can pass into the pleural space but cannot escape on expiration
- Mediastinal shift to the opposite side
- During inspiration, the trachea moves away from the affected side (this does not happen in a simple pneumothorax)
- Patient rapidly deteriorates, owing to decreased venous return and hypoxaemia
- May be iatrogenic, caused by IPPV with high pressure or by PEEP
- Management is by rapid insertion of a hollow, 14 gauge needle into the second intercostal space in the midclavicular line

Traumatic pneumothorax

- Seen after injury to the chest wall and rib fractures
- Compression of lung causes rupture of the alveoli
- In an open pneumothorax, there is communication of the pleural space to the outside
  - If the outside communication is larger than the cross-sectional diameter of the larynx, there is mediastinal shift
  - Should be sealed immediately, followed by surgical closure and insertion of an intercostal drain

Iatrogenic

- Intercostal nerve block
- Percutaneous placement of subclavian catheter
- Thoracocentesis
- Brachial plexus block
- Artificial ventilation

Pneumonia

Definition

- Infection of distal airways and alveoli

Types

- Primary: in previously healthy patients
- Secondary: in immunocompromised patients

Pathological types

- Bronchopneumonia
  - Aetiology and predisposing factors
    - Extremes of age
    - Debilitating disease
    - Cancer
    - Cardiac failure
    - Renal failure
    - COPD
    - Cystic fibrosis
    - Early post-operative period
  - Organisms
    - *Streptococcus pneumoniae*
    - *Haemophilus influenzae*
    - *Staphylococcus aureus* (often a cause of nosocomial pneumonia)
    - Coliforms (often a cause of nosocomial pneumonia)
  - Pathology
    - Patchy distribution
    - Basal changes
    - Bilateral
- Lobar pneumonia
  - Caused by *S. pneumoniae*
  - May occur in post-splenectomy sepsis
  - Clinical features
    - Cough with sputum
    - Fever
    - Chest pain
    - Consolidation of a lobe or part of a lobe
  - Four pathological stages of lobar pneumonia

- Stage of congestion: protein-rich exudate filling the alveoli, with venous congestion
- Stage of red hepatisation: inflammatory cells and red blood cells enter the alveoli, with fibrinous exudate in the pleura
- Stage of grey hepatisation: accumulation of fibrin, with destruction of red blood cells and leukocytes in the alveoli
- Stage of resolution (after 8–10 days): inflammatory cells and fibrin reabsorbed and lung architecture preserved

- Aspiration pneumonia
  - Aetiology
    - Induction of anaesthesia
    - Recovery from anaesthesia
    - Sedation
    - Coma
    - Severe disability
  - Part of lung affected depends on the posture of the patient: the most common site is the apex of the right lower lobe
  - Complications
    - Lung abscess
    - Empyema
  - Organisms
    - *S. pneumoniae*
    - Occasionally anaerobes (in nosocomial aspiration pneumonia)
- Atypical pneumonias
  - Organisms
    - *Mycoplasma pneumoniae*
    - *Coxiella burnetii*
    - *Chlamydia psittaci*
    - *Chlamydia pneumoniae*
  - Affects young adults through droplet infection
  - Treatment
    - Tetracycline
    - Erythromycin

Legionnaire's disease

- Organism: *Legionella pneumophila*
- More common in middle-aged smokers
- Spread by droplet infection
- Can be severe and fatal, with MODS

Intercostal drainage

Indications

- Pneumothorax
- Malignant pleural effusion
- Empyema (non-traumatic)
- Haemopneumothorax
- Post-thoracotomy

Preparation

- Correction of coagulation disorders and platelet defects
- Consent
- Premedication
  - Short-acting benzodiazepines unless contraindicated
  - Midazolam, 1–5 mg, immediately reversed with flumazenil after the procedure
  - Atropine to prevent vasovagal reaction (usual dose is 1 ampoule, containing 0.6 mg)
- Check identity of the patient
- Site and side of the pathology confirmed by clinical examination and chest X-ray
- Lignocaine, 3 mg/kg (20 mL of 1% or 10 mL of 2% lignocaine)

'Safe triangle'

- Anterior border of the latissimus dorsi
- Lateral border of the pectoralis major
- Line superior to the horizontal level of the nipple
- Apex below the axilla
- Advantages
  - No major vessels
  - Muscles are very thin
  - Above the level of diaphragm

Insertion of the drain

- Air and fluid should be aspirated before insertion
- Ultrasound-guided insertion is performed:
  - In empyema
  - For localisation of the diaphragm
  - If there is loculation or pleural thickening
  - In a small effusion
- Size of the tube depends on the age of the patient and the indication
  - A small tube (10–14 Fr gauge) is more comfortable
  - A large tube (28–30 Fr gauge) in acute haemothorax to monitor further blood loss
  - In a child with a bronchopleural fistula, the tube should be smaller than the size of the bronchus, which is roughly equal to size of the little finger of the child

After insertion of the drain

- Chest X-ray
- Nebulisation
- Chest physiotherapy and respiratory exercises
- Analgesia

Findings

- Plenty of air is leaking
  - If lung is expanded: wait and watch
  - If lung is not expanded, this indicates major bronchial injury: thoracotomy needed
- In case of blood, thoracotomy is indicated when there is:
  - > 1500 mL drained on insertion
  - > 200 mL/hour drainage
  - Haemodynamic instability

Massive pleural effusion

- Controlled drainage to prevent re-expansion pulmonary oedema
- Tube clamped for 1 hour after draining each litre, or drainage slowed to 500 mL/hour

Water-seal drainage

- Tip of the tube should be at least 3 cm below water level
- Side vent to allow escape of air
- Disadvantages
  - In-patient management
  - Difficulty in mobilisation
  - Kinking of the tube over the bottle

Removal

- Indication for removal: after bubbling stops
- No role for clamping
- Removed during expiration or when patient performs a Valsalva manoeuvre
- Assistant immediately tightens the knot after removal

Complications of thoracic operations

General complications

- From thoracostomy tubes
  - Bleeding from the intercostal or superior epigastric artery
  - Post-removal pneumothorax
  - Fracture of the chest tube
- Injury to a great vessel
  - Innominate vein: ligation is required
  - Superior vena cava: reconstruction is required
  - Inferior vena cava: reconstruction is required
- Aortic false aneurysm: immediate surgery is required
- Aortic dissection: immediate surgery is required
- Aortic atherosclerotic emboli
- Thoracic duct injury
- Pulmonary embolism
- Wound infection and wound dehiscence

Organ-specific complications

- Heart
  - Atrial fibrillation
  - Atrial flutter
  - Ventricular arrhythmias
  - Conduction disturbances
  - Post-operative myocardial infarction
- Pericardium
  - Constrictive pericarditis
  - Pericardial tamponade
- Lung
  - Pneumothorax
  - Haemothorax
  - Pneumonia
  - Chronic ventilator dependence
  - ARDS
- Phrenic nerve injury
- Kidney
  - Acute renal failure
  - Chronic renal failure
- Peripheral vasculature
  - Bleeding
  - Thrombotic or embolic occlusion
  - False aneurysm
- Gastrointestinal tract
  - Ischaemic phenomena
- Coagulation system
  - Bleeding
- CNS
  - Brachial plexus injury
- Neuropsychiatric changes
  - Behavioural disturbances
  - Sleeplessness

Thyroid gland

Hypothyroidism

- Causes
  - Primary hypothyroidism (common)
    - Autoimmune thyroiditis (Hashimoto's thyroiditis)
    - Treatment of thyrotoxicosis by surgery or radioactive iodine
    - Drugs, e.g. amiodarone, lithium
  - Secondary hypothyroidism
    - Anterior pituitary gland disorder
  - Tertiary hypothyroidism
    - Hypothalamic disorders
- Signs and symptoms
  - Dry skin
  - Tiredness
  - Cold intolerance
  - Coarse hair
  - Weight gain
  - Hoarseness (unrelated to recurrent laryngeal nerve palsy)
  - Constipation

Hyperthyroidism

- Definition: excess production of thyroid hormones
- Causes
  - Primary hyperthyroidism
    - Graves' disease
    - Toxic multinodular goitre
    - Solitary toxic nodule
  - Secondary hyperthyroidism (rare)
    - Exogenous administration of thyroxine
    - Struma ovarii (ectopic hormone production)
    - Choriocarcinoma
  - Unusual cause: the Jod–Basedow phenomenon
    - Excessive release of thyroxine in an iodine-deficient patient on resumption of dietary iodine intake or administration of intravenous contrast
    - Seen in patients with longstanding multinodular goitre

Thyroid cancer

- Classification
  - Differentiated thyroid cancer (DTC)
    - Papillary thyroid cancer
    - Follicular thyroid cancer
  - Medullary thyroid cancer (MTC)
  - Lymphoma
  - Undifferentiated or anaplastic thyroid cancer
- Risk factors
  - Appearance of a new thyroid nodule in patients <20 years or >50 years of age
  - Male sex
  - Clinical features:
    - Consistency
    - Fixation
    - Size
    - Solitary versus multiple nodules
  - History of head and neck irradiation
  - Family history of thyroid malignancy or multiple endocrine neoplasia (MEN) type 2
  - Recurrent laryngeal nerve palsy
  - Cervical lymphadenopathy
- Pre-operative assessment
  - Clinical examination
  - Chest X-ray to exclude metastases
  - Ultrasound to detect gross nodal disease
  - CT or MRI for locally advanced disease
- Surgery
  - Papillary microcarcinoma < 1 cm: lobectomy with isthmusectomy
  - Minimally invasive follicular carcinoma with capsular invasion only: lobectomy with isthmusectomy
  - Differentiated thyroid cancer with extrathyroidal spread: near-total thyroidectomy
  - Bilateral or multifocal differentiated thyroid cancer: near-total or total thyroidectomy
  - Differentiated thyroid cancer with distant metastases: near-total or total thyroidectomy
  - Differentiated thyroid cancer with extensive nodal involvement: near-total or total thyroidectomy

- Post-operative period
  - Lifelong thyroxine therapy
  - Ablation of micrometastases with radioactive iodine
  - Follow-up by thyroglobulin
- Medullary thyroid carcinoma
  - Occurs sporadically or as part of MEN type 1 or type 2
  - Follow-up post-operatively with calcitonin and carcinoembryonic antigen (CEA)
- Lymphoma: core biopsy followed by radiotherapy and/or chemotherapy
- Undifferentiated carcinoma: palliative surgery to relieve symptoms

Thyroidectomy

- Indications
  - Overall assessment of clinical risk factors
  - Fine-needle aspiration cytology suspicious or frankly malignant
  - Pressure symptoms from large nodules, especially in patients from endemic area
  - Retrosternal extension
  - Cosmesis
- Complications
  - Recurrent laryngeal nerve palsy
  - Injury to the external branch of the superior laryngeal nerve
  - Hypoparathyroidism
  - Acute laryngeal oedema
  - Reactive haemorrhage
  - Persistent hyperthyroidism
  - Residual hypothyroidism
  - Wound problems
  - Thyroid storm

Parathyroid gland

Calcium metabolism

- Stores of calcium
  - Bone (mainly)
  - Soft tissue and extracellular fluid (lesser amounts)
- Physiological functions of calcium
  - Bone formation and growth
  - Nerve synapse function
  - Muscle contractility (striated and cardiac muscles)
  - Blood clotting cascade
- Physiological forms of calcium
  - Free ionised form: biologically active
  - Bound form
    - Inactive
    - Bound to albumin (mainly) and also to phosphate and citrate
- Regulation of calcium metabolism
  - Parathyroid hormone
  - Calcitonin
  - 1,25-dihydroxy vitamin D
- Causes of disturbance of calcium balance
  - Disordered hormone balance in hyperparathyroidism
  - Disseminated malignancy
  - Sarcoidosis
  - Vitamin D preparations
  - Milk–alkali syndrome
  - Thyrotoxicosis

Clinical presentation of hypercalcaemia

- Renal calculi
- Polyuria
- Polydipsia
- Pancreatitis
- Bone pains
- Proximal myopathy
- In elderly patients, confusion and personality change
- Pathological fractures (extremely rare)

Calcitonin

- Polypeptide hormone produced in response to hypercalcaemia, by the parafollicular cells of the thyroid
- Inhibits bone resorption by an having an inhibiting effect on osteoclasts
- Increases excretion of calcium in renal tubules, with conservation of magnesium

Hyperparathyroidism

- Classification
  - Primary hyperparathyroidism
    - Adenoma (common)
    - Carcinoma (rare)
  - Familial benign hypocalciuric hypercalcaemia

- – Secondary hyperparathyroidism
- – Tertiary hyperparathyroidism
- – Ectopic hyperparathyroidism
- Findings of investigations
  - – Biochemical
    - Hypercalcuria in the presence of elevated parathyroid hormone
    - Hypophosphataemia
    - Hyperchloraemia
    - Mild acidosis
    - Possible increased alkaline phosphatase
  - – Radiological
    - Generalised demineralisation of bone: ground glass appearance of the skull, loss of lamina dura around the teeth, loss of bone tufts of the terminal phalanges, and bone cysts
    - Renal calculi

Management of hyperparathyroidism

- Surgery
- Pre-operative localisation
  - – Ultrasound
  - – Thallium subtraction scan
  - – Sestamibi scan
  - – CT and MRI
  - – Selective venous sampling
- Total parathyroidectomy and maintenance of the patient on 1-alpha-dihydroxy vitamin D without calcium supplementation

Multiple endocrine neoplasia (MEN) syndromes

MEN type 1

- Parathyroid adenomas
- Pituitary tumours (various types)
- Pancreatic tumours
  - – Insulinoma
  - – Gastrinoma

MEN type 2A

- Medullary thyroid cancer
- Hyperparathyroidism (hyperplasia more common than adenoma)
- Phaeochromocytoma

MEN type 2B

- Medullary thyroid cancer
- Phaeochromocytoma
- Mucosal (mouth) neuroma
- Marfanoid appearance

Pituitary gland

Cushing's disease

- Pituitary (ACTH)-dependent Cushing's syndrome accounts for 70% of all cases
- ACTH-producing pituitary adenoma or microadenoma (< 1 cm in diameter)
- Primary defect is in the hypothalamus with over-production of corticotrophin releasing hormone (CRH)
- Chronically increased levels of ACTH cause adrenal cortical hyperplasia and corticoid excess
- Feedback to ACTH levels is set to a higher point than normal
- Women are affected more commonly than men

Ectopic ACTH syndrome

- From tumours originating from neuroendocrine cells
- Most common type of causative tumour is small cell (oat cell) carcinoma of the lung
- Other causes
  - – Thymoma
  - – Medullary thyroid cancer
  - – Phaeochromocytoma
  - – Pancreatic islet cell tumour
  - – Ovarian cancer
  - – Pancreas, stomach and bronchial carcinoid

Acromegaly

- Caused by excess secretion of growth hormone in an adult

Features

- Local bone growth in the skull and mandible
- Soft tissue proliferation, with increase in the size of the hands, fingers and feet
- Skin becomes thickened and coarse

- Carpal tunnel syndrome
- Hypercalcaemia, hypercalcuria and renal calculi
- Impairment of glucose metabolism and hyperinsulinism

Diagnosis

- Glucose suppression test: increased growth hormone levels even in the presence of increased blood sugar level, i.e. growth hormone secretion not suppressed by giving glucose
- Can be caused by pituitary tumour or ectopic secretion from:
  - Lung cancer
  - Islet cells tumours in the pancreas
  - Carcinoid of the gut

Adrenal gland

Addison's disease

- Causes
  - Primary insufficiency of adrenal cortex due to:
    - Original cause described by Addison was tuberculosis
    - Metastatic disease of the adrenal
    - Haemorrhage into the adrenals
    - Autoimmune
  - Secondary Addison's disease
    - Failure of the pituitary–adrenal axis
    - Exogenous glucocorticoid therapy with suppression of ACTH
- Presentation
  - Acute effects
    - Hypotension and shock
    - Hypoglycaemia
    - Na^+ depletion and dehydration, due to mineralocorticoid deficiency
  - Chronic effects
    - Anorexia and weight loss
    - Muscle weakness
    - Hypotension
    - Skin and mucosal pigmentation

Adrenal causes of hypertension

- Primary aldosteronism
  - Conn's syndrome (the most common)
    - Hypertension
    - Hypokalaemia

- Hypernatraemia
- Decreased plasma renin
  - Bilateral adrenocortical hyperplasia (idiopathic hyperaldosteronism)
  - Aldosterone-producing adrenocortical carcinoma
  - Aldosterone-producing ovarian carcinoma
- Secondary aldosteronism
  - Severe hypertension from cardiovascular or renal disease associated with excessive secretion of aldosterone
  - Hypertensive stimulation of the juxtaglomerular apparatus, leading to secretion of renin, thereby stimulating the renin–angiotensin mechanism
  - Distinguishing factor from primary aldosteronism is an increased plasma renin activity (whereas renin activity is decreased in primary aldosteronism)

Conn's syndrome

- Definition
  - Primary hyperaldosteronism resulting from a Conn's tumour (adrenocortical adenoma)
- Pathology
  - Unilateral or bilateral
  - Adrenocortical hyperplasia
- Clinical features
  - Continuous hypertension in a patient aged 30–50 years
  - More common in women
  - Muscle weakness and cramps
  - Headaches
  - Polyuria and polydipsia
  - Severe hypokalaemia leading to intermittent tetany
- Biochemical investigations
  - Increased plasma aldosterone
  - Decreased plasma renin activity
- Pre-operative localisation
  - CT scan
  - Selective venous catheterisation
- Treatment
  - Excision of adenoma (adrenalectomy) in fit patients
  - Spironolactone therapy in unfit patients

Neoplasms of the adrenal cortex and medulla

- Cushing's syndrome
  - Adrenocortical adenoma
  - Adrenocortical carcinoma
  - Both are aggressive malignancies
- Adrenal neoplasms can be functioning or non-functioning tumours
  - Functioning tumours in children cause:
    - Cushing's syndrome
    - Hyperaldosteronism
    - Virilisation
    - Feminisation
    - Mixed clinical picture
- Treatment: surgical resection

Phaeochromocytoma

- Functioning tumour of catecholamine-producing chromaffin cells
- Can also be extra-adrenal in location
- Called the '10% tumour'
  - 10% are extra-adrenal
  - 10% are malignant
  - 10% are bilateral
  - 10% occur in children
  - 10% are familial
- Associated with MEN and von Recklinghausen's neurofibromatosis
- Clinical features
  - Hypertension with postural drop in blood pressure
  - Sweating
  - Tachycardia
- Diagnosis
  - 24-hour urine for metanephrine and vanillyl mandelic acid
  - Localisation by CT, MRI or iodine-123-meta-iodobenzylguanidine (MIBG) scanning
- Treatment
  - Surgery: excision after pre-operative control of hypertension

Insulinoma

- Accounts for 75% of endocrine tumours of the pancreas
- Most common in the body and tail of the pancreas
- Derived from alpha cells
- Diagnosis by Whipple's triad
  - Hypoglycaemia caused by fasting
  - Decreased blood glucose during symptomatic episodes
  - Relief of symptoms by intravenous glucose
- Majority of tumours are solitary
- 10% are malignant
- Localisation
  - Angiography
  - Pancreatic ultrasound and CT scanning
  - Endoscopic ultrasound
- Treatment is by surgery
  - If localised: enucleation
  - If deep: distal pancreatectomy or Whipple's procedure
  - For MEN type 1 with multiple tumours: subtotal pancreatectomy

Gastrinoma

- Originates in the pancreas
- Multiple in 50% of cases
- Malignant in 60% of cases
- Most common tumour occurring in extrapancreatic locations, e.g. duodenum
- Results in Zollinger–Ellison syndrome
  - Gastric hypersecretion
  - Widespread peptic ulceration
  - Diarrhoea
- Can be a part of MEN syndrome
- Treatment
  - Medical: antisecretory agents
  - Surgical: tumour enucleation from pancreas
  - Total gastrectomy is not done

Carcinoid tumour

Definition

- Apudomas arising from enterochromaffin cells throughout the gut
- Associated with MEN type 1 or type 2

Site

- Appendix (the most common)
- Small bowel (the second most common)

Clinical features

- May be asymptomatic
- Acute appendicitis

- Obstruction, pain and bleeding from the small bowel
- Carcinoid syndrome

Carcinoid syndrome

- Caused by metastasis from a carcinoid tumour to the liver
- Clinical features
  - Cutaneous flushing
  - Diarrhoea
  - Bronchoconstriction and wheezing
  - Pulmonary stenosis, due to collagen deposition
- Active substance is 5-hydroxytryptamine
- Diagnosis
  - Measurement of 5-hydroxyindoleacetic acid in the urine as a diagnostic marker
- Management of liver metastases
  - Segmental lobar resection
  - If resection is not possible, hepatic artery embolisation
  - Thermal ablation
  - Cryotherapy
  - Infusion of 5-fluorouracil through the hepatic artery

Rare endocrine tumours

VIPomas

- Associated with production of vasoactive intestinal polypeptide (VIP)
- Clinical features
  - Watery diarrhoea
  - Hypokalaemia
  - Achlorhydria

Glucagonoma

- Arises from pancreatic alpha cells
- 25% are benign
- Causes hypersecretion of glucagon and secondary diabetes
- Clinical features
  - Anaemia
  - Weight loss
  - Characteristic rash: necrolytic migratory erythema

Somatostatinoma

- Derived from pancreatic delta cells
- Clinically causes diabetes mellitus, cholelithiasis and steatorrhoea

Splenic functions

Haemopoietic function

- In the embryo: the spleen is the only source of blood cells until the fifth month of gestation
- After birth: spleen produces blood cells in certain haematological disorders, e.g. haemoglobinopathies, myelodysplastic syndromes

Mechanical filtering function

- Occurs in the red pulp
- Removal of old or abnormal red blood cells
- Removal of abnormal leucocytes
- Removal of normal and abnormal platelets and cellular debris

Immunologic functions

- Occurs in the white pulp (malpigian capsule)
- Opsonisation, mainly for poorly opsonised or encapsulated organisms
- Production of:
  - Opsonin: essential for opsonisation
  - Properdin (factor P): essential for the alternative pathway of the complement cascade
  - Tuftsin, which influences antibody formation
  - Antibodies (B lymphocytes)

Hyposplenism

- Decreased functions of spleen
- Causes
  - Splenectomy: elective or traumatic
  - Auto-splenectomy of sickle cell anaemia, due to multiple splenic infarcts
  - Bone marrow transplantation
    - Splenic irradiation
    - Chronic graft-versus-host disease
  - Asplenia: congenital absence of the spleen associated with cardiac anomalies and biliary atresia

Hypersplenism

- Splenomegaly, associated with:
  - Any combination of anaemia, leucopenia or thrombocytopenia
  - Compensatory bone marrow hyperplasia
- Improvement occurs after splenectomy

Splenomegaly

- Enlarged spleen
- Needs to be up to three times the normal size to be palpable clinically

Causes

- Infections (infectious splenomegaly)
  - Bacterial infections
    - Splenic abscess
    - Tuberculosis
    - From subacute bacterial endocarditis
  - Viral infections
    - Infectious mononucleosis (glandular fever)
    - Viral hepatitis
  - Parasitic infestations
    - Malaria
    - Kala-azar (visceral leishmaniasis)
    - Schistosomiasis
- Haematological disorders (hyperplastic splenomegaly)
  - Haemolytic anaemias
    - Thalassaemia
    - Sickle cell anaemia
    - Congenital spherocytosis
  - Leukemias: acute and chronic
  - Lymphomas: Hodgkin's disease, non-Hodgkin's lymphoma, primary splenic lymphoma
  - Polycythaemia rubra vera
  - Essential thrombocytopenia
  - Macroglobulinaemia
  - Myelofibrosis
- Connective tissue disorders (inflammatory splenomegaly)
  - Rheumatoid arthritis

- Felty's syndrome
- Systemic lupus erythematosus
- Polyarteritis nodosa
- Infiltrative disorders (infiltrative splenomegaly)
  - Amyloidosis
  - Sarcoidosis
  - Splenic metastases
- Metabolic disorders
  - Gaucher's disease
  - Niemann–Pick disease
  - Glycogen-storage disease
  - Mucopolysaccharidosis
- Congestive disorders (congestive splenomegaly: Banti's syndrome)
  - Right heart failure
  - Splenic vein thrombosis
  - Portal hypertension
    - Budd–Chiari syndrome
    - Cirrhosis
- Other disorders
  - Histiocytosis X (Letterer–Siwe disease)
  - Splenic cysts: hydatid or dermoid
  - Splenic tumours: haemangioma or haemangiosarcoma

Clinical features

- Mass in the left upper quadrant of the abdomen
- Characteristics of the mass
  - Moves with respiration
  - Directed towards the right iliac fossa
  - It is not possible to insinuate fingers between it and the costal margin, i.e. the upper border is under the ribs
  - Splenic notch may be felt
  - Dull to percussion

Investigations

- Laboratory investigations
  - Full blood count, with platelet count
  - Erythrocyte sedimentation rate (ESR)
  - Liver function tests
- Imaging
  - Abdominal ultrasound
  - CT scan
  - MRI
  - Splenoportography
  - Angiography
  - Splenic scan

- Biopsy
  - Liver biopsy
  - Bone marrow biopsy
  - Lymph node biopsy

Splenectomy

- Becoming rarer because non-invasive diagnostic procedures and medical management have improved

Indications

- Splenic rupture
  - Spontaneous rupture
  - Traumatic rupture
    - Blunt trauma
    - Penetrating trauma
    - Motorcycle accident in which one end of the handlebar strikes the abdomen
- To control or stage disease
  - Immune haemolytic anaemia
  - Immune thrombocytopenia
  - Hodgkin's disease, as part of staging laparotomy (rarely done nowadays)
- To correct chronic or severe hypersplenism
  - Hairy cell leukemia
  - Myeloid metaplasia
  - Felty's syndrome
  - Gaucher's disease
  - Splenic vein thrombosis
  - Haemolytic splenomegaly
    - Thalassaemia major
    - Splenic sickle cell sequestration crisis
    - Congenital erythropoietic porphyria

Procedure

- Open procedure or laparoscopic procedure
- Total splenectomy or partial splenectomy

Haematological consequences

- Thrombocytosis
  - Fairly acute
  - Platelet count may be $> 1000 \times 10^9/L$
  - Risk of thromboembolism
  - Platelet count drops within 1–2 weeks, but may stay at levels of $400 \times 109/L$ to $500 \times 10^9/L$ for over a year

- Leukocytosis
  - Initially, polymorphonuclear leucocytes (granulocytes) are elevated
  - Then lymphocytes are elevated
  - Lastly monocytes are elevated
- Reticulocytosis: reticulocyte count > 20%
- Red blood cell changes, with formation of:
  - Target cells
  - Howell–Jolly bodies
  - Heinz bodies
  - Siderocytes

Complications

- Early complications
  - Infection: subphrenic abscess
  - Thrombosis: aspirin is given until the platelet count returns to normal
- Late complications
  - Infective: overwhelming post-splenectomy infection (OPSI) or overwhelming post-splenectomy sepsis (OPSS)

OPSI and OPSS

- Fulminant life-threatening infection representing major long-term sequel
- Relative risks
  - 0.4%/year
  - Greatest in 1st 2 years post-splenectomy but remains for life
  - More in children (splenectomy is contraindicated in children <5)
  - More after elective splenectomy
- Common pathogens
  - *Streptococcus pneumoniae* (in 50–90% of cases)
  - *Haemophilus influenzae* type B
  - *Neisseria meningitides* type B
  - Group A streptococci

- Caused by loss of opsonisation and decreased B-lymphocytes
- Clinical presentation
  - Non-specific, flu-like prodrome followed by rapid evolution to full-blown bacteraemic septic shock with disseminated intravascular coagulation (true emergency)
- Management
  - Early recognition of patients at risk
  - Aggressive intervention
    - Fluid resuscitation
    - Empiric antibiotics, e.g. cefotaxime, ceftriaxone or vancomycin
- Prophylaxis
  - Immunoprophylaxis
    - Pneumovax 23, given 2 weeks before or after an elective splenectomy or 2 weeks after an emergency splenectomy, with a booster every 5 years
    - *Haemophilus* B conjugate vaccine: for children only, with a booster every year
    - Meningococcal vaccine: should be given pre-splenectomy (three doses for infants, two doses for young children, and one dose for older children and adults)
  - Chemoprophylaxis (given lifelong)
    - Penicillin V
    - Amoxicillin
    - Erythromycin
- General measures
  - Medi-alert bracelet
  - 'No-spleen' card

Chapter 19 — Gastrointestinal system

Gastrointestinal physiology

Gastrointestinal innervation

Enteric nervous system
- Myenteric plexus (Auerbach's plexus)
  - Between the outer longitudinal and the inner circular muscles
  - For motility
- Submucous plexus (Meissner's plexus)
  - Between the middle circular and mucosal layers
  - For secretion
- Contents
  - Motor neurones, which innervate smooth muscle
  - Secretory neurones, which regulate endocrine and exocrine secretion in the mucosa
  - Sensory neurones, which respond to stretch, tonicity and the presence of glucose and amino acids
  - Interneurones
- Substances secreted
  - Acetylcholine
  - Serotonin
  - Gamma-aminobutyric acid (GABA)
  - Polypeptides (see below)

Extrinsic innervation
- Function of the autonomous nervous system
- Parasympathetic cholinergic innervation
  - Increases smooth muscle activity
- Sympathetic noradrenergic innervation
  - Decreases smooth muscle activity
  - Decreases sphincter contraction

Effects of polypeptides secreted by neurones
- Polypeptides secreted by motor neurones
  - Vasoactive intestinal peptide (VIP): relaxation of smooth muscles and sphincters
  - Substance P: contraction of smooth muscle
  - Cholecystokinin: inhibition of gastric emptying
  - Somatostatin: inhibition of intestinal motility
  - Neurotensin: relaxation of circular smooth muscle
  - Encephalin:
    - Relaxation of intestinal smooth muscle
    - Pyloric contraction
  - Galanin: contraction of intestinal smooth muscle
- Polypeptides secreted by secretory neurones
  - Gastrin releasing peptide (GRP): release of gastrin
  - Calcitonin gene-related peptide (CGRP): release of somatostatin
  - Somatostatin: inhibition of acid and intestinal secretion
  - VIP: stimulation of intestinal secretion
  - Substance P: inhibition of acid and stimulation of pepsin secretion
- Polypeptides secreted by sensory neurones
  - CGRP
  - Substance P

Gastric motility and emptying
- Receptive relaxation when food enters stomach
- Peristaltic contraction, which mixes food and releases it into the duodenum at a controlled rate
  - Gastric slow wave or basic electric rhythm, which is the pacemaker for antral peristalsis
  - Plays a major role in control of gastric emptying
- Peristalsis occurs even when the stomach is empty; it gradually increases in intensity and is felt as painful hunger contractions

Regulation of gastric motility and secretion

- Neural regulation
  - Local autonomic (cholinergic) regulation
  - From the CNS via the vagus nerve
  - Humoral regulation
    - Gastrointestinal hormones
- Actions of vagal stimulation
  - Increased gastric secretion caused by release of GRP, leading to increased acidity
  - Releases acetylcholine, which acts directly to release acid and pepsin
- Phases of regulation
  - Cephalic phase
    - Presence of food in the mouth leads to stimulation of gastric secretion via the vagus nerve
    - The sight, smell and thought of food stimulate acid secretion
    - Regulatory centre is in the hypothalamus
    - Anger and hostility increases secretion
    - Fear and depression decreases secretion
  - Gastric phase
    - By food in the stomach
    - Receptors in the wall of stomach respond to stretch and amino acids via Meissner's plexus
    - Stimulates parietal cells to increase acid secretion
    - Reflexes are totally within the wall of the stomach
  - Intestinal phase
    - Fats, carbohydrates and acid in the duodenum inhibit gastric acid and pepsin secretion and gastric motility
  - Other influences
    - Hypoglycaemia through the brain and vagal efferents: increases acid and pepsin secretion
    - Alcohol and caffeine by direct effect on the mucosa: increase secretion
- Gastric emptying
  - Food rich in carbohydrate empties faster than protein, which is in turn faster than fat
  - Hyperosmolality of duodenal contents decreases gastric emptying (probably neural in origin)
  - Enterogastric reflex: products of protein digestion and H^+ ions in the duodenum decrease gastric emptying
  - Vagotomy decreases gastric emptying

Factors preventing oesophagogastric reflux

- Anatomical factors
  - Valvular effect of angle of His (oesophagogastric angle)
  - Pinch-cock action of the right diaphragmatic crus
  - Rosette-like folds of gastric mucosa at the cardia
  - Presence of a 2 cm length of intra-abdominal oesophagus
  - Sling band of muscle on the fundus that accentuates the angle of His
- Physiological factors
  - High-pressure zone at the oesophagogastric junction

Diagnosis of oesophageal disorders

Typical symptoms

- Dysphagia
  - Mechanical: for solids
  - Functional (globus hystericus): for liquids
- Regurgitation
  - Reflux disease
  - May lead to aspiration pneumonitis
- Odynophagia
  - Oesophagitis
    - Reflux
    - Radiation
    - Viral infection
    - Fungal infection
- Chest pain and heartburn
  - Reflux
  - Increased at night
- Waterbrash: reflux

Atypical clinical features

- Anaemia, due to chronic blood loss
- Haematemesis
- Pulmonary symptoms

Investigations for oesophageal disease

Summary of investigations for oesophageal disease		
Category	Test	Indications
Radiological	Chest X-ray	Aspiration pneumonitis, oesophageal perforation
	Barium swallow	Dysphagia, perforation, motility disorders
	Fluoroscopy	Motility disorders, reflux
	CT	Staging of malignancy
Ultrasound	External	Motility disorders, reflux
	Endoscopic	Staging of malignancy
Radio-isotope		Oesophageal transit, reflux
Endoscopy + biopsy		All patients with dysphagia
Physiological	Manometry	Reflux, motility disorders, non-cardiac chest pain
	24 hour pH	Reflux

Gastrointestinal motility waves

Distal two thirds of stomach

- Propulsive and retropulsive waves
  - Start in the mid-stomach and move distally to the pylorus
  - Since the waves move faster than gastric contents, retropulsion occurs
  - Purpose is for thorough mixing and digesting of food and to enable controlled release into the duodenum
- Migrating motor complex
  - From the stomach to the terminal ileum during fasting state

Small intestine

- Migrating motor complex: during the fasting state
- Propulsive waves: during the fed state, in aboral direction

Colon

- Proximal colon
  - Disorganised contraction waves to:
    - Mix contents
    - Allow maximum absorption of water

- Distal colon
  - Mass movements: to move luminal contents aborally
  - Segmental contractions to slow the forward movement of contents

Rectum

- Faster segmental contraction to slow the influx of material
- Upon filling, distension initiates the rectal sphincteric reflex and causes the desire for defaecation
- Voluntary control of the external anal sphincter causes accommodation of the rectal vault and the termination of the rectal sphincteric reflex

Gastro-oesophageal reflux disease

- Physiological phenomenon normally occurring in the post-prandial period
- Becomes pathological if the duration of exposure is long (> 5% of 24 hours), when it causes mucosal sensitisation

Factors that resist reflux and damage

- Competence of lower oesophageal sphincter
  - Sling-like muscle arrangement
  - Length of the intra-abdominal segment of the oesophagus (minimum of 2 cm)
  - Diaphragmatic crural mechanism
  - Acute angle of His
- Oesophageal clearance of refluxate
  - Peristalsis
  - Neutralisation by swallowed saliva
- Mucosal resistance by submucosal glands that produce HCO_3^-
- *Helicobacter pylori* infection, which is protective against gastro-oesophageal reflux disease

Factors that promote reflux and damage

- Dysfunctional gastro-oesophageal sphincter
  - Primary weakness of smooth muscle
  - Short length of intra-abdominal oesophagus
  - Increased transient oesophageal relaxations
  - Presence of hiatus hernia
- Gastric distension and gastric outlet obstruction
- Refluxate
  - Pure acid and pepsin
  - Mixed acid and duodenal juices (more harmful)

Clinical features

- Heartburn, which increases on bending and stooping
- Regurgitation, which increases on bending and stooping
- Dysphagia, which increases on bending and stooping
- Aspiration syndromes

Classification

- Savary–Miller classification (endoscopic)
  - Grade 1: single erosion
  - Grade 2: multiple erosions
  - Grade 3: circumferential erosion
  - Grade 4: chronic lesion
  - Grade 5: columnar epithelium

Complications

- Reflux oesophagitis
- Deep ulceration with peri-oesophagitis
- Strictures and webs
- Columnar metaplasia (Barrett's oesophagus)

Treatment

- Change of lifestyle
  - Dietary changes
    - Small frequent meals
    - Avoidance of smoking
  - Postural changes
    - Sleeping propped up
- Medical therapy
  - Antacids
  - Histamine-2 blockers
  - Proton pump inhibitors
  - Prokinetics
- Surgical therapy
  - Nissen fundoplication (complete or partial)
  - Posterior gastropexy
  - Angelchik's prosthesis (split ring around the gastro-oesophageal junction)

Oesophageal motility disorders

Classification

- Primary disorders
  - Specific conditions
    - Achalasia
    - Diffuse oesophageal spasm
    - 'Nutcracker' oesophagus (high-amplitude peristalsis)
  - Non-specific conditions
    - High pressure at the lower oesophageal sphincter
    - Hypoperistalsis or aperistalsis
- Secondary disorders
  - Systemic sclerosis
  - Systemic lupus erythematosus
  - Rheumatoid arthritis
  - Diabetes mellitus

– Chagas' disease (achalasia caused by *Trypanosoma cruzi*)

Achalasia

- Aetiology: decrease or loss of myenteric ganglion cells
- Pathogenesis
  - Loss of propulsive peristalsis
  - Stasis, leading to progressive dilatation and lengthening
  - Mucosal inflammation and ulcers
- Clinical features
  - Dysphagia for solids
  - Regurgitation with halitosis
  - Chest pain
  - Respiratory complications
    - Pneumonia
    - Bronchiectasis
    - Lung abscess
- Investigations
  - Contrast radiology: shows fluid levels and 'parrot-beak' appearance
  - Endoscopy
  - Manometry
- Treatment
  - Long-acting nitrates to decrease lower oesophageal pressure
  - Injection of botulinum toxin
  - Pneumatic dilatation of the lower oesophageal sphincter
  - Surgical myotomy (open or laparoscopic)

Diffuse oesophageal spasm

- Multiple spontaneous contractions of long duration, alternating with normal peristalsis
- Aetiology
  - Cholinergic
  - Emotional stress
  - Olfactory stimuli
- Clinical features
  - Substernal chest pain
  - Odynophagia
  - Dysphagia
- Treatment
  - Medical therapy
    - Long-acting nitrates
    - Anticholinergics
    - Psychotropics

– Surgery
  - Long myotomy from the aortic arch to the oesophagogastric junction

'Nutcracker' oesophagus

- Hypercontractile peristalsis
- Treatment
  - Long-acting nitrates
  - Anti-secretory therapy
  - Calcium channel blockers
  - Long myotomy

Oesophageal foreign body

- Most commonly impacted material is food, which usually signifies underlying disease
- Investigations
  - Plain X-ray
  - Contrast X-ray may make endoscopy difficult
- Management
  - Removal by flexible endoscopy
  - Usually removed with grasping forceps, snare or basket
  - An over-tube is used in case of sharp objects
  - Button cells should never be pushed into the stomach as it corrodes the mucosa
  - Food bolus
    - Patient given fizzy drinks to break up the bolus
    - The cause of the obstruction is then investigated

Oesophageal carcinoma

- Incidence: 2%

Causes

- Increased dietary intake of tannic acid (strong tea)
- Vitamin A deficiency
- Riboflavin deficiency
- Zinc deficiency
- Fungal contamination of food
- Opium ingestion
- Thermal injury
- Smoking
- Drinking of spirits
- Human papilloma virus (HPV) infection

- Barrett's oesophagus
- Oesophageal stasis
  - Stricture
  - Web
  - Achalasia
- Post-cricoid carcinoma as part of Plummer–Vinson syndrome

Classification

- Squamous cell carcinoma
  - Ulcerated
  - Annular (causing dysphagia)
- Adenocarcinoma
  - – Usually in the lower third of the oesophagus

Spread

- Lymphatic spread
- Local spread
  - To the mediastinum
  - Tracheo-oesophageal fistula
  - To the aorta (causing fatal haemorrhage)
- Haematogenous
  - To the liver
  - To the lungs

Prognosis

- Poor
- 5-year survival: 5%

Macroscopic types

- Polypoid
- Stenosing
- Ulcerative

Associated oncogenes and tumour-suppressor genes

- EGF DNA
- EGF receptor
- TGF-alpha
- *hst* 1 and *int* 2
- *p53* mutations
- *CDK N2* deletion

Clinical features

- Progressive dysphagia

Investigations

- CT scan
- Endoscopic ultrasound
- Bronchoscopy

TNM staging

- TNM staging of oesophageal cancer (AJCC)
  - TX – primary tumour cannot be assessed
  - T0 – no evidence of primary tumour
  - T_{IS} – carcinoma-in-situ
  - T1a – tumour invades lamina propria
  - T1b – tumour invades sub-mucosa
  - T2 – tumour invades muscularis propria
  - T3 – tumour invades adventitia
  - T4 – tumour invades adjacent structures
  - NX – regional lymph nodes cannot be assessed
  - N0 – no regional lymph nodes
  - N1 - lymph nodal mets
  - MX – distant metastases cannot be assessed
  - M0 – no distant metastases
  - M1 – distant metastases
- Stage grouping
  - Stage 0 – T_{IS} N0 M0
  - Stage I – T1 N0 M0
  - Stage IIA – T2 N0 M0; T3 N0 M0
  - Stage IIB – T1,2 N1 M0
  - Stage III – T3 N1 M0, T4, any N, M0
  - Stage IV – any T, any N, M1
- 5-year survival
  - T1 – 46.1%
  - T2 – 29%
  - T3 – 21.7%
  - T4 – 70%

Treatment

- Nutritional therapy pre-operatively
- Surgery
  - Oesophagectomy with nodal resection
  - Oesophagogastrectomy
- Minimally invasive procedures
  - Endoscopic mucosal resection
  - Laser therapy
  - Photodynamic therapy
- Chemoradiation therapy
  - Neo-adjuvant chemoradiation
  - Palliative chemoradiation
- Radiotherapy
  - External-beam radiation
  - Intra-luminal brachytherapy
- Chemotherapy
  - 5-fluorouracil and cisplatin

- Intubation
  - Celestin tube
  - Self-expanding metal stents
- Photodynamic therapy
- Electrocoagulation

Oesophageal diverticula

Classification

- Congenital diverticulum, due to incomplete duplication
- Acquired diverticulum
  - Pulsion diverticulum, caused by increased intraluminal pressure
  - Traction diverticulum: inflammatory adhesions with mediastinal strictures
  - Pseudodiverticulum, caused by dilatation of the oesophageal glands

Clinically important diverticula

- Pharyngo-oesophageal diverticulum (Zenker's diverticulum): accounts for 65% of cases
- Mid-thoracic diverticulum (15% of case)
- Epiphrenic diverticulum (20% of cases)

Zenker's diverticulum

- Pulsion variety, secondary to cricopharyngeal diverticulum
- Site: the posterior aspect of pharyngo-oesophageal junction, on the left
- Aetiology: failure of the cricopharynx to relax with swallowing
- Complications
  - Pneumonitis
  - Lung abscess
  - Bleeding
  - Perforation (iatrogenic)
  - Carcinoma (in 0.3% of cases)
- Clinical features
  - More common in males
  - More common in the middle-aged and elderly
  - Dysphagia, chronic cough and recurrent chest infections
  - If large, it is clinically palpable on the left side of the neck
- Investigations
  - Barium swallow
  - Manometry

- Treatment
  - Surgery
    - Cricopharyngeal myotomy
    - Diverticulectomy
    - Diverticulopexy

Other diverticula

- Mid thoracic diverticulum
  - Secondary to oesophageal spasm
  - Complications
    - Inflammation and perforation
    - Tracheobroncho-oesophageal fistula
  - Surgery: excision and layered closure
- Epiphrenic diverticulum
  - Secondary to increased intraluminal pressure
  - Ulceration leads to haematemesis
  - Treatment
    - If small, they are managed conservatively
    - If large, they are treated by excision and correction of the underlying motility disorder

Peptic ulcer

Definition

- Breach in the epithelial surface of the gastrointestinal tract caused by attack by acid and pepsin

Sites

- Stomach
- Duodenum
- Lower oesophagus
- Gastrojejunal anastomosis
- Meckel's diverticulum with gastric mucosa

Classification and aetiology

- Acute peptic ulcer
  - Acute gastritis
    - Drugs
    - Alcohol
  - Severe hyperacidity
    - Zollinger–Ellison syndrome
  - Stress ulceration
    - Sepsis
    - Pancreatitis
    - Trauma
    - Head injury (Cushing's syndrome)
    - Burns (Curling's ulcer)
    - Mucosal ischaemia

- Chronic peptic ulcer
  - Normal mucosal barrier consists of an HCO_3^- barrier and the surface epithelium
  - Ulceration is due to:
    - Destruction of the mucosa
    - Loss of the epithelium
  - Examples
    - *H. pylori* gastritis
    - Drug-induced ulceration by non-steroidal anti-inflammatory drugs
    - Smoking-related ulceration
    - Diet-related ulceration
    - Alcohol-related ulceration
    - Stress-related ulceration
- Other predisposing factors
  - Uraemia
  - Hyperparathyroidism
  - Hypercalcaemia
  - Chronic obstructive pulmonary disease (COPD)
  - Alcoholic cirrhosis

Complications

- Perforation, leading to peritonitis
- Bleeding as a result of erosion of a vessel at the base of the ulcer
- Penetration into the liver or pancreas
- Scarring, leading to pyloric stenosis
- Malignant change
  - Rare in gastric ulcers
  - Never in duodenal ulcers

Carcinoma of the stomach

Aetiology and associations

- Diets rich in nitrates
  - Smoked fish
  - Spicy foods
- Blood group A
- Pernicious anaemia
- Atrophic gastritis
- Previous gastric surgery
- Benign gastric ulcer
- *H. pylori* infection
- Genetic associations
  - Changes in tumour suppressor genes: *p53*, k-*ras*, *APC*
  - Over-expression of oncogenes: c-*myc*
- Type III intestinal metaplasia

Classification

- Japanese classification
  - Early (involving the mucosa with or without the submucosa)
    - Protruding
    - Superficial
    - Excavating
  - Advanced (beyond the muscularis propria)
- Lauren or 'DIO' classification
  - Diffuse: worse prognosis, e.g. linitis plastica
  - Intestinal: well differentiated
  - Others

Prognosis

- Good in:
  - Early gastric cancer
  - Cases in which few nodes are involved
  - Well-differentiated tumours

Microscopic classification

- Intestinal: glands with mucus-secreting cells (signet ring)
- Diffuse: poorly demarcated, invasive margin

Spread

- Direct spread, to adjacent organs, e.g. the pancreas
- Lymphatic spread
  - Local lymph nodes along the right and left gastric arteries
  - To the coeliac nodes
  - To the porta hepatis nodes, causing obstructive jaundice
  - To distant nodes, notably to the left supraclavicular nodes (Virchow's nodes), causing Troisier's sign
- Haematogenous spread, via the portal vein to the liver
- Trans-coelomic spread, producing a Krukenberg tumour

Staging

- TNM (UICC) staging (T – tumour, N – nodes, M – metastases, P – peritoneal deposits, H – hepatic deposits)
  - Tx – unknown
  - T_{IS}

- Tumour-in-situ
- No breach of basement membrane
- Intra-epithelial tumour without invasion of lamina propria
- T1 – up to lamina propria/sub-mucosa
- T2 – up to muscularis propria/sub-serosa
- T3 – serosal penetration
- T4 – diffuse infiltration of gastric wall
- N0 – no nodes
- Nx – nodal status unknown
- N1
  - Peri-gastric nodes, within 3 cm of edge of tumour
  - In case of pyloric growth, juxtapyloric is N1, whereas in cardiac growth, juxtapyloric is N2
- N2
  - Peri-gastric >3 cm from edge of tumour
  - Nodes along left gastric, common hepatic, splenic or celiac vessels
- There is no N3; beyond N2, it becomes M1
- M0 – no metastases
- M1
  - Distant metastases
  - Liver, ovary
  - Nodes beyond regional
- P0 – no peritoneal metastases
- P1 – peritoneal metastases to adjacent but not distant peritoneum
- P2 – a few metastases to distant peritoneum
- P3 – numerous metastases to distant peritoneum
- H0 – no hepatic deposits
- H1 – deposits limited to one lobe
- H2 – a few metastases in both lobes
- H3 – numerous metastases in both lobes
- Staging based on TNM
  - Stage I A – T1
  - Stage I B – T1 N1 / T2 N0
  - Stage II – T1 N2 / T2 N1 / T3 N0
  - Stage III A – T2 N2 / T3 N1/ T4 N0
  - Stage III B – T3 N2 / T4 N1
  - Stage IV – T4 N2 / M1
  - If N2 – it is minimum stage II
  - If T3 – it is minimum stage II
  - If T4 – it is minimum stage III A
  - If M1 – it is stage IV
- Stage grouping

Stage grouping

		P0 H0 M0				P0 H1 N0,1,2
		N0	N1	N2	N3	
P0 H0 M0	T1	Ia	Ib	II	IIIa	IVa
	T2	Ib	II	IIIa	IIIb	
	T3	II	IIIa	IIIb	IVa	
	T4	IIIa	IIIb	IVa		
P1 H0 T1,2,3	IVa					

- Staging by Japanese Research Society for Gastric Carcinoma
  - Serosal penetration of primary tumour (Ps)
    - SSY – sub-serosal invasion; serosa clear
    - Se – serosal invasion
    - Si – serosal invasion through all layers
    - Sei – serosal invasion ± neighboring structures
  - Peritoneal spread
    - P0 – none
    - ↓
    - P3 – multiple nodules below meso-colon or on diaphragm
  - Hepatic spread
    - H0 – none
    - ↓
    - H3 – multiple, both lobes
  - Nodal spread
    - N0 – no nodes
    - N1-3 – stations 1–3 involved
    - N4 – beyond station 3

Complications

- Weight loss
- Anaemia
- Dysphagia in lesions of the cardia
- Gastric outlet obstruction in lesions of the antrum
- Bleeding: haematemesis, malaena
- Jaundice, hepatomegaly and ascites in advanced carcinoma

Sequelae of gastric surgery

- Recurrence of the disease
- Nutritional sequelae
  - Weight loss
  - Anaemia
    - Iron deficiency
    - Vitamin B12 deficiency
  - Milk intolerance
  - Bone disease
  - Dumping syndromes
  - Reactive hypoglycaemia
  - Bile vomiting
  - Diarrhoea
  - Small stomach syndrome
- Mechanical sequelae
  - Afferent or efferent loop obstruction
  - Jejunogastric intussusception
  - Gastro-oesophageal reflux
- Other sequelae
  - Cholelithiasis
  - Bezoar formation

Peristalsis

Definition

- Reflex response initiated by the gut wall being stretched by its contents, occurring in all parts of gastrointestinal tract

Constituents

- Gut wall stretching initiates circular contraction behind the stimulus and relaxation in front of it
- Wave of contraction moves caudally, propelling the food at 2–25 cm/second
- Peristalsis can be increased or decreased by the autonomic nervous system but is independent of extrinsic innervation

Polypeptides involved

- Stretch is sensed by neurones containing CGRP
- Circular contraction is produced by acetylcholine and substance P
- Relaxation in front of the stimulus is produced by VIP

Ileus

- Definition: decrease in intestinal motility

Causes

- Trauma to intestines causes direct inhibition of smooth muscle
- Irritation of peritoneum causes increased discharge of noradrenergic fibres in the splanchnic nerves

Effects

- Contents are not propelled into the colon
- Bowel becomes irregularly distended by pockets of gas and fluid

Return of peristalsis after laparotomy

- Small bowel: 6–8 hours
- Stomach: 8 hours
- Colon: 2–3 days

Treatment of adynamic ileus

- Nasoenteric tube aspiration

Gut hormones

Classification

- Gastrin family
  - Gastrin
  - Cholecystokinin
- Secretin family
  - Secretin
  - Glucagon
  - Glicentin (GLI)
  - VIP
  - Gastric inhibitory polypeptide (GIP)

Gastrin

- Produced by G-cells (APUD cells, or amine precursor uptake and decarboxylation cells) in the gastric antral mucosa
- TG cells also produce gastrin and are found throughout stomach and GIT
- Gastrin is found in pancreatic islets in fetal life – persistence of the cells in adult life leads to gastrinoma
- Actions
  - Stimulation of gastric acid and pepsin secretion
  - Stimulation of growth of the mucosa of the stomach, small and large intestines (trophic action)
  - Stimulation of gastric motility

- Stimulation of insulin and glucagon secretion after a protein meal
- Factors that increase gastrin secretion
  - Luminal factors
    - Action of peptides and amino acids
    - Distension
  - Neural factors
    - Increased vagal discharge
  - Blood-borne factors
    - Calcium
    - Adrenaline
- Factors that decrease gastrin secretion
  - Luminal factors
    - Acid
  - Blood-borne factors
    - Secretin
    - GIP
    - VIP
    - Glucagon
    - Calcitonin

Cholecystokinin

- Also known as pancreozymin
- Secreted by cells in the mucosa of the upper small intestine
- Actions
  - Contraction of the gallbladder
  - Secretion of pancreatic juice rich in enzymes
  - Augmentation of action of secretin in producing alkaline pancreatic juice
  - Inhibition of gastric emptying
  - Increased secretion of enterokinase
  - Enhancement of motility of the small intestine and colon
  - Augmentation of contraction of the pyloric sphincter to prevent duodenogastric reflux (together with secretin)
- Factors that increase secretion
  - Contact of intestinal mucosa by products of digestion (peptides and amino acids)
  - Presence of fatty acids in the duodenum
- Factors that decrease secretion
  - Movement of products of digestion to the lower gastrointestinal tract

Secretin

- Secreted by S cells in the upper small intestine

- Actions
  - Increased secretion of HCO_3^- by the biliary and pancreatic duct, leading to alkalinisation of pancreatic juice
  - Augments the action of cholecystokinin in producing pancreatic juice
  - Gastric acid secretion
  - Contraction of the pyloric sphincter
- Factors that increase secretin
  - Products of protein digestion
  - Acid in the upper small intestine, which causes alkaline pancreatic juice (by a feedback mechanism)

Gastric inhibitory peptide (GIP)

- Produced by K cells in the mucosa of the duodenum and jejunum
- Increased by glucose and fat in the duodenum
- Actions
  - Inhibition of gastric secretion and motility
  - Stimulation of insulin secretion

Vasoactive intestinal peptide (VIP)

- Found in nerves of the gastrointestinal tract
- Actions
  - Increases intestinal secretion of electrolytes and water
  - Relaxation of intestinal smooth muscles, including sphincters
  - Dilatation of peripheral blood vessels
  - Inhibition of gastric acid secretion

Other gastrointestinal hormones

- Motilin
  - Secreted by enterochromaffin cells of the duodenal mucosa
  - Causes contraction of intestinal smooth muscle cells
- Neurotensin
  - Produced by mucosal cells of the ileum
  - Inhibits gastrointestinal motility and increases ileal blood flow
- Substance P
  - Increases motility of the gastrointestinal tract

- GRP
  - Present in vagal nerve endings
  - Increases gastrin secretion
- Somatostatin
  - Secreted by D cells of the pancreatic islets and the gastrointestinal mucosa
  - Inhibits secretion of gastrin, VIP, GIP, secretin and motilin
  - Also inhibits acid secretion, pancreatic exocrine secretion, gastrointestinal motility and gallbladder contraction
- Glucagon
  - Secreted by A cells of the pancreatic islets and by the gastric and duodenal mucosa
  - Plays a role in the hyperglycaemia of diabetes

Functions of the liver

- Production of bile
- Storage
  - Glycogen
  - Vitamins A, D, E and K
  - Vitamin B12
- Metabolism of proteins, fats and carbohydrates
- Detoxification and inactivation of hormones, drugs and toxins
- Reticuloendothelial function, via Kupffer cells
- Haemopoiesis in the fetus

Energy sources and supply

- From metabolites received from the gut
- From peripheral tissues during fasting
  - Fatty acids and glycerol from adipose tissue
  - Lactate and pyruvate from erythrocytes
  - Lactate, pyruvate and keto acids from skeletal muscles
- Conversion of energy to glucose
  - Glycogenolysis
  - Gluconeogenesis
  - Both contribute to energy supply

Synthesis and metabolism of nitrogenous compounds

- Ammonia from proteins and urea
- Protein synthesis
  - Integral membrane proteins
  - Secretory proteins

- Albumin
- Immunoglobulin
- Clotting factors
- Proteases
  - Acute phase proteins
    - C-reactive protein (CRP)

Lipoprotein synthesis and lipid metabolism

- Chylomicrons
- Very low-density lipoprotein (VLDL)
- High-density lipoprotein (HDL)
- Low-density lipoprotein (LDL)
- All of these molecules transport excess cholesterol from the peripheral circulation to the liver for bile acid synthesis

Control of blood coagulation and fibrinolysis

- Synthesis of clotting factors
- Synthesis of inhibitors of coagulation
  - Antithrombin III
  - Protein C
  - Protein S
  - C1 inhibitor
  - alpha-1 antitrypsin
- Synthesis of antiplasmin (which is fibrinolytic)
- Clearance and catabolism of activated clotting factors and plasminogen activators by Kupffer cells

Detoxification of harmful metabolites and drugs

- Oxidation–reduction by cytochrome p450
  - Insulin
  - ADH
  - Growth hormone
  - Steroids
  - Catecholamines
- Conjugation
  - Morphine
  - Propranolol
  - Dopamine
  - Adrenaline
- Hydrolysis

Metabolism of haem and bile pigments

- Breakdown of haem through cleavage of the porphyrin ring by the enzyme haem

oxygenase in the spleen and Kupffer cells to form biliverdin
- Biliverdin is reduced to bilirubin by bilirubin reductase
- Bilirubin conjugates to monoglucoronides and diglucoronides (bile pigments) in the liver

Enterohepatic circulation
- See below

Bile secretion causes fat absorption
- Bile secretion causes fat absorption

Immune surveillance by Kupffer cells
- Phagocytosis of bacteria
- Clearance of endotoxins

Haemopoiesis
- Liver has a haemopoietic function in the fetus up to 20th week of gestation

Extrahepatic (enteropathic) circulation of bile salts
- 95% of bile acids entering the gut are reabsorbed by receptors in the terminal ileum
- Primary bile acids, e.g. cholic acid and chenodeoxycholic acid, enter the gut
- They are converted to secondary bile acids (deoxycholic acid and lithocholic acid) in the proximal colon by dehydroxylation
- They circulate back to liver, where lithocholic acid is sulphated and the rest enter back into intestines unchanged
- Sulphated lithocholic acid is excreted in faeces and others are recycled, six to eight times a day
- Purpose
  - Conservation of bile acids by recycling: hepatic synthesis of bile acids is only 5% to replace daily losses; 95% are recycled

Portal hypertension
Causes
- Pre-hepatic portal hypertension (obstruction of the portal vein)

  - Congenital atresia or stenosis
  - Portal vein thrombosis
  - Extrinsic compression, e.g. from a tumour
- Hepatic portal hypertension (obstruction to portal flow within the liver)
  - Cirrhosis (the most common cause in the UK)
  - Hepatoportal sclerosis
  - Schistosomiasis (the most common cause in many parts of the world
  - Sarcoidosis
- Post-hepatic portal hypertension
  - Budd–Chiari syndrome (idiopathic hepatic venous thrombosis)
  - Other causes of hepatic venous thrombosis
    - Polycythaemia
    - Oral contraception
    - Congenital obliteration of hepatic veins
    - Tumour invasion of hepatic veins
  - Constrictive pericarditis

Portal vein pressure
- Normal portal vein pressure: 7–10 mmHg
- In portal hypertension: > 10 mmHg; average: 20–25 mmHg

Sites of portosystemic anastomosis
- Oesophageal branch of the left gastric vein → oesophageal tributaries of azygos system (lower end of the oesophagus)
- Superior rectal branch of inferior mesenteric vein → the inferior rectal veins
- Portal tributaries of mesenteric → retroperitoneal veins
- Veins of the abdominal wall and veins accompanying the ligamentum teres and falciform ligament
- Veins of the diaphragm in relation to bare area of liver

Associations of portal hypertension
- Hypersplenism
  - Haemolytic anaemia
  - Leukopenia
  - Thrombocytopenia
- Ascites

- Gastrointestinal haemorrhage from oesophageal varices:
  - Balloon tamponade
    - Sengstaken–Blakemore tube
    - Linton tube
  - Endoscopic sclerotherapy
  - Endoscopic ligation
  - Drugs
    - Vasopressin plus nitroglycerin
    - Octreotide
  - Surgery
    - Portosystemic shunts (portocaval, splenorenal or mesocaval): may lead to encephalopathy
    - Transjugular intrahepatic portosystemic stent shunt (TIPSS)

Gallstones

Types

- 80% are mixed stones, 10% of which contain calcium
- 10% are pure cholesterol stones

Aetiology

- Following Crohn's disease of the terminal ileum and terminal ileal resection
- Oestrogen increases hepatic synthesis of cholesterol in women of childbearing age
- Diet high in animal fat and low in fibre
- Decreased motility of the gallbladder
  - Pregnancy
  - Starvation and total parenteral nutrition
- Pure pigment stones
  - Thalassaemia and sickle cell disease
  - Hereditary spherocytosis
  - Infection with *Escherichia coli* or *Bacteroides* species

Consequences of gallstones

- Inflammation of the gallbladder
  - Acute cholecystitis
  - Chronic cholecystitis
  - Acute-on-chronic cholecystitis
- Obstructive jaundice leading to secondary biliary cirrhosis
- Ascending cholangitis
- Empyema of the gallbladder
- Mucocele of the gallbladder

- Gallstone ileus
  - Fistula between the gallbladder and duodenum
  - Large stone enters the duodenum through the fistula, causing obstruction at the terminal ileum
- Pancreatitis: associated with multiple small stones
- Carcinoma of the gallbladder
- Perforation of the gallbladder

Treatment options

- Cholecystectomy
- Cholecystolithotomy
- Dissolution by methyl-tert-butyl ether (MTBE) and percutaneous lithotripsy
- Extracorporeal shock wave lithotripsy (ESWL)
- Oral bile-salt therapy
- Chemical sclerosis

Obstructive jaundice

Definition

- Hyperbilirubinaemia caused by obstruction to the extrahepatic biliary system

Aetiology

- Common causes
  - Stones in the common bile duct (CBD)
  - Carcinoma of the head of the pancreas
  - Malignant porta hepatis nodes
- Infrequent causes
  - Ampullary carcinoma
  - Pancreatitis
  - Liver secondaries
- Rare causes
  - Benign strictures
    - Iatrogenic strictures
    - Traumatic strictures
  - Recurrent cholangitis
  - Mirizzi's syndrome
  - Sclerosing cholangitis
  - Cholangiocarcinoma
  - Biliary atresia
  - Choledochal cyst

Comparison of urinalysis findings in haemolytic, obstructive and hepatocellular jaundice			
	Haemolytic	Obstructive	Hepatocellular
Conjugated bilirubin	Normal	Increased	Normal
Urobilinogen	Increased	Nil	Normal

Investigations

- Aim: to differentiate between hepatocellular and obstructive jaundice
- Conjugated bilirubin: > 35 mmol/L
- Alkaline phosphatase (ALP) and gamma-glutamyl transferase (GGT) are increased more than aspartate aminotransferase (AST) and alanine aminotransferase (ALT)
- Albumin may be reduced
- Prolonged prothrombin time (PT)
- Urinalysis shows increased conjugated bilirubin and no urobilinogen (see table)
- Other investigations
  - All patients should undergo:
    - Spiral CT scanning
    - Endoscopic retrograde cholangiopancreatography (ERCP) or magnetic resonance cholangiopancreatography (MRCP)
    - Laparoscopy if biliary or pancreatic cancer is suspected
  - Ultrasound
    - Normal CBD diameter: < 8 mm
    - In obstructive jaundice, common bile duct diameter: > 9 mm
    - Diameter may increase with age and after previous biliary surgery
  - CT scan
    - For visualising lower end of the CBD
    - For staging malignancies
  - ERCP
    - Enables biopsy and brush cytology specimen to be taken
    - Stone extraction may be possible
  - Percutaneous transhepatic cholangiography (PTC)
    - Rarely done nowadays
    - 22 gauge Chiba needle is used
    - Allows biliary drainage and stenting
  - Image-guided biopsy
  - Endoscopic ultrasound

Complications

- Ascending cholangitis
  - Charcot's triad
    - Pain
    - Fever
    - Jaundice
- Clotting disorders
  - Deficiency of factors II, VII, IX and XI (the vitamin K-dependent factors)
- Hepatorenal syndrome
- Disordered drug metabolism
  - Half-life of some drugs are prolonged, e.g. morphine
- Impaired wound healing

Pre-operative preparation

- Parenteral administration of vitamin K and normalisation of PT
- Intravenous hydration and bladder catheterisation
- Forced natriuresis by mannitol or a loop diuretic
- Antibiotic prophylaxis against Gram-negative aerobes
- Pre-operative biliary decompression in long-standing jaundice

Biliary strictures

Benign strictures

- Causes
  - Operative bile duct injury (iatrogenic)
  - Penetrating and non-penetrating abdominal injuries
  - Chronic duodenal ulcer
  - Chronic pancreatitis
  - Recurrent pyogenic cholangitis and parasitic infestations
  - Sclerosing cholangitis

- Bismuth's classification
  - Type I: low CBD stricture with > 2 cm stump
  - Type II: middle CBD stricture with < 2 cm stump
  - Type III: high CBD stricture, no stump available, but bile duct confluence is preserved
  - Type IV: involvement of the bile duct confluence (Klatskin's tumour)
  - Type V: combined stricture of the common hepatic duct and an aberrant right hepatic duct
- Strasberg's classification
  - Type A: leak from a minor duct in continuity with the CBD
  - Type B: occlusion of an aberrant CBD
  - Type C: leak from a duct not in continuity with the CBD, e.g. transection of the common hepatic duct
  - Type D: lateral injury to the CBD in continuity
  - Type E: disconnection of a major duct (the common hepatic duct or the CBD)
- Aetiology
  - Wrong identification of duct at operation
  - Flush ligation for bleeding
  - Excessive dissection and compromise of blood supply
  - Trauma during exploration
  - Injury caused by diathermy or laser
- Treatment
  - If identified at operation:
    - Major injury: roux-en-Y hepaticojejunostomy
    - Minor injury: primary repair with T-tube
  - If identified post-operatively:
    - Roux-en-Y hepaticojejunostomy
    - Endoscopic sphincterotomy or balloon dilatation

Malignant strictures

- Caused by scirrhous cholangiocarcinoma
- Confined to the proximal (hilar) ducts
- Treatment
  - Resection in operable cases
  - Percutaneous transhepatic or endoscopic stenting in inoperable cases

Functions of the pancreas
Exocrine functions

- Proteolysis
  - Via conversion of trypsinogen to trypsin by enterokinase in duodenum
  - Release is triggered by cholecystokinin
  - Activated trypsin converts more trypsinogen to trypsin
  - Acts on long protein chains and splits them into smaller polypeptides
- Carbohydrate digestion
  - By amylase
  - Acts on starch and glycogen, converting them to glucose
- Fat digestion
  - By lipase
  - Acts on triglycerides to produce monoglycerides and free fatty acids

Endocrine functions

- Islets of Langerhans secretions
  - Insulin, secreted by beta cells
  - Glucagon, secreted by alpha cells
  - Somatostatin, secreted by gamma cells
  - Pancreatic polypeptide, secreted by delta cells
- Insulin
  - Regulates blood sugar by promoting cellular uptake of glucose, especially in liver and muscle, and its storage as glycogen (glycogenesis)
  - Increases glucose uptake into fat cells and increases triglyceride synthesis from glucose (lipogenesis)
  - Increases uptake of amino acids by skeletal muscle cells
  - Increases K^+ uptake by cells
- Glucagon
  - Promotes glycolysis with production of glucose
  - Responsible for homoeostatic maintenance of blood sugar
  - Stimulates gluconeogenesis and production of ketone bodies in the liver
- Somatostatin
  - Inhibits growth hormone
  - Delays gastric emptying
  - Reduces gastric secretion
  - Reduces pancreatic exocrine secretion

Acute pancreatitis

Definition

- Acute inflammatory process of the pancreas caused by the effects of enzymes released from the pancreatic acini (autodigestion)

Aetiology

- Gallstone disease (in 50% of cases)
- Chronic alcoholism
- Infection
  - Mumps
  - Coxsackievirus infection
  - Typhoid fever
- Hypercalcaemia, e.g. in hyperparathyroidism
- Trauma
- Post-operative, after upper GI surgery with handling of pancreas
- Hyperlipidaemia
- Drugs
  - Corticosteroids
  - Oestrogen-containing oral contraceptives
  - Azathioprine
  - Thiazide diuretics
- Hypothermia
- Vascular insufficiency
  - Shock
  - Polyarteritis nodosa
- Scorpion bites
- Iatrogenic, e.g. after ERCP

Pathogenesis

- Duct obstruction (common channel theory)
  - Reflux of bile into pancreatic duct or increased intraductal pressure damages the acini and causes leakage
- Direct acinar damage by viruses, bacteria or drugs

Consequences

- Protease release
  - Widespread destruction of the pancreas
  - Further release and destruction ensues
- Lipase release
  - Fat necrosis
  - White flecks on the pancreas, mesentery and omentum
- Elastase release
  - Destruction of blood vessels, leading to haemorrhage
  - Acute haemorrhagic pancreatitis

Clinical signs

- Caused by seepage of haemorrhagic fluid along fascial planes
- Cullen's sign: bluish discoloration of the peri-umbilical skin
- Grey Turner's sign: bluish discoloration of the loins

Biochemical changes

- Increased serum amylase
  - Seen in the first 24 hours
  - Later falls to normal
- Hypocalcaemia, due to deposition of calcium in areas of fat necrosis
- Hyperglycaemia, due to damage to the pancreatic islets
- Increased bilirubin and ALP, due to bile duct oedema

Plain abdominal X-ray findings

- Intestinal distension in the region of the pancreas
  - Sentinel jejunal loop
  - Colon cut-off
  - Duodenal ileus
- Generalised paralytic ileus
- Haziness and obliteration of psoas outline, due to retroperitoneal fluid collection
- Elevation of left diaphragm, due to basal atelectasis
- Sub-diaphragmatic fluid collection

Classification according to severity

- Acute oedematous pancreatitis: mild and self-limiting
- Acute persistent pancreatitis: unresolving and leading to complications
- Acute haemorrhagic pancreatitis: necrotising and fulminant

Ranson's criteria for severity prediction

- At admission, a greater severity is suggested by:
  - Age > 55 years

- Leucocyte count $>16 \times 10^9$/L
- Glucose > 11.1 mmol/L
- Lactate dehydrogenase (LDH) > 350 units/L
- AST > 250 units/L
- After 48 hours, a greater severity is suggested by:
  - Haematocrit > 10
  - Urea > 5 mmol/L
  - $Ca^{2+} < 2$ mmol/L
  - $p_aO_2 < 60$ mmHg
  - Base deficit > 4
  - Fluid requirement > 6 L

Other severity scores

- Glasgow criteria
- The Acute Physiology and Chronic Health Evaluation (APACHE)

Other markers

- Trypsin-activated peptide
- CRP
- Tumour necrosis factor (TNF) and interleukins (ILs)

Management

- Medical therapy
  - Correction of hypovolaemia
  - Nasogastric suction and parenteral feeding
- Indications for surgery
  - Doubtful diagnosis
  - Failure to improve
  - Known stone disease

Complications

- Pancreatic pseudocyst: localised fluid collection in the lesser sac
- Pancreatic abscess
- Stress-induced gastric erosions
  - Haematemesis
  - Malaena
- Acute renal failure
- Toxic psychosis
- Multiple organ failure
- Chronic pancreatitis

Prognosis

- Mortality: 10–20%
- In haemorrhagic pancreatitis, mortality is 50%

Chronic pancreatitis

Definition

- Relapsing disorder that arises insidiously following repeated attacks of acute pancreatitis

Causes

- Chronic alcohol consumption (the most common cause)
- Cystic fibrosis
- Hypercalcaemia
- Hyperlipidemia
- Familial pancreatitis (rare)

Pathology

- Parenchymal destruction
- Fibrosis
- Loss of acini
- Calculi
- Duct stenosis and post-stenotic dilatation ('chain of lakes' appearance on ERCP)

Gross appearance

- Hard, irregular organ
- Parenchymal calcification

Management

- Maintenance of adequate nutrition
- Enzyme replacement
- Insulin supplements
- Indications for surgery
  - Intractable pain
  - Complications

Complications

- Lower bile duct obstruction
  - Suppurative cholangitis
  - Secondary biliary cirrhosis
  - Carcinoma must be ruled out
- Vascular involvement
  - Multiple pseudo-aneurysms
  - Sectorial portal hypertension
- Duodenal obstruction
  - Caused by enlargement of the head of the pancreas
  - Cancer must be ruled out
- Pancreatic cysts and pseudocysts
- Ascites and pleural effusions
- Dominant mass leading to suspicion of cancer

Surgical treatment

- Roux-en-Y pancreaticojejunostomy, if the duct is dilated
- Whipple's pancreaticoduodenectomy, if carcinoma is suspected

Carcinoma of the pancreas

Pathological classification

- Duct cell in origin
  - Adenocarcinoma (accounts for 90% of cases)
  - Giant cell carcinoma
  - Micro-adenocarcinoma
  - Mucinous colloid carcinoma
  - Cystadenocarcinoma (mucinous)
- Acinar cell in origin
  - Acinar cell carcinoma
  - Acinar cell cystadenocarcinoma
- Connective tissue in origin
  - Leiomyosarcoma
  - Hemangiopericytoma
  - Malignant fibrous histiocytoma
- Miscellaneous
  - Pancreaticoblastoma
  - Papillary and cystic neoplasms
  - Mixed duct and islet cell neoplasms
  - Neuroblastoma
  - Lymphoma

Aetiology

- High-protein, high-fat diet
- Cigarette smoking
- Industrial carcinogens
  - Beta-naphthylamine
  - Benzidine
- Molecular basis
  - Oncogene: k-ras
  - Tumour suppressor genes:
    - *p53*
    - *p16*
    - *DPC4*
    - *RB*-1
- Diabetes mellitus
- Alcoholism

Clinical features

- Involvement of the head of the pancreas
  - Obstructive jaundice
  - Pain, anorexia and weight loss
  - Haematemesis and malaena
  - Ascending cholangitis
  - Palpable gallbladder (Courvoisier's sign)
- Involvement of the body and tail of the pancreas
  - Pain and weight loss
  - Migrating thrombophlebitis (Trousseau's sign)
  - Blumer's shelf
  - Left supraclavicular nodes (Troisier's sign)

Investigations

- CT scan
- ERCP with cytology
- Endoscopic ultrasound
- Percutaneous needle biopsy (in inoperable cases)
- Transduodenal biopsy
- Laparoscopy and direct-vision biopsy

Surgical treatment

- Only for relatively fit patients under the most favourable circumstances
- Options
  - Whipple's procedure
  - Pylorus-preserving pancreaticoduodenectomy
  - Total pancreatectomy
  - Regional pancreatectomy

Consequences of terminal ileal resection

Malabsorption pattern: terminal ileopathy

- Vitamin B12 malabsorption, leading to megaloblastic anaemia
- Bile salt malabsorption, leading to increased risk of gallstones
- Watery diarrhoea
- Steatorrhoea, which produces insoluble Ca^{2+} soaps, which leads to increased oxalic acid absorption and to urinary calculi and hyperoxaluria
- Malabsorption of vitamins A, D, E and K, and of the minerals magnesium, zinc and Ca^{2+}

Common causes of terminal ileopathy

- Ileal resection
- Ileal utilisation for urinary diversion
- Radiation injury

Management

- For deficiencies of vitamin B12, A, D, E and K: intramuscular injections
- For watery diarrhoea: codeine phosphate or loperamide
- For bile salt malabsorption: cholestyramine
- For steatorrhoea: medium-chain triglycerides (absorbed without previous emulsification)
- Low fat diet
  - Spares bile salts
  - Decreases faecal water and fat
  - Reduces hyperoxaluria

Ulcerative colitis

Definition

- Chronic non-specific inflammatory disease that involves whole or part of colon
- Confined to the mucosa
- Nearly always involves the rectum

Aetiology

- Immunological, due to changes in epithelial antigen presentation resulting from acquired expression of class II MHC molecules, which activate T-helper cells to induce a sustained mucosal immune reaction
- Dietary causes
- Genetic causes
  - Familial clustering
  - Association with HLA-DR2
  - Increased incidence in monozygotic twins
  - Associated with other genetic disease, e.g. ankylosing spondylitis and sclerosing cholangitis

Pathology

- Initially mucosal
- Abscesses in the crypts of Lieberkühn
- Raised margins of ulcer (pseudopolyps)

- Backwash ileitis, leading to involvement of the terminal ileum

Complications

- Toxic dilatation of the colon
- Haemorrhage
- Stricture of the colon
- Perforation of the colon
- Rare complications
  - Perianal suppuration
  - Giant inflammatory polyposis
  - Carcinoma (in long-standing cases)
    - Onset of ulcerative colitis in childhood
    - Total colonic involvement
    - Continual rather than intermittent symptoms
- Extra-colonic complications
  - Sero-negative arthritis: sacro-ileitis, ankylosing spondylitis
  - Sclerosing cholangitis
  - Cirrhosis
  - Pericholangitis
  - Iritis
  - Uveitis
  - Episcleritis
  - Erythema nodosum
  - Pyoderma gangrenosum
  - Aphthous stomatitis
  - Amyloidosis (rare)

Treatment

- Medical therapy
  - 5-aminosalicylic acid derivatives given by enema, orally or intravenously
  - Corticosteroids
- Surgery
  - Indications for emergency surgery
    - Severe disease
    - Perforation
    - Bleeding
  - Indications for elective surgery
    - Failure of medical treatment
    - Growth retardation
    - Malignant transformation
- Surgical procedures
  - Colectomy and ileostomy with preservation of rectal stump
  - Colectomy with ileorectal anastomosis
  - Proctocolectomy with permanent ileostomy
  - Proctocolectomy with ileoanal pouch

Complications of ileostomy

- Stenosis
- Prolapse
- Peristomal irritation
- Fistula
- Para-ileostomy hernia
- Ileostomy diarrhoea

Crohn's disease

Definition

- Chronic inflammatory disorder of unknown aetiology

Sites

- Mainly small bowel but can affect any part of the gastrointestinal tract

Characteristics

- Transmural inflammation
- Caseating granulomas
- Thickened and fissured bowel, leading to intestinal obstruction and fistula formation

Aetiology

- May be genetic
  - HLA-DR 1
  - HLA-DQW 5
  - HLA-B 27
- Environmental
  - Diet high in refined carbohydrates
  - Smoking
  - Oral contraceptives
- Infective
  - Yeast infections
  - Chlamydial infections
  - *Pseudomonas maltophilia*
  - *Mycobacterium paratuberculosis*
- Immunological
  - Defective cell-mediated immunity
  - Possibly autoimmune in origin
- Vasculitis
  - May be due to multifocal gastrointestinal infection

Pathology

- Segmental pattern
  - Involved small bowel separated by normal bowel, known as skip lesions

- Longitudinal ulcers, progressing to fissures
- Fibrosis, leading to narrowing of the lumen (Cantor's string sign in barium enema)
- Cobblestone appearance, due to mucosal oedema

Complications

- Malabsorption syndrome, due to widespread involvement
- Short-bowel syndrome, due to extensive surgery
- Fistula formation
  - Internal fistulae
    - Enterovesical fistula
    - Ileocolonic fistula
  - External fistulae
    - Enterocutaneous fistula
    - Perianal fistula
- Anal lesions
- Acute complications
  - Obstruction
  - Perforation
  - Haemorrhage
  - Toxic dilatation (rare)
- Increased risk of carcinoma
- Gallstones and renal calculi, due to malabsorption
- Extra-alimentary manifestations
  - Finger clubbing
  - Erythema nodosum
  - Pyoderma gangrenosum
  - Uveitis
  - Amyloidosis (rare)

Clinical syndromes

- Pseudo-appendicitis
- Small bowel obstruction
- Abscess formation: right iliac fossa to pelvis to psoas to groin
- Fistula formation
- Diarrhoea
- Growth retardation
- Portal venous gas: rare and fatal

Tests for disease activity

- Erythrocyte sedimentation rate (ESR)
- Serum alpha-1 glycoprotein level
- CRP
- OKT-9 lymphocyte positivity

Difference between ulcerative colitis and Crohn's disease

Ulcerative colitis versus Crohn's disease		
	Ulcerative colitis	**Crohn's disease**
Clinical features		
Rectal bleeding	Very common	Usual
Abdominal pain	Infrequent	Common
Abdominal mass	Rare	Sometimes
Spontaneous fistula	Very rare/never	Sometimes
Perianal infection	15%	30-40%
Rectal involvement	95%	50%
Carcinoma	Yes	No
Radiology		
Distribution	Continuous with rectum	Discontinuous along and around colon
Rectum	Involved	Normal
Strictures	Rare	Often present
Mucosa	Granular, shallow ulcers, pseudopolyps	Fissuring, deep ulcer, cobblestone appearance
Small bowel	Backwash ileitis	Skip lesions
Gross pathology		
Site	Confined to the colon 60% rectum and sigmoid, 25% splenic flexure; occasional backwash ileitis in extensive cases	Any part if GIT, mouth to anus. 50% ileum and colon, 30% ileum only
Lesion	Continuous proximal spread from the rectum. No skip lesions	Skip lesions of abnormal areas between normal
Thickness	Confined to the mucosa	Involves the whole of bowel wall
Acute phase	Swollen red and ulcerated bowel	Swollen red and ulcerated bowel
Chronic phase	Regeneration of the epithelium with inflammatory pseudopolyp formation	Nose pipe thickening with fibrosis, luminal narrowing and obstruction
Mucosa	Atrophic with pseudopolyps	Cobblestone appearance

Continued opposite

Continued

Serosa	Not affected	Fatty encroachment
Ulcers	Shallow and small	Very deep, longitudinal and fissuring leading to adhesions and fistulas
Histopathology		
Inflammation	Mucosal	Transmural
Vascularity	Intense	Seldom prominent
Focal lymphoid hyperplasia	Mucosa/submucosa	Transmural
Mucus secretion	↓↓	↓
Microscopic appearance	Nontypical granulomas. Inflammation confined to lamina propria. Crypt abscess and distortion. Metaplasia and dysplasia. Shallow ulcers	Noncaseating epithelioid granulomas. Transmural inflammation. Crypt distortion. Lymphoid follicles. Deep fissuring ulcers

Treatment

- Medical therapy
  - Dietary modifications
    - Correct deficiencies
    - Total parenteral nutrition if required
  - Drugs
    - 5-aminosalicylic acid derivates
    - Corticosteroids
  - Antibodies against TNF-alpha
  - Broad-spectrum antibiotics, e.g. ciprofloxacin
- Surgery
  - Resection
  - Bypass surgery
  - Stricturoplasty
  - Repair of fistulae
  - Short-bowel syndrome surgery
    - Home total parenteral nutrition
    - Small bowel transplantation

Diverticulosis of the colon

Definition

- Herniation of mucosa through the colonic wall

Sites

- Occurs at weak points where blood vessels pierce the bowel wall

Pathology

- Diverticular wall is made up of mucosa and submucosa
- Pulsion diverticula are those that are pushed out by increased intraluminal pressure
- Most common in the sigmoid colon

Aetiology

- Low-fibre diet and consequent small, hard stools

Complications

- Inflammation leading to diverticulitis
- Perforation
  - Local perforation causes paracolic abscess
  - Perforation into the general peritoneal cavity causes faecal peritonitis
  - Perforation into an adjacent viscus causes fistula formation
    - Colovesical fistula
    - Vaginocolic fistula
    - Ileocolic fistula
- Bleeding, due to erosion of the underlying vessel
- Obstruction, due to fibrosis and narrowing from repeated diverticulitis and stricture

Differential diagnosis

- Congenital diverticular disease has the full thickness of bowel wall in it, e.g. in Meckel's diverticulum

Clinical features

- Chronic abdominal pain in the left iliac fossa
- Distension relieved by flatus
- Constipation

Diagnosis

- Barium enema shows sacculations

Treatment

- For pain: a high-fibre diet and antispasmodics
- For diverticulitis:
  - Intravenous fluids and antibiotics
  - Percutaneous drainage of abscess
  - Sigmoid colectomy with Hartmann's procedure
- For stricture: sigmoid colectomy
- For fistula: resection and anastomosis
- For bleeding: mesenteric angiography plus resection or subtotal colectomy

Colonic polyps

Definition

- Protuberant growths into the bowel lumen
- If > 100 polyps are present, it is called polyposis

Types

- Sessile or pedunculated
- Benign or malignant
- Mucosal, submucosal or muscular

Classification

- Neoplastic polyps
  - Benign (adenomatous) polyps
    - Tubular polyps
    - Tubulovillous polyps
    - Villous polyps
  - Malignant polyps
    - Polypoid adenocarcinoma
    - Carcinoid polyps
- Inflammatory polyps: pseudopolyps of ulcerative colitis

- Hamartomatous polyps
  - Peutz–Jeghers polyps (multiple)
  - Juvenile polyps (solitary)
- Unclassified: metaplastic (hyperplastic) polyps
- Mesenchymal polyps
  - Benign polyps
    - Lipoma
    - Fibroma
    - Leiomyoma
    - Hemangioma
  - Malignant polyps
    - Sarcoma
    - Lymphoma

Malignant potential of adenoma

- 1% if < 1 cm in diameter
- 10% if 1–2 cm in diameter
- 40% if > 2 cm in diameter
- 5% if tubular
- 20% if tubulovillous
- 40% if villous
- Sessile polyps have a greater chance of malignant change than pedunculated polyps

Specialised polyps

- Familial adenomatous polyposis
  - Autosomal-dominant condition
  - Hundreds of polyps in the colon and rectum
  - Carcinomatous change before the age of 40 years
  - FAP gene in the long arm of chromosome 5
- Gardner's syndrome
  - Familial adenomatous polyposis plus:
    - Desmoid tumour
    - Osteomas of mandible or skull
    - Sebaceous cysts

Complications

- Malignant change
- Bleeding
  - Haematochezia
  - Chronic bleeding, which can lead to iron-deficiency anaemia
- Diarrhoea and/or tenesmus
- Intestinal obstruction

Aetiology

- May have environmental causes
- Dietary causes
  - Decreased dietary fibre and antioxidants
  - Increased meat, fat and alcohol
  - Ca^{2+} and folate are protective
- Genetic causes
  - Familial adenomatous polyposis has an autosomal-dominant inheritance (APC gene)
  - Gardner's syndrome
  - Peutz-Jeghers syndrome
  - Hereditary non-polyposis colorectal cancer (HNPCC) has an autosomal-dominant inheritance
  - Cowden's disease

Treatment options

- Endoscopic polypectomy
- Colectomy
  - If large polyps
  - If resection margins are positive for malignancy
  - In polyposis (> 100 polyps)
- Transanal endoscopic microsurgery
- Total proctectomy with coloanal anastomosis

Hamartomatous polyps

- Definition of hamartoma: a benign, tumour-like lesion, the growth of which is co-ordinated with that of the individual, and that consists of mature, well-differentiated tissue types

Peutz-Jeghers syndrome

- Inherited autosomal-dominant condition
- Jejunal and/or ileal polyps plus mucocutaneous pigmentation
- Rarely involves the stomach, duodenum or large bowel
- Clinical features
  - Intestinal colic
  - Acute intestinal obstruction from intussusceptions or luminal polyp
  - Bleeding
    - Acute gastrointestinal haemorrhage
    - Chronic iron-deficiency anaemia
  - Pigmentation of the lips and buccal mucosa

- Complication
  - Malignant transformation (in 2–3% of cases)
- Treatment
  - If polyp > 2 cm in diameter, it is excised
  - Surgical treatment of complications
    - Obstruction
    - Haemorrhage

Juvenile polyps

- Affects infants and children
- Familial tendency
- Single in 70% of cases, though can be multiple
- The rectum and distal sigmoid colon are involved in 70% of cases

Colorectal carcinoma

Aetiology

- Inherited genetic factors
  - Familial adenomatous polyposis: autosomal-dominant gene on chromosome 5
  - HNPCC
    - Autosomal-dominant inheritance
    - Two types: Lynch 2 HNPCC and Lynch 1 HNPCC
    - Lynch 2 HNPCC is a familial cancer syndrome with early onset (at 20–30 years), and is associated with endometrial carcinoma
    - Lynch 1 HNPCC causes extracolonic carcinoma; sometimes known as hereditary non-site-specific colon cancer
- Environmental factors
  - High economic status
  - Dietary factors
    - Low-fibre diet, leading to increased bowel transit time
    - High-fat diet, leading to increased bile acid production
- Inflammatory bowel disease
- Colorectal polyps: adenoma–carcinoma sequence
- Schistosomal colitis
- Exposure to irradiation
- Ureterocolostomy
- Cholecystectomy, which causes increased bile acid secretion

- *H. pylori*-induced hypergastrinaemia
- Long-standing inflammatory bowel disease

Genetics

- Activation of oncogenes
  - K-*ras*
  - C-*myc*

- Loss of mutation of tumour-suppressor genes
  - *APC* on chromosome 5
  - *p53*
- Over-expression of inhibitors of apoptosis: *bcl*-2

Distribution within the colon and rectum

- Rectum: 30%
- Sigmoid colon: 20%
- Ascending colon: 25%
- Descending colon: 15%
- Transverse colon: 10%

Staging

- Duke's staging
- TNM

Spread

- Direct spread
  - Encircling of bowel wall
  - Into neighbouring structures
- Blood-borne spread
  - To the liver
  - To the lungs
- Lymphatic spread
- Trans-coelomic spread

Complications

- Obstruction
- Perforation
  - Direct perforation: at the tumour site
  - Perforation of the caecum: in closed loop obstruction
  - Perforation into an adjacent organ, leading to fistula formation

Investigations

- Blood tests
  - Full blood count
  - Liver function tests
  - Carcinoembryonic antigen (CEA)

- Endoscopy
  - Sigmoidoscopy
  - Colonoscopy
- Radiology
  - Double-contrast barium enema
- Staging investigations
  - Chest X-ray
  - Liver ultrasound
    - External ultrasound
    - Intra-operative contact ultrasound
  - CT and/or MRI
  - Endorectal ultrasound

Surgical treatment

- Surgery for tumour
  - Radical excision of affected section of colon, along with its vascular pedicle and accompanying lymphatic drainage
  - Transverse colectomy
    - Not done nowadays
    - Either extended right or left depending on position of tumour
  - Left hemicolectomy: subtotal colectomy is preferred
  - For local spread: en-bloc curative resection along with involved organs
  - For rectal carcinoma: mesorectal excision is always done
- Surgery for obstruction
  - Three-stage procedure
    - Proximal defunctioning colostomy
    - Resection and anastomosis
    - Closure of colostomy
  - Two-stage procedure
    - Hartmann's procedure
    - Reversal of Hartmann's procedure
  - Single-stage procedure
    - On-table lavage with primary anastomosis
    - Subtotal colectomy with ileo-colonic anastomosis
  - Recently, endoscopic insertion of an expanding metal wall stent has been performed
- Surgery for metastases
  - Resection of liver metastases
  - Laparoscopy-assisted

Chemotherapy

- Adjuvant:
  - 5-fluorouracil and folinic acid

- Palliative:
  - 5-fluorouracil and folinic acid
  - Regional 5-fluorouracil via the hepatic artery

Radiotherapy

- May be curative (as suggested by practice in France)
- Adjuvant radiotherapy can be combined with chemotherapy
- Palliative radiotherapy may lead to radiation proctocolitis

Faecal incontinence

Causes

- Trauma
  - Obstetrical procedures
  - Surgery
  - Accidental trauma
- Anorectal disease
  - Haemorrhoids
  - Carcinoma of the anal canal
  - Crohn's disease
- Diarrhoea
  - Irritable bowel syndrome
  - Malabsorption
- Congenital causes
  - Treated imperforate anus
  - Hirschsprung's disease
  - Spina bifida
- Neurological causes
  - Pudendal nerve damage
  - Stroke
  - Spinal cord damage
- Miscellaneous causes
  - Behavioural
  - Faecal impaction
  - Co-existing urinary incontinence, which suggests a neuropathological cause; digital rectal examination should be done to assess sphincter tone

Investigations

- Sigmoidoscopy
- Anorectal manometry
- Pudendal nerve latency
- Ultrasound of the anal canal

Treatment

- Conservative management
  - Anti-diarrhoeal agents
  - Pelvic floor exercises
  - Anal plug
- Surgery
  - Anterior sphincter repair
  - Post-anal repair
  - Total pelvic floor repair
  - Gracilis neosphincter
  - Gluteus maximus transposition
  - Artificial sphincter insertion
  - If intractable: colostomy

Haemorrhoids

Definition

- Abnormalities of the vascular cushions of the anus

Anal cushions

- Three spaces filled by arteriovenous communication and supported by a fibrous matrix
- Degeneration of fibroelastic tissue causes them to prolapse into anal canal

Clinical features

- Bright red bleeding per rectum that is painless
- Swelling
- Pruritus
- Minor soiling

Grades

- First degree: only bleeding
- Second degree: prolapses on defaecation and reduces spontaneously
- Third degree: requires manual reduction
- Fourth degree: irreducibly prolapsed

Investigation

- Sigmoidoscopy and colonoscopy to rule out other proximal conditions

Complications

- Thrombosis
- Massive haemorrhage
- Faecal incontinence

Treatment

- Outpatient management
  - Sclerotherapy
  - Banding
  - Laser photocoagulation
- Surgery
  - Haemorrhoidectomy
  - Stapled anopexy (excision of the circumferential strip of mucosa above the dentate line)
- For thrombosis: cold compresses

Rectal prolapse

Definition

- Protrusion of the rectum through the anal canal

Classification

- Partial or incomplete: prolapse of mucosa only (seen in children)
- Complete: prolapse of the entire thickness (seen in the elderly)

Aetiology

- Laxity of tissue in the rectal submucosa, leading to abnormal mobility of rectal mucosa on the circular muscle
- Laxity of pelvic floor musculature

Clinical features

- In children
  - Mucosa visible
  - Mucus and blood in stools
  - No sphincter abnormality
- In adults
  - Sphincteric tone is deficient
  - Loops of small bowel felt anteriorly in the rectovesical pouch or the pouch of Douglas

Diagnosis

- Clinical diagnosis
- Defaecating proctography
- Barium enema to exclude colonic pathology

Complications

- Faecal incontinence
- Irreducibility leading to gangrene

Treatment

- In children
  - Self-limiting condition
  - Sclerosant injection into the lower rectal mucosa
- In adults
  - For partial prolapse: stapled anopexy
  - For complete prolapse
    - Perineal approach
    - Trans-abdominal approach
  - Perineal approach
    - Thiersch wiring: obsolete
    - Delorme's procedure: excision of cuff of mucosa and plication of muscle layer
    - Perineal proctosigmoidectomy: excision of prolapsed portion and coloanal anastomosis
  - Trans-abdominal approach
    - Rectopexy: rectal wall fixed to the sacrum by suture, mesh or Ivalon sponge
    - Resection rectopexy: resection of the sigmoid colon and colorectal anastomosis

Perianal sepsis and fistula-in-ano

Aetiology

- Crohn's disease
- Malignancy
- Tuberculosis
- Pilonidal sinus
- Trauma
- Idiopathic

Pathogenesis

- Infection of anal glands in the inter-sphincteric plane
- Pus tracks:
  - Downwards, causing a perianal abscess
  - Upwards, causing an inter-sphincteric abscess
  - Through the external sphincter, causing fistulae

Classification of fistula

- Intersphincteric fistula
- Trans-sphincteric fistula

- Suprasphincteric fistula
- Extra-sphincteric fistula

Intersphincteric fistulae

- Accounts for 50% of cases
- Tracks between dentate line and skin
- Can have an internal opening

Trans-sphincteric fistula

- Accounts for 30% of cases
- Tracks through the external sphincter
- May be low or high

Suprasphincteric fistula

- Tracks above the puborectalis muscle and then down through the levator ani into the ischiorectal fossa

Clinical features

- Abscess: pain and fever
- Fistula: pruritus and discharge

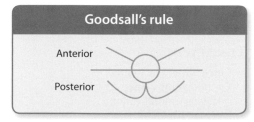

Goodsall's rule

Anterior

Posterior

- External fistulous opening anterior to a transverse line drawn across the anus is more likely to have a straight-line track with a corresponding internal opening
- External fistulous opening posterior to a transverse line is more likely to have a curved track with an internal opening in the posterior midline
- Bilateral posterior external opening is more likely to be a horse-shoe fistula with a single internal opening

Diagnosis

- Examination under anaesthetic and probing
- Fistulography
- MRI, in complete fistula with secondary extensions and abscesses

Treatment

- For an abscess
  - Incision and drainage

- For a fistula
  - Laying open the track
  - Curetting the granulation tissue
  - Leaving the wound to granulate
- For a high fistula
  - Seton, loosely tied and removed after 3 weeks
  - Fistulectomy and advancement flap repair
  - Fibrin glue application after fistulotomy
- For a high trans-sphincteric fistula
  - Temporary colostomy
  - Lay open the fistula
  - Sphincter repair after fistula healing
- For Crohn's disease
  - Long-term seton
  - Defunctioning colostomy

Fissure-in-ano

Definition

- Linear ulcer in the anal canal just distal to the dentate line

Causes

- Primary
- Secondary
  - Crohn's disease
  - Trauma

Aetiology

- High resting anal pressure caused by increased internal sphincter tone, leading to:
  - Decreased blood flow and O_2 tension in the skin of the anal canal
  - Watershed of blood supply
    - Anterior and posterior midline in females
    - Posterior midline in males

Clinical features

- Pain on defaecation associated with bright red bleeding
- Pruritus ani and mucus discharge
- Examination reveals skin tag and fissure

Diagnosis

- Examination under anaesthetic and biopsy to exclude Crohn's disease or malignancy

Treatment

- The principle of treatment is to decrease the resting anal sphincter tone
- For patients with minimal symptoms
  - Local anaesthetic
  - Bulk laxatives
- For more severe symptoms
  - Glyceryl trinitrate cream, 2%
- Surgery
  - Lateral sphincterotomy up to the dentate line (a minor degree of incontinence may be present)

Pilonidal sinus and abscess

Definition

- Multiple subcutaneous sinuses and abscess cavities containing hair in the natal cleft of young males

Aetiology

- Frictional forces generated in the depths of the natal cleft drive hairs inside, where they develop a foreign body reaction
- Secondary infection leads to abscess formation

Clinical features

- May be asymptomatic
- Pain and discharge
- Variable number of pits, with or without pus

Treatment

- For asymptomatic cases
  - No treatment is needed
- For an abscess
  - Incision and drainage
- For chronic discharge
  - Wide excision down to the deep fascia and removal of all sinuses and nests of hair
  - May be left open to granulate or primarily closed
  - Coring out of extensions if present
  - Recurrence rate: 20%

Pruritus ani

Definition

- Perianal itching

Aetiology

- Idiopathic in the majority of cases
- Anorectal disease
- Dermatological disease
- Primary cause is minor anal leakage resulting from internal sphincter dysfunction, leading to irritation, which is exacerbated by cleansing and scratching

Clinical features and assessment

- Perianal excoriation and ichthyosis
- Digital rectal examination to assess sphincter tone
- Proctoscopy to look for haemorrhoids
- Biopsy of lesions
- Fungal smears
- For *Enterobius* infestation: Cellotape test

Treatment

- Cause should be treated
- For idiopathic cases
  - Dietary modification
  - Good hygiene
  - Avoidance of scratching
  - Cream containing antifungal agents and corticosteroids

Anal cancer

- Accounts for 5% of all bowel cancers
- Usually squamous cell in type
- Rarely an adenocarcinoma or a malignant melanoma

Classification

- Squamous cell carcinoma
- Basaloid carcinoma
- Muco-epidermoid carcinoma

Spread

- Local spread
  - Proximal spread to the rectum
  - Radial spread to the sphincters
- Lymphatic spread
  - Peri-rectal spread
  - To the inguinal canal
- Distant spread
  - To the liver
  - To the lungs
  - To the bones

Aetiology

- HIV infection
- HPV infection

Clinical features

- Anal pain
- Rectal bleeding
- Anal mass
- On examination, a malignant ulcer at the anal margin

Investigations

- Examination under anaesthetic and biopsy
- Ultrasound to assess sphincters
- Fine-needle aspiration of the inguinal nodes

Treatment

- For small, mobile lesions
  - Local excision
- For larger lesions
  - Radiotherapy plus chemotherapy (5-fluorouracil and mitomycin)
- For recurrence
  - Abdominoperineal resection
  - Colostomy during radiotherapy or chemotherapy
- For lymph node metastases
  - Radical dissection

Anatomy and physiology of the kidneys

Proximal convoluted tubules

- Active transport of Na^+
- Cl– follows passively
- Osmotic gradient draws water
  - Net absorption of all three
  - Volume of filtrate decreases, but no change in osmolality

Loop of Henle

- Thin descending limb, permeable to solutes and water
  - Filtrate is concentrated and reduced in volume
- Thick ascending limb, impermeable to water, actively transports Na^+
  - Osmolality of medullary fluid increases
  - Tubular fluid is diluted

Distal convoluted tubule

- Remaining Na^+ is actively reabsorbed

Collecting ducts

- Water is reabsorbed

Control of reabsorption

- Aldosterone
  - Produced in the adrenal cortex
  - Increases Na^+ and water reabsorption from the distal convoluted tubule
  - Depends on release of renin
  - Increases secretion of K^+ in the distal convoluted tubule
- ADH
  - Synthesised by the paraventricular nucleus of the hypothalamus
  - Released from the posterior pituitary by:
    - Decreased circulating blood volume (volume receptors)
    - Decreased arterial pressure, mediated by baroreceptors
    - Increased osmolality of the extracellular fluid (ECF), mediated by osmoreceptors
  - Results in:
    - Increased permeability of collecting ducts to water, causing increased ECF volume
    - Direct vasoconstriction, causing increased blood pressure; ADH is otherwise called vasopressin
- Atrial natriuretic hormone (ANP)
  - Released from atria by increased ECF volume
  - Increases glomerular filtration rate (GFR)
  - Inhibits tubular reabsorption of Na^+
  - Causes increased excretion of Na^+ and water
- Therefore, aldosterone and ADH increase the ECF volume, whereas ANP decreases the ECF volume

Functions of the kidneys

Elimination (excretion) of metabolic waste products

- Water-soluble waste products of body metabolism
  - Urea from amino acids
  - Creatinine from muscle protein
  - Uric acid from nucleic acids
  - Bilirubin from haemoglobin
  - Metabolites of hormones
- Foreign substances
  - Breakdown products of drugs, toxins and food additives
  - Myoglobin from rhabdomyolysis

Maintenance and regulation

- Water and electrolyte balance is achieved by adjusting the excretion according to the intake
- Acid–base balance is achieved by regulating the body fluid buffer stores and by the excretion of sulphuric acid and phosphoric acid

Glucose synthesis

- From amino acids and other precursors (gluconeogenesis), during prolonged fasting, rivalling the liver

Hormone production

- Renin–angiotensin system, renin secreted from the juxtaglomerular apparatus
- Kallikrein from the distal convoluted tubules
  - Produced in response to volume expansion
  - Causes renal vasodilatation and decreased Na$^+$ and water reabsorption
- 1-alpha-hydroxylase
  - Produced in response to decreased Ca^{2+}
  - Converts 25-hydroxy-cholecalciferol to 1,25-dihydroxy-cholecalciferol
  - Increases Ca^{2+} reabsorption from the intestines
- Erythropoietin
  - Produced in response to hypoxia
  - Causes increased red blood cell destruction and vasoconstriction
  - Stimulates increased production of nucleated red cells (reticulocytes)
- Prostaglandins, from endothelium – prostaglandin (PG) -I2 – and renal intestinal cells – PG-E2
  - Produced in response to reduced renal perfusion
  - Leads to renal vasodilatation and decreased Na$^+$ and water reabsorption

Renin–angiotensin mechanism

- Renin released from the juxtaglomerular apparatus by:
  - Decreased afferent arterial pressure
  - Decreased Na$^+$ in filtrate as a result of hyponatraemia or decreased GFR
- Renin causes conversion of angiotensinogen to angiotensin I in the kidney
- Angiotensin I is converted to angiotensin II by angiotensin converting enzyme (ACE) in the vascular endothelium of the lung
- Angiotensin II
  - Stimulates release of aldosterone
  - Causes systemic vasoconstriction
  - Causes release of ADH
  - Causes central stimulation of thirst
- Aldosterone increases ECF volume by increasing Na$^+$ and water reabsorption at the distal convoluted tubule

- ADH increases the permeability of the collecting ducts to water, and thus increases reabsorption of water

Renal autoregulation

Physical factors

- Renal blood flow (for both kidneys)
  - Total: 1.2 L/minute: 20–25% of cardiac output
  - This is 400 mL/minute per 100 g of kidney for each kidney
  - Renal perfusion fraction (RPF): 660 mL/minute
  - GFR: 120 mL/minute (20% of RPF)
- Regulation
  - Intrinsic autoregulation
    - Acts between mean arterial pressure (MAP) of 80 and 180 mmHg
    - If MAP < 80 mmHg, renal blood flow stops
    - Glomerular filtration stops at a MAP of < 40–50 mmHg
    - Results from the intrinsic myogenic response of the afferent arterioles (vasoconstriction or vasodilatation) in response to changes in blood pressure
  - Local intra-renal autoregulation
    - Through the release of intrinsic vasodilator prostaglandins (PG-I2 and PG-E2) in response to decreased renal perfusion in hypotension, which increases renal blood flow
    - This mechanism is severely blunted by non-steroidal anti-inflammatory drugs and aspirin
- GFR
  - Normal GFR: 120 mL/minute (20% of RPF)
  - Filtration fraction is 20%, i.e. the percentage of RPF that is filtered by the glomeruli (GFR divided by RPF)
  - Regulation
    - Decrease in RPF leads to activation of the renin–angiotensin system and release of angiotensin II
    - Causes selective vasoconstriction of the post-glomerular (efferent) arteriole and generation of back pressure

- This maintains the filtration pressure in the glomerular capillary despite the decreased flow
- This mechanism is severely blunted by ACE inhibitors, e.g. enalapril and captopril, and by angiotensin receptor antagonists

Physical factors that regulate tubular function

- Tubuloglomerular feedback
  - Increased GFR increases flow rate in the ascending limb of the loop of Henle and decreases NaCl reabsorption
  - This increases NaCl concentration in the distal convoluted tubule, which evokes a signal to the glomerulus through the macula densa (sensor) in the juxtaglomerular apparatus
  - This decreases GFR in the same nephron, and vice versa
  - May be due to:
    - Renin–angiotensin system releasing angiotensin II, which causes constriction of the glomerular mesangium and a decrease in filtration surface area, which results in a decreased ultrafiltration coefficient (Kf) and a decreased GFR
  - Release of adenosine causes vasoconstriction of the pre-glomerular (afferent) arteriole, which leads to a decrease in glomerular hydrostatic pressure and so a decreased GFR
  - This mechanism is responsible for a further decrease in GFR in acute renal failure, where tubular damage leads to impaired absorption capacity and increased NaCl concentration in the distal convoluted tubule, with consequent activation of the tubuloglomerular feedback
  - Feedback mechanism is blocked by diuretics
  - Glomerulotubular balance
    - Increased GFR leads to increased oncotic pressure of the blood in the peritubular capillaries and

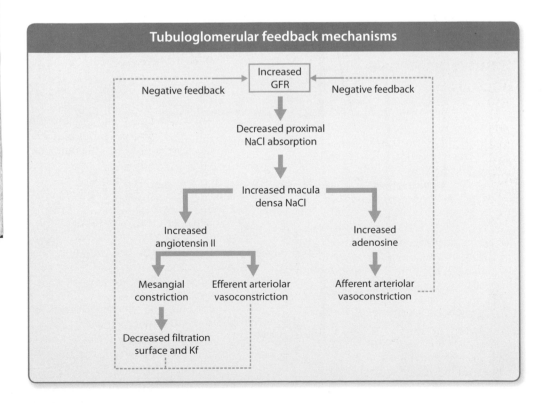

Tubuloglomerular feedback mechanisms

Increased GFR

Negative feedback ← → Negative feedback

Decreased proximal NaCl absorption

Increased macula densa NaCl

Increased angiotensin II

Increased adenosine

Mesangial constriction   Efferent arteriolar vasoconstriction

Afferent arteriolar vasoconstriction

Decreased filtration surface and Kf

Summary of regulation of renal function

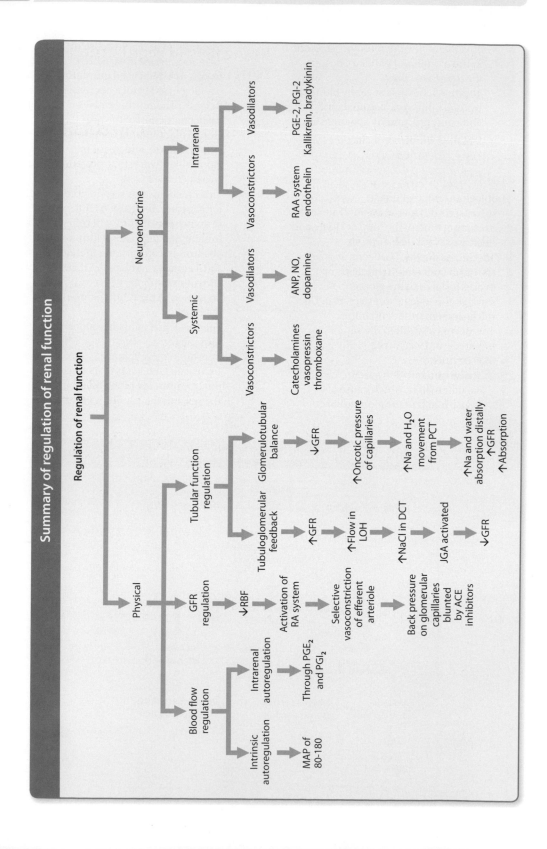

movement of Na⁺ and water out of the proximal tubular lumen, which increases Na⁺ and water absorption distally

- Therefore, increased GFR causes increased absorption
- It buffers the effect of changes in GFR on the urine output rate, regulating the delivery of filtrate to more distal absorption sites of the nephron and maintaining the concentration of urine

Neuroendocrine factors

- Primarily systemic factors
  - Vasoconstrictors, which increase Na⁺ and water reabsorption
    - Catecholamines
    - Vasopressin
    - Thromboxane
  - Vasodilators, which decrease Na⁺ and water reabsorption
    - Nitric oxide
    - Dopamine
    - ANP
- Local intrarenal factors
  - Vasoconstrictors, which increase Na⁺ and water reabsorption:
    - Renin–angiotensin–aldosterone system
    - Endothelin
  - Vasodilators, which decrease Na⁺ and water reabsorption
    - Prostaglandins: PG-I2 and PG-E2
    - Kallikrein
    - Bradykinin

Summary of regulation of renal function

- See figure opposite

Countercurrent mechanism

- The countercurrent mechanism is a concentrating mechanism that depends on the maintenance of increasing osmolality along the medulla
- Produced by countercurrent multipliers in the loop of Henle and maintained by countercurrent exchangers in the vasa recta
- The countercurrent system is where the inflow runs parallel to, counter to and in close proximity to the outflow for some distance
- In kidneys, it acts as a concentrating mechanism, which maintains medullary hypertonicity

Countercurrent multiplier

- Thin ascending limb
  - Permeable to solutes and water
  - Filtrate is concentrated and reduced in volume
- Thick ascending limb
  - Impermeable to water
  - Actively transports solutes
  - Increases osmolality of medullary fluid

Countercurrent exchanger

- Na⁺ and urea from the interstitium diffuse into the descending vessels and out of the

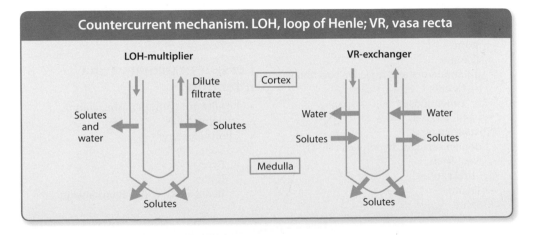

Countercurrent mechanism. LOH, loop of Henle; VR, vasa recta

ascending vessels
- – Maintains medullary osmolality
- – Recirculates solutes
- Water diffuses out of the descending vessels and into the ascending vessels
  - – Excess water is removed

Net effect

- The creation of an efficient way of concentrating urine over a relatively short distance along the nephron, with minimal energy expenditure
- Medullary hypertonicity is maintained

Haematuria

Classification

- Macroscopic haematuria
- Microscopic haematuria (< 5 red blood cells per high-power field)
- Chemical haematuria (assessed by dipstick)

Causes

- Renal causes
  - – Glomerular diseases
  - – Polycystic kidneys
  - – Carcinoma
  - – Stone
  - – Trauma (including renal biopsy)
  - – Tuberculosis
  - – Embolism
  - – Renal vein thrombosis
  - – Vascular malformation
- Ureteric causes
  - – Stone
  - – Neoplasia
- Bladder causes
  - – Carcinoma
  - – Stone
  - – Trauma
  - – Inflammatory and infective conditions
    - • Cystitis
    - • Tuberculosis
    - • Bilharziasis
- Prostatic causes
  - – Benign prostatic hyperplasia (BPH)
  - – Neoplasm
- Urethral causes
  - – Trauma
  - – Stone

- – Urethritis
- – Neoplasm
- General causes
  - – Anticoagulants
  - – Thrombocytopenia
  - – Haemophilia
  - – Sickle cell disease
  - – Malaria
  - – Factitious disease

Investigations

- Ultrasound
- Kidneys, ureters and bladder (KUB) X-ray
- Cystoscopy
- Urine cytology
- Intravenous urography (IVU)

Urinary tract infection

Clinical features

- May be asymptomatic
- Dysuria
- Urinary frequency

Organisms

- Commonly derived from bowel, e.g. *Escherichia coli*
- Uncommon organisms
  - – *Mycobacterium tuberculosis*
  - – *Schistosoma species*

Investigations

- Urinalysis
- Upper tract assessment
  - – KUB X-ray
  - – Cystoscopy
- In men
  - – Ultrasound with post-void residual picture
  - – Flow rate

Persistent urinary tract infection

- Results from reflux causing chronic pyelonephritis
- Clinical features
  - – Loin pain
  - – Pyrexia
  - – Rigors
  - – Renal abscess in diabetes mellitus

- Obstructed tract with infection requires urgent decompression via nephrostomy
- Xanthogranulomatous pyelonephritis: chronically obstructed tract with upper tract infection, associated with stone disease
- Tuberculous infection causes a persistent sterile pyuria
- Schistosomiasis causes chronic irritation of bladder, leading to squamous metaplasia, calcification and squamous carcinoma

Urinary stone disease

Precipitating factors

- Diet
- Dehydration
- Stasis
- Infection
- Hyperparathyroidism
- Idiopathic hypercalcuria
- Milk–alkali syndrome
- Hypervitaminosis D
- Cystinuria
- Inborn errors of purine metabolism
- Gout
- Chemotherapy leading to excess uric acid levels
- Anatomical abnormalities producing stasis

Types of calculi

- Calcium oxalate
- Phosphate
- Urate
- Cysteine
- Xanthine and pyruvate

Clinical features

- Acute ureteric colic: loin to groin pain

Sites of impaction

- Vesico–ureteric junction
- Pelvic brim
- Pelvi–ureteric junction
- Necks of the calyces

Investigations

- Urinalysis
- Plain abdominal radiography
- Ultrasound
- IVU
- Spiral CT scan

Treatment

- For an acute episode
  - Non-steroidal anti-inflammatory drugs
  - If stone < 4 mm in diameter
    - Allow spontaneous passage
    - Forced diuresis
  - If stone is big
    - Nephrostomy
    - Stenting
    - Extracorporeal shock wave lithotripsy (ESWL)
- Interval treatment
  - ESWL
  - Uretero-renoscopy and stenting
  - Percutaneous nephrolithotomy
- Prevention of recurrences : increased fluid intake

Tumours of the urinary tract

Renal tumours

- Adenocarcinoma (Grawitz's tumour, hypernephroma, renal cell carcinoma):
  - Aetiology
    - Smoking
    - Coffee drinking
    - Industrial exposure to cadmium, lead, asbestos or aromatic hydrocarbons
    - In renal cysts and end-stage renal disease
    - von Hippel–Lindau disease
  - Clinical features
    - Haematuria
    - Loin pain
    - Palpable mass
    - Paraneoplastic syndrome: hypertension due to renin secretion, polycythaemia due to erythropoietin secretion, and hypercalcaemia due to ectopic parathyroid hormone secretion
  - Spread
    - Direct spread to perinephric tissue, adjacent organs, the renal vein and the inferior vena cava

- Lymphatic spread to the para-aortic nodes
- Haematogenous spread to the liver, brain, bone and lungs (cannon-ball lesions)
- Wilms' tumour
  - Most common intra-abdominal malignancy in children
  - More common in those < 3 years old
  - Clinical features
    - Abdominal mass
    - Haematuria
    - Abdominal pain
    - Hypertension
    - Intestinal obstruction
  - Metastases
    - Liver
    - Lungs
    - Regional nodes
  - Treatment
    - Surgical excision
    - Chemotherapy and radiotherapy
  - Cure rate: 80–90%

Carcinoma of the renal pelvis

- Cell types
  - Transitional cell (common)
  - Squamous cell: in areas of squamous metaplasia
- May involve the renal vein
- Aetiology
  - Analgesic abuse
  - Exposure to aniline dyes in rubber, plastics and gases
  - Squamous metaplasia resulting from chronic irritation
    - Calculi
    - Infection
- Prognosis is poor

Urothelial tumours

- Transitional epithelium extends from the tip of the papillae to the navicular fossa in men, and to half-way down the urethra in women
- Sites of carcinoma
  - Bladder in 90% of cases
  - Renal pelvis in 9% of cases
  - Ureter in 1% of cases
- Aetiology
  - Smoking
  - Industrial carcinogens

- Presenting features
  - Painless microscopic haematuria
  - Recurrent urinary infection
  - Signs and symptoms of persistent cystitis
- Investigations
  - Cystoscopy
  - Urine cytology
  - IVU
  - CT scan
- Transitional cell carcinoma of the bladder
  - Involves the posterior and lateral walls
  - Predisposing factor is a diverticulum
  - Carcinoma *in situ* develops into a poorly differentiated tumour
  - Treatment
    - Cystoscopic resection
    - Intravesical chemotherapy
    - Bacille Calmette–Guérin (BCG)

Carcinoma of the prostate

- Incidence
  - Commonest in the sixth to seventh decades
  - Develops as an adenocarcinoma in the peripheral zone
- Spread
  - Local extension through the prostate capsule to the bladder and seminal vesicle
  - Lymphatic spread
    - To pelvic nodes
    - To para-aortic nodes
  - Haematogenous spread via the prostatic plexus to:
    - The spine
    - The lungs
    - The liver
- Clinical presentation
  - Urinary symptoms
  - Rectal examination reveals a prostatic mass
  - Bone pain
- Diagnosis
  - Prostate-specific antigen (PSA): low sensitivity and specificity
  - Transrectal biopsy
- Treatment
  - Radical prostatectomy, if life span is expected to be at least 10 years and if the tumour is confined

- Hormonal therapy, if the tumour is locally advanced:
  - Anti-androgens
  - Luteinising hormone releasing hormone (LHRH) agonists

Carcinoma of the testis

- Classification
  - Seminoma
  - Teratoma (the most common type)
  - Combined seminoma and teratoma
  - Malignant lymphoma
  - Interstitial (Leydig's cell) tumour
  - Sertoli's cell tumour
- Clinical features
  - Unilateral painless enlargement of the testis
  - Secondary hydrocoele
  - Retroperitoneal mass
  - Lymph node metastases
    - Para-aortic nodes
    - Supraclavicular nodes
  - Gynaecomastia
- Investigations
  - Ultrasound
  - Markers
    - Alpha-fetoprotein
    - Human chorionic gonadotropin (hCG)
- Treatment
  - Radical orchidectomy through an inguinal approach
  - Radiotherapy and chemotherapy
- Cure rate: close to 100%

Carcinoma of the scrotum

- Uncommon
- Mainly seen in the elderly
- Carcinogens
  - Soot of chimney sweeps
  - Lubricating mineral oil
- Cell type: squamous
- Spreads to inguinal lymph nodes
- Treatment is by wide excision

Carcinoma of the urethra

- Rare tumour
- Associated with chronic irritation within the urethra leading to stricture
- Treatment is by radical excision

Carcinoma of the penis

- Rare; unknown in circumcised men
- Aetiology
  - Poor hygiene
  - Accumulation of smegma
  - Balanoposthitis
- Histology: squamous cell carcinoma
- Spreads to the inguinal lymph nodes
- Erythroplasia of Queyrat: an intra-epidermal carcinoma of the glans penis

Infections and inflammations of the testis and epididymis

Epididymitis

- Presents along with orchitis
- Aetiology
  - In children and the elderly: bacterial urinary tract infection
  - In young adults: sexually transmitted urethritis, e.g. gonorrhoea
  - Systemic infection or inflammation
    - Tuberculosis
    - Sarcoidosis
    - *Cryptococcus* species infection
- Diagnosis
  - Differential diagnosis is acute torsion of the testis
  - Urine contains pus cells and bacteria
  - If in doubt, prompt surgical exploration is required
- Complications
  - Abscess: ultrasound-guided drainage
  - Testicular infarction
  - Chronicity
  - Obstruction of sperm transport and subfertility
- Management
  - Antibiotics, based on culture and sensitivity
  - Bed rest, analgesia and elevation

Orchitis

- Infection spreads by direct extension from the vas and epididymis or by blood-borne spread from septicaemia
- Non-bacterial causes
  - Viruses: mumps

- Chemicals, parasites, trauma and tuberculosis cause granulomatous orchitis

Other non-malignant testicular swellings

- Epididymo-orchitis
- Torsion of the testis
- Hematocoele
  - Testicular trauma from sports or violence
  - Bleeding into layers of tunica vaginalis
- Sperm granuloma (spermatocoele)
  - Extravasation of sperm from tubules into the interstitium
  - Follows vasectomy
  - Causes a painful lump on the testis
  - Treatment is by excision
- Torsion of the testicular appendage
  - Causes sudden pain, oedema and congestion
  - Mistaken for testicular torsion
  - Treatment is by excision

Testicular torsion

Pathology

- Torsion of intravaginal or extravaginal spermatic cord
- Compression of testicular veins and then the arterial supply, leading to pain
- Ischaemic testicular damage occurs within 6 hours

Anatomical abnormalities that predispose to torsion

- Abnormally long spermatic cord
- Presence of a long mesorchium
- Maldescent of the testis (a horizontal lie on clinical examination)
- High insertion of the tunica vaginalis ('bell clapper deformity'), leaving a length of cord free within the tunica vaginalis

Clinical features

- Common at puberty
- Causes sudden pain in the scrotum, groin and lower abdomen
- On examination, high-placed testis may be found

- Differential diagnoses are infection and tumour

Treatment

- Prompt surgical exploration through a scrotal incision
- After untwisting:
  - If the testis is viable, it should be fixed
  - If the testis is non-viable, it should be removed
  - Other testis should be fixed

Scrotal skin conditions

Necrotising fasciitis (Fournier's gangrene)

- Infection with more than one organism
  - Coliforms
  - *Bacteroides* species
  - Diphtheroids
  - *Pseudomonas* species
- Has a sudden onset, with severe constitutional upset
- Inflammation leads to patchy necrosis of the scrotal skin, progressing to extensive sloughing
- Treatment is with antibiotics and wide surgical debridement
- Recovery is complete

Carcinoma of the scrotum

- Occupational exposure to carcinogens (chimney sweepers)
- Treatment is by wide local excision and inguinal lymph node dissection if the nodes are involved

Urinary retention

Definition

- Lack of ability to urinate

Signs and symptoms

- Poor stream with intermittence
- Straining
- Sense of incomplete voiding
- Urgency
- Incontinence
- Nocturia
- Increased frequency

Sequelae

- Bladder stones
- Loss of detrusor muscle tone
- Hydronephrosis
- Hypertrophy of the detrusor muscle
- Diverticula of the bladder wall

Causes

- BPH
- Prostatic carcinoma and pelvic malignancies
- Congenital urethral valve abnormalities
- Detrusor muscle dyssynergia
- Circumcision
- Urethral stricture

Investigations

- Uroflowmetry
- Post-void urethral scan
- PSA for prostatic carcinoma
- Renal function testing for backflow kidney damage

Treatment

- Acute retention
  - Urinary catheterisation
  - Suprapubic catheterisation
- Chronic retention: treatment depends on the cause
- For BPH
  - alpha-1 blockers
  - 5-alpha-reductase inhibitors
  - Prostatectomy
  - Transurethral resection of the prostate (TURP)

Benign prostatic hyperplasia (BPH)

Clinical diagnosis

- Obstructive symptoms
- Reduced urine flow
- Increased residual urine volume
- Enlarged prostate without evidence of malignancy on rectal examination and transrectal ultrasound

Risk factors

- Age > 60 years
- Western diet
- Hypertension
- Diabetes mellitus

Pathophysiology

- Increase in both glandular and stromal elements
- Affects periurethral tissue (transition zone)
- Investigation is the same as for urinary retention

Management

- Conservative management: watchful waiting
- Pharmacotherapy
  - Phytotherapy: plant extracts
  - 5-alpha-reductase inhibitors: finasteride
  - Alpha-1 blockers
    - Prazosin
    - Indoramin
- Surgery
  - Open prostatectomy
  - TURP
  - Parasurgical therapy
    - Balloon dilatation
    - Stenting
    - Laser coagulation
    - Transurethral needle ablation

Carcinoma of the prostate

Aetiology

- High-calorie diet rich in saturated fat, red meat and vitamin A
- Vitamin E
- Phyto-oestrogens, e.g. lignans and isoflavonoids, have a protective effect

Pathology

- Arises from the peripheral zone
- Adenocarcinoma from glandular elements in 98% of cases
- Prostatic intraepithelial neoplasia (PIN) is a premalignant condition

Screening

- By PSA
- Normal PSA: < 4 ng/L
- Intermediate elevation (4–20 ng/L): probability of cancer is 25–35%

- High elevation (> 10 ng/L): probability of cancer is 50–60%
- Strongest predictor (>80%): PSA > 10 micrograms/L and hard prostate on rectal examination

Diagnosis

- Digital rectal examination
- PSA
- Imaging
  - Plain X-ray: osteosclerotic bone secondaries
  - Transrectal ultrasound (TRUS)
  - Bone scan for metastases
  - CT and/or MRI to assess local extent
- Biopsy: TRUS-guided

Staging

- TNM
  - T1: PIN
  - T2: tumour confined within prostate
  - T3: tumour through the capsule
  - T4: tumour invading adjacent structures
  - N1: regional nodes involved
  - M1: distant metastases

Signs and symptoms of metastatic disease

- Bone pain
- Renal failure
- Anaemia
  - Renal failure
  - Bone marrow infiltration
- Leg swelling
  - Lymphatic obstruction
  - Venous obstruction
- Paraplegia
- Pathological fracture
- Proptosis

Treatment options

- TURP for early disease
- Radical prostatectomy
- Radiotherapy
  - Curative
  - Adjuvant
  - Palliative
- Hormonal therapy
  - Orchidectomy
  - LHRH agonists

- Anti-androgens, e.g. cyproterone acetate
- Chemotherapy yields no response
- Palliative treatment
  - TURP
  - Stenting

Other prostatic disorders

Prostatitis

- Acute prostatitis
  - Severe constitutional symptoms
  - May lead to abscess formation
  - Drained by transurethral resection
- Recurrent subacute prostatitis
  - Treated with antibiotics and alpha-blockers
- Chronic non-bacterial prostatitis
  - May be due to infection with *Chlamydia*
  - Treated with quinolone antibiotics and alpha-blockers
- Prostatodynia
  - Pain without inflammation
  - Treated with alpha-blockers and non-steroidal anti-inflammatory drugs
  - Associated with depression and neurosis

Acute renal failure

Definition

- Rapid onset of renal impairment that results in accumulation of nitrogenous waste products (urea and creatinine) within the body
- Acute tubular necrosis: intrinsic, but reversible, damage to the kidney

Causes

- Pre-renal acute renal failure
  - Decreased cardiac output
    - Acute myocardial infarction
    - Cardiac arrest
    - Cardiac failure
    - Cardiac tamponade
  - Decreased circulatory volume
    - Sepsis
    - Haemorrhage
    - Hypoalbuminaemia

- Decreased ECF volume
  - Diarrhoea, vomiting
  - Excessive diuresis
  - Sweating
  - Burns
- Vascular disease
  - Renal artery embolism or thrombosis
  - Renal artery stenosis
  - Valvular heart disease
- Renal (intrinsic) acute renal failure
  - Ischaemia, which can be due to all pre-renal causes
  - Ischaemia and toxin
    - Hypercalcaemia
    - Hepatorenal syndrome
  - Renotoxic agent
    - Primary acute tubular necrosis: aminoglycosides and paracetamol
    - Tubular obstruction in myeloma
    - Myoglobinuria in muscle injury
    - Haemoglobinuria from mismatched blood transfusion
  - Acute interstitial nephritis
    - Antibiotics: penicillin
    - Non-steroidal anti-inflammatory drugs
    - Thiazide diuretics
- Post-renal acute renal failure
  - Obstructive uropathy

Differentiation of pre-renal ARF and renal ARF

Characteristics of pre-renal and renal acute renal failure		
Characteristic	Pre-renal ARF	Renal ARF
Urinary sodium (mmol/L)	<10	>20
Urinary urea (mmol/L)	>150	<150
Urine/plasma osmolality	>1.1	<1.1
Urine/plasma urea	>8	<3

Renal replacement therapy

Indications in acute renal failure

- Uraemia (significant retention of nitrogenous waste products with associated clinical signs): urea > 30 mmol/L
- Metabolic acidosis (pH < 7.2)
- Hyperkalaemia (K^+ > 6 mmol/L)
- Significant fluid overload with pulmonary oedema
- Creatinine clearance < 10 mL/min
- Encephalopathy

Types

- Haemodialysis
  - Based on diffusion
  - Removes small molecules
  - Cost-effective
- Haemofiltration
  - Based on convection
  - Removes larger molecules
- Haemodiafiltration
  - Combination of both haemodialysis and haemofiltration
  - Less cost-effective

Patterns of therapy

- Intermittent: for stable and uncomplicated acute renal failure
- Continuous for patients with:
  - Cardiovascular instability
  - Cerebral oedema
  - Hypoxia

Complications of dialysis

- Disequilibrium syndrome
  - Caused by rapid filtration of urea
  - Causes cerebral oedema and seizures
- Hypotension, caused by sudden decrease in intravascular volume
- Immune reaction and hypoxia, caused by filtration membrane and extracorporeal circuit
- Line sepsis
- Line disconnection, causing:
  - Air embolism
  - Haemorrhage

Urological trauma

Renal trauma

- Blunt trauma from road traffic accidents
- Penetrating trauma
  - Stab wounds
  - Gunshot wounds
  - Iatrogenic trauma
    - Percutaneous nephrostomy
    - Renal biopsy
- Classification
  - Contusion: subcapsular haematoma
  - Minor laceration: single tear, communicating with renal pelvis
  - Major laceration: multiple tears, communicating with renal pelvis
  - Major vascular: avulsion
  - Injury to renal pelvis: avulsion
- Complications
  - Haemorrhage
    - Primary
    - Secondary
  - Urinary extravasation
    - Fistula
    - Urinoma
    - Hydronephrosis
  - Infection
    - Pyelonephritis
    - Infected urinoma
    - Septicaemia
  - Infarction
    - Segmental
    - Total
  - Hypertension due to infarction
  - Death from associated injuries
- Clinically suspected from haematuria following trauma
- Diagnosis
  - IVU
  - CT scan
  - Angiography
  - Renal ultrasound
- Management
  - Conservative management
  - Surgery
    - Renal reconstruction
    - Renorrhaphy
    - Partial nephrectomy

- Vascular reconstruction
- Nephrectomy

Ureteric trauma

- Penetrating wounds
  - Gunshot wounds
  - Difficult pelvic surgeries
  - Ureteroscopy
- Complications (if missed)
  - Ileus
  - Urinoma, causing infection and abscess formation
  - Uretero–vaginal fistula
  - Healing by fibrosis may lead to stricture
- Diagnosis
  - IVU
  - Retrograde pyelogram
- Treatment
  - Ureteronephrostomy
  - Ureteroureterostomy
  - Stenting

Bladder injuries

- Aetiology
  - Traumatic injuries
    - Blunt trauma: extraperitoneal or intraperitoneal
    - Penetrating trauma: gunshot and stab wounds
  - Iatrogenic trauma
    - Open surgeries
    - Endoscopic procedures
- Extraperitoneal: usually due to road traffic accidents, and associated with pelvic fractures
- Complications
  - Urinary ascites
  - Urinary fistula
  - Pelvic abscess
- Clinical presentation
  - Unable to void
  - No urethral injury
  - Impalpable bladder
- Investigations
  - Ascending cystogram
  - CT scan
  - IVU
    - Extraperitoneal: extravasation confined to the pelvis

- Intraperitoneal: extravasation throughout the peritoneum
- Management
  - Extraperitoneal
    - Non-operative: catheterisation and antibiotics
  - Intraperitoneal
    - Operative closure

Urethral injuries

- Aetiology
  - Trauma
    - Membranous urethral injury
    - Bulbar urethral injury
    - Penile urethral injury
  - Iatrogenic trauma
- Classification
  - Mucosal tear
  - Partial rupture
  - Major distraction
- Complications
  - Stricture
  - Erectile dysfunction
  - Incontinence
  - Fistula formation
  - Periurethral complications

- Extravasation
- Abscess formation
- Necrotising fasciitis of the perineum
- Diagnosis
  - Suprapubic cystostomy
  - IVU
- Management
  - Mucosal and partial: conservative therapy
  - Complete: urethroplasty

Injuries to the external genitalia

- Penetrating trauma
  - Gunshot wounds
  - Combined urethral, scrotal, penile and testicular injuries are repaired separately
- Fractured penis
  - Urethrogram
  - Urgent surgical exploration
- Testicular trauma
  - Scrotal ultrasound
  - Exploration if there is a large hematocoele

Principles of paediatric and neonatal surgery

Maintenance of body temperature

- Large surface in relation to weight
- Skin is thinner and capillary beds are closer to surface
- Temperature-regulating centres in the brain are immature
- Mechanisms of heat conservation, e.g. vasoconstriction and shivering, are absent
- Treatment of hypothermia
  - Provision of a draught-free environment
  - Avoidance of unnecessary exposure
  - Covering with foil
  - Active methods to provide heat, e.g. incubator, warm blanket and hot-air blower

Assessment of respiratory and cardiovascular function

- Respiratory function
  - Child is always kept flat and on its side for clearance of the pharynx soon after birth
  - Higher position of larynx causes predominantly nasal breathing, leading to occlusion and rapid respiratory depression
  - Diaphragm is the main muscle of respiration; if it is impaired, e.g. in increased intra-abdominal pressure, ventilation is compromised
  - Normal respiratory rate is 30 breaths/minute; if it is increased, metabolic acidosis rapidly ensues
  - Immature central respiratory control, and therefore apnoeic spells are common
    - Treatment: intravenous aminophylline
    - If persistent: mechanical ventilation

- Cardiovascular function
  - Cardiovascular system is unstable during the transition period from fetal to adult type of circulation
  - Hypoxia, hypercapnia and acidosis may cause pulmonary vasoconstriction, leading to increased pulmonary vascular resistance and resulting in reversion to the fetal type of circulation and a shunting of deoxygenated blood from right to left

Metabolic status

- Blood glucose
  - Normal stores decreased in premature neonates
  - Control is disrupted in illness and in children of diabetic mothers
  - Hypoglycaemia causes hypotonia, lethargy, convulsions and apnoeic spells
  - Intragastric and intravenous glucose supplements given
  - In emergency situations, intraperitoneal or even subcutaneous infusion can be given
- Red cell mass
  - Polycythaemia at birth
  - Haemoglobin drops to 11 g/L at 3 months of age
  - Haematinics, and occasionally blood transfusion, may be required
- Hypocalcaemia
  - Results in twitching and convulsions
  - Excessive blood transfusion is one of the causes
  - Treatment: 30 ng/kg of calcium gluconate, i.e. 0.3 ml/kg of 10% calcium gluconate
- Jaundice
  - Normal, mild jaundice in the first 3–7 days of life is caused by temporary enzyme deficiency

- In premature neonates there is an increased risk of kernicterus (deposition of unconjugated bilirubin in the basal ganglia)
- Treatment
  - Hydration
  - Phototherapy
  - Repeat blood transfusion
- Feeding
  - Neonates not fed orally, i.e. those with a nasogastric tube or gastrostomy, will lose the will to feed, and so should be sham fed
  - Breast-feeding

Fluid and electrolytes

- Replacement of fluid deficit
  - Mild deficit: 2.5% of body weight (weight × 25, e.g. for a 3 kg child a mild deficit is replaced by 75 mL of fluid infusion)
  - Moderate deficit: 5% of body weight (weight × 50)
  - Severe deficit: 8% of body weight (weight × 80)
- Normal requirement
  - 100 mL/kg/day for the first 10 kg
  - 50 mL/kg/day for the next 10 kg
  - 25 mL/kg/day thereafter
- Parenteral nutrition
  - Normal requirement: 85 kcal/kg/day
  - Central-vein care is needed

Vascular access

- Short-term access
  - 22–26 gauge cannula plus infusion pumps for volume delivery
  - Should be visible and constantly monitored
- For nutrition
  - Subclavian vein or internal jugular vein is used
  - Open access to external or internal jugular vein or saphenofemoral junction
- Arterial access
  - Right or left radial arteries
  - Avoided if hand anomaly is present
  - Alternatives: anterior or posterior tibial artery, femoral artery or axillary artery
  - Umbilical artery is avoided, owing to the high incidence of aortic thrombosis and embolism

Neural tube defects

- Neural tube is formed from fusion of the edges of the neural groove

Spina bifida

- Caused by failure of the posterior vertebral arch to fuse (common in the lumbosacral region)

Spina bifida occulta

- Spinal cord is normal and no neurological deficit
- Skin dimple at the site of defect
- Subtle neurological abnormalities, e.g. enuresis and incontinence, may persist

Meningocoele and meningomyelocoele

- Bulging of meninges through a defect
- If only the meninges bulge, the defect is a meningocoele
- If the spinal cord and nerve roots bulge along with meninges, the defect is a meningomyelocoele
- Can result in hydrocephalus (Arnold–Chiari malformation)
- Diagnosed prenatally by increased alpha-fetoprotein
- Clinical manifestations
  - Limb weakness
  - Sensory loss
  - Joint dislocation and contracture
  - Urinary disorder
- Treatment: surgical closure of the defect with a ventricular–caval shunt within 48 hours of birth

Congenital heart disease

- Incidence: 0.8% of live births

Cyanotic heart defects

- Complete transposition of the great vessels
- Aortic atresia
- Mitral valve atresia
- Tetralogy of Fallot
  - Pulmonary stenosis
  - Transposition of aorta
  - Ventricular septal defect (VSD)
  - Right ventricular hypertrophy
- Pulmonary stenosis with atrial septal defect (ASD)

Acyanotic heart defects

- ASD
- VSD
- Patent ductus arteriosus (PDA)
- Pulmonary stenosis
- Coarctation of the aorta

Indications for surgery

- Severe cyanosis, hypoxia
- Deleterious effects on growth and development
- Reduced life expectancy caused by heart failure and subacute bacterial endocarditis

Diaphragmatic hernia

Types

- Bochdalek's hernia: posterolateral hernia, through the foramen of Bochdalek
- Morgagni's hernia: anterior parasternal location, through the foramen of Morgagni

Cause

- Physiological herniation of bowel occurs in fetal life; this is retracted at 10–12 weeks' gestation as a result of closure of diaphragm
- Failure of closure leads to bowel herniation into the chest, causing a hypoplastic lung

Clinical features

- Respiratory distress within 24–48 hours of birth
- Bowel sounds on affected side of the chest
- X-ray shows air-filled loops of bowel within the chest

Treatment

- Intestinal decompression
- Reduction of hernia
- Primary diaphragmatic repair

Congenital anomalies of the gastrointestinal system

Classification

- Mechanical anomalies
  - Atresia: interruption of continuity
  - Stenosis: narrowing of the lumen
  - Intraluminal obstruction: meconium ileus
- Functional anomalies
  - Absent neurones: Hirschsprung's disease
  - Abnormal neural networks: neuronal intestinal dysplasia
  - Abnormal smooth muscle: megacystic megacolon
- Unknown aetiology
  - Chronic idiopathic intestinal pseudo-obstruction

Oesophageal atresia and tracheo-oesophageal fistula

- Chromosomal anomalies: trisomy 13 and 18
- Types
  - Pure oesophageal atresia: no tracheo-oesophageal fistula
  - Tracheo-oesophageal fistula from upper pouch
  - Multiple tracheo-oesophageal fistulae
  - Tracheo-oesophageal fistula from an intact oesophagus (H-type)
  - Missing oesophageal segment (the most common type)
- Associations
  - Imperforate anus
  - ASD
  - Aplasia of the hands
  - Single kidney
- Clinical features
  - Inability to swallow
  - Insertion of a nasogastric tube is not possible
- X-ray
  - Air in the bowel indicates tracheo-oesophageal fistula
- Timing of surgery: within 24–36 hours of birth
- Complications
  - Anastomotic leak
  - Long-term stricture

Pyloric stenosis

- Marked hypertrophy of the pyloric musculature
- Common in first-born males
- Occurs 4–6 weeks after birth

- There may be a genetic predisposition
- Clinical presentation
  - Hungry child
  - Projectile vomiting
  - Vomitus not bile-stained
  - Visible gastric peristalsis
  - Dehydration and/or weight loss
  - Palpable pylorus when the child is fed ('olive tumour')
- Management
  - Correction of fluid and electrolyte loss and resulting imbalances (a hypokalaemic hypochloremic metabolic alkalosis)
  - Surgery only after biochemistry has returned to normal
  - Ramstedt's pyloromyotomy
    - Splits the hypertrophic muscle at the submucosal plane from the stomach to the duodenum
    - Performed through a circum-supraumbilical incision or through a laparoscopy
  - Normal feeding after recovery
  - Discharge in 24–72 hours

Duodenal atresia

- Commonly at the second part of duodenum at the level of ampulla
- Bile-stained vomiting
- May be associated with Down's syndrome
- X-ray shows double-bubble appearance (gastric and duodenal bubbles)
- Treatment: duodenoduodenostomy

Small bowel atresia

- Caused by internal hernia in the antenatal period, infarction, absorption and loss of bowel length
- Surgery: resection of dilated bowel and anastomosis

Malrotation

- Normal rotation occurs at the sixth to 10th week of gestation
- Bowel undergoes a 270° counter-clockwise rotation
- Failure, arrest or abnormal rotation leads to midgut volvulus
- If occurs antenatally, the bowel gets absorbed, resulting in a short bowel state

- If occurs postnatally, sudden onset of duodenal obstruction ensues
- Treatment: urgent operation, derotation and release of Ladd's bands

Meconium ileus

- Occurs in cystic fibrosis, an autosomal-recessive inheritance
- High levels of Na+ and Cl– in the sweat
- Pancreas undergoes fibrocystic dysplasia, leading to loss of enzymes and thick meconium, which causes lower ileal obstruction
- Contrast X-ray shows a microcolon containing pellets
- Surgery: resection of thickened, meconium-filled loops and anastomosis
- Long-term management
  - Pancreatic supplements
  - Care of respiratory tract
  - Gene therapy
- Counselling of family members

Intussusception

- Definition: invagination of the bowel into itself
- Pathology
  - Progression
  - Compression of mesentery within the intussusception, leading to vascular congestion and bowel strangulation
  - If occurs antenatally, the sterile infracted bowel is resorbed, leading to intestinal atresia
- Age: 9–18 months
- Occurs in a previously well child
- Causes
  - Hyperplasia of lymph tissue in the Peyer's patch
  - Meckel's diverticulum
  - Mucosal polyps
  - Peutz–Jeghers syndrome
  - Foreign bodies
- Clinical features
  - Spasms of severe abdominal colic
  - Bile-stained vomiting as a result of intestinal obstruction
  - Rectal oozing of mucus and blood ('redcurrant jelly' stool)
  - Sausage-shaped mass in the right hypochondrium

- Treatment
  - Contrast enema reduction if the child is stable
  - Surgery if enema reduction fails
    - Push-back
    - Resection if gangrene is present

Colonic atresia

- Less common than small bowel atresia
- Causes a rapid massive distension
- Treatment: surgical resection and end-to-end anastomosis

Hirschsprung's disease (congenital aganglionosis)

- Rectosigmoid is involved in 75% of cases
- Association with Down's syndrome
- Caused by failure of intra-uterine migration of ganglion cells from the neural crest
- Within the aganglionic segment, there is proliferation of nerve fibrils
- Bowel immediately proximal becomes markedly dilated and hypertrophic
- Clinically presents as failure to pass meconium, bile-stained vomiting, and explosive evacuation following digital rectal examination
- Diagnosis by rectal biopsy
  - Absence of ganglia
  - Hypertrophy and proliferation of nerve fibrils
  - Increased acetyl cholinesterase in Auerbach's plexus and Meissner's plexus
- Treatment
  - Bowel evacuation
  - Elective curative surgical resection

Imperforate anus

- Associated with abnormalities of the urinary tract, lumbosacral spine and associated nerves
- Types
  - Anal stenosis
  - Absent anal canal and dimple
  - Recto–urethral fistula and dimple
- Diagnosis is by invertogram
- Treatment: colostomy followed by repair

Congenital inguinal hernia

- More common in males
- Indirect variety: via processus vaginalis
- Organs that are found in a hernia sac
  - Ileum
  - Appendix
  - Ovary and fallopian tube in females
  - Uterus in females
  - Bladder
- Presence of gonad in the sac of a child with normal female genitalia raises the suspicion of testicular feminisation (androgen insensitivity) syndrome
- Clinical features
  - Non-tender
  - Spontaneous reduction when child is asleep
  - Compression of testicular vessels or vas leads to testicular infarction and/or vas occlusion
- Surgery
  - Simple cases: herniotomy
  - If excessively large or there is major disruption of the inguinal canal: herniorrhaphy

Anterior abdominal wall anomalies

Types

- Exomphalos minor
- Exomphalos major
- Gastroschisis

Exomphalos minor

- Intact hernia sac passing into the umbilical cord through an expanded umbilical port, which contains loops of small bowel and a patent vitello-intestinal duct opening at its apex
- Surgery
  - Resection of the vitello-intestinal duct
  - Umbilical cicatrisation

Exomphalos major

- Supra-umbilical midline hernia of at least 5 cm
- Intact or ruptured sac

- Wide divarication of rectus abdominis muscles and the anterior fibres of the diaphragm
- Treatment
  - Surgery: primary, staged, delayed closure
  - If rupture is present, resuscitation and cardiovascular support is required, followed by closure

Gastroschisis

- No hernia sac
- Whole midgut is extruded, along with the sigmoid colon, bladder, ovary and testis
- Treatment: same as ruptured exomphalos major

Urological abnormalities

Hypospadias

- Caused by under-virilisation in an otherwise normal male child
- Types
  - Glandular hypospadias
  - Penile hypospadias with chordee
  - Perineal hypospadias with chordee
- May be associated with maldescended testis
- Surgery: before 3–4 years

Congenital adrenal hyperplasia

- Autosomal-recessive inheritance: chromosome 6 abnormality
- Caused by a deficiency of the enzyme 21-hydroxylase
- Uninhibited stimulation of the adrenals by the pituitary with excessive androgens
  - Virilisation of female external genitalia
  - Inability to mount normal stress response, owing to mineralocorticoid deficiency, leading to vomiting, dehydration and circulatory collapse
- Diagnosis: deficiency of 17-hydroxy-progesterone

- Treatment
  - Lifelong replacement therapy with hydrocortisone and mineralocorticoids
  - Reduction clitoroplasty and vulvovaginoplasty

Hydrocoele

- Common in males
- Non-tender, bluish swelling in the inguinal region and scrotum
- Becomes large and tense following physical activity
- Cord and testicle lie posteromedial to the sac
- Initial management: conservative, awaiting spontaneous fusion of processus vaginalis during the first 6 months after birth
- Indications for surgery
  - Persistent patency
  - Discomfort from its size
- Surgery: herniotomy

Undescended testis

- Incidence
  - At full term: 4%
  - At 6 months: 1.4%
  - Much higher in premature infants
- More common on the right side because of later descent on this side
- Scrotum on the ipsilateral side is hypoplastic
- Types
  - Incompletely descended: testis found along the pathway of descent
  - Ectopic testis
    - Groin crease
    - Overlying the femoral vessels
    - At the base of the penis
    - In the perineum
  - See table opposite
- Complications
  - Hernia resulting from a patent processus vaginalis
  - Unstable lie of the testis, leading to torsion

Comparison of incompletely descended testis with ectopic testis	
Incompletely descended testis	**Ectopic testis**
Patent processus vaginalis	Closed processus vaginalis
Fibrotic cremaster	Normal cremaster
Smaller volume	Normal volume
Histologically abnormal (higher content of potentially neoplastic dysgenetic tissue)	Histologically normal
Normal vas deferens	Normal vas deferens
Testicular vessels of normal length	Testicular vessels of normal length

- Loss of spermatogonia
- Increased risk of malignancy
- Treatment
  - Before 6 months of age
  - Orchidopexy
    - Processus vaginalis ligated and divided
    - Testis brought down through to the subdartos pouch
  - Short vessels: microvascular anastomosis

Urinary tract anomalies

- Kidney anomalies
  - Anomalies of rotation
  - Single kidney
  - Ectopic, pelvic kidney
  - Horse-shoe, duplex kidney
  - Agenetic, multicystic, cystic or dysplastic kidney
- Pelvi calyceal system: pelviureteric junction obstruction
- Ureter anomalies
  - Vesicoureteric obstruction
  - Vesicoureteric reflux
  - Duplex ureter
  - Ureterocoele
- Bladder anomalies
  - Neurogenic bladder
  - Bladder diverticulum
- Obstructive uropathy: hydroureteronephrosis

Pain management

Definition of pain

- Unpleasant sensory or emotional experience associated with actual or potential tissue damage

Physiological processes in pain

- Transduction: at the level of peripheral nerve endings
- Transmission: at the level of the spinal cord
- Modulation: at the level of the spinal cord
- Perception: by the patient

Post-operative pain

- Adverse effects of post-operative pain
  - Respiratory: effects restriction of respiratory movements causing decrease in vital capacity and functional residual capacity
    - Retention of secretions
    - Atelectasis
    - Pneumonia
  - Cardiovascular effects
    - Tachycardia
    - Hypertension
    - Increased catecholamines
    - All causing increased myocardial oxygen demand, leading to increased risk of myocardial infarction
  - Neuroendocrine effects
    - Increased catecholamines
    - Increased catabolic hormones
    - Both causing increased Na^+ and water retention
  - Delayed mobilisation: increased risk of deep venous thrombosis
- Methods available to tackle post-operative pain
  - Pre-operative counseling
  - Trans-cutaneous electrical nerve stimulation (TENS)
  - Opioids
    - Pethidine
    - Morphine
  - Local anaesthetics, e.g. lignocaine 3 mg/kg with adrenaline 5 mg/kg
    - Local infiltration
    - Nerve block
    - Epidural block
  - Non-steroidal anti-inflammatory drugs
  - Pre-emptive analgesia (given pre-operatively)
  - Patient-controlled analgesia (PCA)
    - Set dose
    - Lock-out period
- Monitoring
  - Of pain:
    - Visual analogue score (1–10)
    - Verbal rating score (1–4, corresponding to no pain, mild pain, moderate pain and severe pain)
  - Of sedation and respiration

Pain of malignancy

- Common causes
  - Bone pain
    - Local infiltration
  - Visceral pain
    - Soft tissue infiltration
    - Stretching of capsule
    - Stretching of hollow organ
  - Nerve pain
    - Irritation
    - Infiltration
    - Compression
  - Myofascial pain
  - Superficial, e.g. pressure sore
- Steps in management
  - Step 1: non-opioid analgesia plus adjuvant measures
  - Step 2: weak opioid plus adjuvant measures
  - Step 3: strong opioid plus adjuvant measures
- Nerve blocks useful in:
  - Unilateral pain
  - Localised pain
  - Involvement of one or two nerve roots
  - Upper abdominal pain
  - Rib pain

Rehabilitation

Definition

- The achievement of the optimum mental and physical state necessary to overcome a disability incurred by trauma or ablative surgery for disease, thereby enabling independence and active involvement in family life and society and a return to gainful employment

Clinical outcomes

- Disease-specific or corrected survival
- Disease-free survival
- Recurrence-free survival
- Length of hospital stay

Quality of life

- Physical quality of life
- Social quality of life
- Psychological quality of life

Rehabilitation team

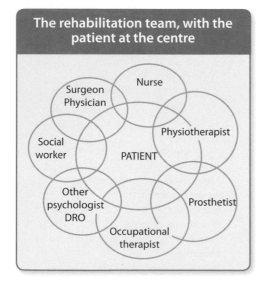

The rehabilitation team, with the patient at the centre

Principles of organ donation

Basic issue

- Donor shortage, resulting in:
  - Longer waiting times for patients on the list
  - Increase in number of patients dying while waiting for an organ

Strategies to minimise donor shortage

- Organ-procurement organisations
- Marginal donors
  - Older donors
    - Pre-transplant biopsy
    - Assessment for vascular disease
  - Paediatric donors
    - To children if possible, but can also be to adults
  - Non-heart-beating donors
    - Flush after heart has stopped beating
    - Cooling and removing: same as brain-dead donors
- Living donors
  - Related donors
    - Improved long-term function
    - Shorter waiting time
  - Unrelated donors
    - Ethical issues should be addressed
    - Buying and selling of organs is unacceptable
- Application of brain-death criteria
- Presumed consent
  - Assumes that every brain-dead person is an organ donor without family consent
  - Not successful in all countries
- Xeno-transplantation
  - Latest development
  - Requires immunosuppression
  - From transgenic animals
  - Risk of viral transmission
  - Ethical issues arise

Index